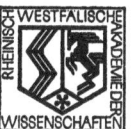

ABHANDLUNGEN
DER RHEINISCH-WESTFÄLISCHEN AKADEMIE DER WISSENSCHAFTEN

BAND 87

Sixth Münster International
Arteriosclerosis Symposium

New Aspects of Metabolism and Behaviour of Mesenchymal Cells
during the Pathogenesis of Arteriosclerosis

Sixth Münster International
Arteriosclerosis Symposium

New Aspects of Metabolism and Behaviour of Mesenchymal Cells during the Pathogenesis of Arteriosclerosis

Under the Protectorate of
Rheinisch-Westfälische Akademie
der Wissenschaften

Werner H. Hauss, Robert W. Wissler,
Hans-Joachim Bauch

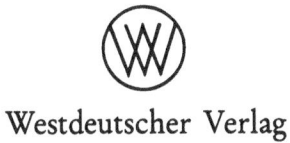

Westdeutscher Verlag

Von der Klasse für Natur-, Ingenieur- und Wirtschaftswissenschaften
in die Reihe der Abhandlungen aufgenommen
am 6. Dezember 1989.

Die Deutsche Bibliothek – CIP-Einheitsaufnahme

**New aspects of metabolism and behaviour of mesenchymal
cells during the pathogenesis of arteriosclerosis** / Sixth
Münster International Arteriosclerosis Symposium. Werner H.
Hauss; Robert W. Wissler; H.-J. Bauch. [Hrsg. von der
Rheinisch-Westfälischen Akademie der Wissenschaften]. –
Opladen: Westdt. Verl., 1991
(Abhandlungen der Rheinisch-Westfälischen Akademie der
Wissenschaften; Bd. 87)
NE: Hauss, Werner H.; Wissler, Robert W.; Bauch, H.-J.; Münster
International Arteriosclerosis Symposium < 06, 1990 > ; Rheinisch-
Westfälische Akademie der Wissenschaften < Düsseldorf > :
Abhandlungen der Rheinisch-Westfälischen...
ISBN 978-3-322-99114-0   ISBN 978-3-322-99112-6 (eBook)
DOI 10.1007/978-3-322-99112-6

Herausgegeben von der
Rheinisch-Westfälischen Akademie der Wissenschaften

Der Westdeutsche Verlag ist ein Unternehmen der Verlagsgruppe
Bertelsmann International.

© 1991 by Westdeutscher Verlag GmbH Opladen
Herstellung: Westdeutscher Verlag
Satz: I. Junge, Düsseldorf

ISSN 0171-1105
ISBN 978-3-322-99114-0

Contents

SESSION II: DISORDERS IN MESENCHYMAL CELLS IN THE EARLY
PHASE OF ATHEROGENESIS

POSTER PRESENTATIONS

Sixth Münster International Arteriosclerosis Symposium:
"New Aspects of Metabolism and Behaviour of Mesenchymal
Cells during the Pathogenesis of Arteriosclerosis"
Münster/Westfalen, October 8th to October 10th, 1990

Under the Protectorate of
Rheinisch-Westfälische Akademie
der Wissenschaften

Supported by
Rheinisch-Westfälische Akademie der Wissenschaften, Düsseldorf
Ministerium für Wissenschaft und Forschung
des Landes Nordrhein-Westfalen, Düsseldorf
Deutsche Forschungsgemeinschaft, Bonn

Scientific Committee
W.H. Hauss, Münster
R.W. Wissler, Chicago
G. Assmann, Münster
E. Buddecke, Münster
U. Gerlach, Münster
H.-J. Bauch, Münster

Organized by
Institut für Arterioskleroseforschung
an der Universität Münster

Speakers and Chairmen

Bauch, H.-J., Institut für Arterioskleroseforschung an der Universität Münster, Domagkstr. 3, D-4400 Münster (Germany)

Bender, F., em. Univ.-Professor, Parkallee 38, D-4400 Münster (Germany)

Betz, E., Physiologisches Institut I der Universität Tübingen, Gmelinstraße 5, D-7400 Tübingen (Germany)

Born, G.V.R., The William Harvey Research Institute, St. Bartholomew's Hospital, Medical College, Charterhouse Square, GB-London EC1M 6BQ (England)

Breithardt, G., Medizinische Klinik und Poliklinik der Universität Münster, Albert-Schweitzer-Str. 33, D-4400 Münster (Germany)

Brodde, O.-E., Zentrum für Innere Medizin, Abt. für Nieren- und Hochdruckkranke, Universitätsklinikum Essen, Hufelandstr. 55, 4300 Essen 1 (Germany)

Buddecke, E., Institut für Physiologische Chemie und Pathobiochemie der Universität Münster, Waldeyerstraße 15, D-4400 Münster (Germany)

Gerlach, U., Med. Klinik und Poliklinik – Innere Medizin B – der Universität Münster, Albert-Schweitzer-Str. 33, D-4400 Münster (Germany)

Hansson, G.K., Dept. of Clinical Chemistry, Sahlgren's Hospital, Gothenburg University, S-413 45 Gothenburg (Sweden)

Haudenschild, C.C., Mallory Institute of Pathology, Cardiovascular Research Laboratory, 784 Massachusetts Avenue, Boston, MA 02118 (USA)

Junge-Hülsing, G., Medizinische Klinik der Städtischen Krankenanstalten Osnabrück, Natruper-Tor-Wall 1, D-4500 Osnabrück (Germany)

Kienast, J., Medizinische Klinik und Poliklinik der Universität Münster, Albert-Schweitzer-Str. 33, D-4400 Münster (Germany)

Kling, Physiologisches Institut 1 der Universität Tübingen, Gmelinstr. 5, D-7400 Tübingen (Germany)

Kuhl, H., Experimentelle Endokrinologie, Univ.-Frauenklinik, Johann-Wolfgang-Goethe-Universität, Theodor-Stern-Kai 7, D-6000 Frankfurt (Germany)

Lee, K.T., Kosin Medical College, Graduate School, 34 Amnam-Dong, Suh-Ku, Pusan 602-030 (Korea)

Libby, P., Vascular Medicine and Atherosclerosis Unit, Brigham and Women's Hospital and Harvard Medical School, 221 Longwood Avenue, Boston, MA 02115 (USA)

Lichtlen, K., Medizinische Klinik der Medizinischen Hochschule Hannover, Postfach 61 01 80, D-3000 Hannover 61 (Germany) *van de Loo, J.*, Medizinische Klinik und Poliklinik der Universität Münster, Albert-Schweitzer-Str. 33, D-4400 Münster (Germany)

Numano, F., Internal Medicine Tokyo Medical & Dental University, 5-45, Yushima, 1-Chome, Bunkyo-Ku, Tokyo (Japan)

Orekhov, A.N., Institute of Experimental Cardiology, USSR Cardiology Research Center, 3rd Cherepkovskaja Street 15 A, Moscow 121552 (USSR)

Rahn, K.-H., Medizinische Poliklinik — Innere Medizin D — der Universität Münster, Albert-Schweitzer-Str. 33, D-4400 Münster (Germany)

Raidt, H., Nephrologisches Institut an der Universität Münster, Fliednerstr. 44, D-4400 Münster (Germany)

Robenek, H., Institut für Arteriosleroseforschung an der Universität Münster, Domagkstr. 3, D-4400 Münster (Germany)

Robert, L., Laboratoire de Biochimie du Tissu Conjonctif Faculté de Médecine Université Paris XII, 8, rue du Général Serrail, F-94010 Créteil Cedex (France)

Roessner, A., Gerhard-Domagk-Institut für Pathologie der Universität Münster, Domagkstr. 17, D-4400 Münster (Germany)

Seiffert, D., Research Inst. of Scripps Clinik CVB 3, 10666 North Torrey Pines Rd., La Jolla, CA 92037 (USA)

Siegrist, J., Medizinische Soziologie, Fachbereich Humanmedizin der Universität, Bunsenstraße 2, D-3550 Marburg (Germany)

Smirnov, V.N., Institute of Experimental Cardiology, USSR Cardiology Research Center, 3rd Cherepkovskaja Street 15A, Moscow 121552 (USSR)

Scheld, H.H., Klinik und Poliklinik für Thorax-, Herz- u. Gefäßchirurgie der Universität Münster, Albert-Schweitzer-Str. 33, D-4400 Münster (Germany)

Tanaka, K., Department of Pathology Faculty of Medicine Kyushu University, 3-1-1 Maidashi, Higashi-Ku, Fukuoka 812 (Japan)

Wissler, R.W., The University of Chicago Medical Center, Department of Pathology, 5841 S. Maryland Avenue, Chicago, IL 60637 (USA)

DINNER SPEECH

Epic Poem of Celebration
to Honor the 20th Anniversary of the
Highly Successful Institute for Atherosclerosis Research in Munster

Robert W. Wissler, Ph.D., M.D.

In days gone by when I was young
I never dreamed about
Working days as full of fun
As this night is, no doubt

I never dreamed that one day I
Would stand before a crowd
Of famous folk of repute high
To read a poem aloud.

And later on when studies took
Me into Earlham College
Professor Charles gave me a book
To teach me German knowledge.

I read a lot and learned the rules
And loved the German songs,
But even in this best of schools
My words were filled with "wrongs."

And so tonight I seek your time
To sit and not to fret
My message is not a German rhyme
It's English that you'll get.

So what I'll try to do tonight
For those of you who're here
Is offer you a little bite
Of dessert sweet and dear.

This evening I will try to trace
A fruitful twenty years
Of progress at the swiftest pace
As science shifted gears.

In 1969 I know
That Herr Professor Hauss
Urged all his friends to strike a blow
"Munster's not a mouse."

Research will move big stones he said
That block the open door
Preventing many being dead
Of heart disease and more.

He called for effort big and strong
To tackle heart diseases
Applying lessons brought along
By recent research breezes.

"Unspecific mesenchymal reaction"
Or "UMR" he stated
Will be the path for fastest action
To progress unabated.

For ills Westphalians endure
Research will be the drum
To find solutions real and sure
And march to overcome.

With help from Doctor Leo Brandt
The minister of research
The first one mil Deutsch Marks advanced
The first big forward lurch.

In 1970 on 10th of March
Came President Kuhn's report
The Institute began research
With Landesamt support.

This LVA* Westphalian progress
Like the conquest of TB
Predicts the Institute's success
It's marvelous to see.

* (LVA = Landesversicherungsanstalt)

Advisory boards began to show
For two important reasons
One which helps the system go
And monitors science's seasons.

To be as sure as sure can be
That balance is achieved
Between clinicians' basic science free
And no one is deceived.

With Hauss directing forward motion
Progress was very great
His scientific staff showed great devotion
In nineteen-seventy-eight.

Increased from 16 in seventy-one
to 50 scientists strong
And space and proffered space was won
Increased to 1737 m^2 wide and long —

Furthermore the DM support
Also increased 5 fold
From Land Nordrhein-Westphal source
Plus other grants of gold.

And all this effort has paid off
And yielded great results
So now we all our hats do doff
The Institute exults.

So most of what we see each time
Is progress on risk factors
On how the cells of mesenchyme
React to these bad actors.

To hypertension and to high blood fats
And nicotine abuse
The multifunctional mesenchymal cells of rats
Were caught in a big noose.

The Procam studies ever clear
Have yielded world wide praise
They offer facts we need to hear
To lift our hopes for days.

And so the early plan persists
And Werner should be proud
Clinicians make with scientists
A joyful noise out loud.

So on this great occasion now
Celebrating twenty
Professor Hauss should take a bow
For progress there is plenty —

The Institute is going strong
And many studies show
The worth of working hard and long
On fats and cells, and so

We wish you all a long, long time
Of research very nifty
And maybe then another rhyme
When celebrating 50.

With apologies to all real epic poets, Robert W. Wissler, 8 October 1990

GREETINGS

Hans Schadewaldt

I am very honoured to welcome all participants of the 6th International Münster Symposium on Arteriosclerosis, once again under your direction, but also under the auspices of the Rheno-Westphalian Academy of Sciences, organized in this beautiful restored old Westphalian metropolis. As announced in your program you will use two official congress-languages, English and German. But since the first three sessions will be held in English, I beg your pardon that I too use now the Latinum novum for medicine. I confess that I would prefer naturally as a medico-historian the old fashioned Latin language, utilized since many centuries as the language of scientists all over the world, but in our century English has replaced Latin as the new international common medical language, which will be understood in nearly all parts of our globe.

Our Rheno-Westphalian Academy has two sections, one for humanities, the other for natural, engineering and economic sciences. It is its mission to encourage research in our country by promoting interdisciplinary symposia. I as medico-historian belong as historian to the humanities, but being in the same time doctor in medicine, an M.D., I feel that my interests are also in the medical progress. So I am especially happy that I can welcome you at this occasion as president of our Academy. You will treat many actual problems of special interest and I can establish with satisfaction, that you will discuss as well as cellular pathological questions, thought until the field of molecular biology, and humoral pathological ideas, which affect the problem of the formation of arteriosclerosis.

Now as before the nosological entities continue to be a problem, not yet completely investigated by the scientific medicine, and scientists of many parts of our world, coming from Tokyo, Moscow, Göteborg and London until the New World, were coming here together to discuss jointly the important questions of our time.

That your papers and the discussions too, as it is the tradition of our Academy, will be published in our proceedings is a great satisfaction for me. By these publications of the deliberations will be reached also public outside the strictly speaking specialists. I personally regret, that I could not assist to the last night dinner speech of Professor Wissler of Chicago on "Twenty years Institute of Arteriosclerosis Research: History and Accomplishments". I am sure, that unfortunately a very important part of contemporary medical history has slipped away.

But at the end I could not at all deny to renounce totally of my beloved Latin language and therefore I recite as an historian of nautical medicine the verses of the Roman poet VERGIL in his "Aeneis":
"Nunc, nunc insurgite remis",
in English "All men rewing!"

U. Witting

Herzlich begrüße ich Sie im Namen der Medizinischen Fakultät der Westfälischen Wilhelms-Universität Münster zum 6. Internationalen Arteriosklerose-Symposium. Den von weit her angereisten Wissenschaftlern aus USA, Japan, Schweden, UdSSR, Großbritannien und Korea, die ihre neuesten Forschungsergebnisse zu Pathogenese der Arteriosklerose vorstellen werden, gilt mein besonderer Willkommensgruß.

Sie alle, meine Damen und Herren, werden mit Ihren Vorträgen und Diskussionen dazu beitragen, daß unser Verständnis über Funktion und Stoffwechsel der Mesenchymzelle vertieft und unsere Vorstellungen über deren Rolle in der Pathogenese der Arteriosklerose erweitert werden. Insoweit wird konsequent weiterverfolgt, was der Gründer und jetzige Ehrenvorsitzende des Instituts für Arterioskleroseforschung, Herr Prof. Hauss, als Ziel aller Bemühungen in seiner Begrüßungsrede zum vorhergehenden, dem 5. Internationalen Symposium, so formuliert hat:
"Noch vor der Therapie steht die Prophylaxe und vor diese hat der liebe Gott die Klärung der Pathogenese gestellt".

Wenn nun mit immensem Aufwand an molekularbiologischer Forschung Erkenntnisfortschritte über die Entstehungsmechanismen der Arteriosklerose erzielt werden, so eröffnen sich — bei entsprechendem wissenschaftlichen Konsens — auch gezielte Ansätze für eine wirksame Prävention von Herz-Kreislauf-Erkrankungen.

Die Auswirkungen dieser mit großem Leid verbundenen Erkrankungen belasten aber auch in erheblichem Maße das System unserer sozialen Sicherung. Nach den Ausführungen des 1. Direktors der LVA Westfalen, Herrn Dr. Riehemann, erfordern allein die Herz-Kreislauf-Erkrankungen einen Rentenaufwand von jährlich ca. 900 Millionen Mark. Dieser Aspekt berührt aber nur einen Teil der sozial-ökonomischen Bedeutung dieser Erkrankungen, deren Prävention wesentliches Motiv Ihrer wissenschaftlichen Aktivitäten darstellt. Mit Blick auf diese von Herrn Professor Hauss so prägnant formulierte Zielsetzung wünsche ich Ihrer Tagung einen erfolgreichen Verlauf.

Ladies and Gentlemen,

to conclude, I would like to wish all of you a successful meeting and a productive and fruitful exchange of scientific experiences. Besides your scientific

activities, I hope you will find some time to visit Münster's beautiful city with
its typical Westphalian pubs and restaurants.

Thank you very much.

Ich danke Ihnen für Ihre Aufmerksamkeit.

Fritz Krüger

20 Jahre erfolgreiche Arterioskleroseforschung in Münster, 6. Internationales
Symposium des Institutes für Arterioskleroseforschung der Universität Münster,
dazu möchte ich die Teilnehmer, Gäste und Besucher im Namen des Rates und der
Verwaltung der Stadt Münster herzlich willkommen heißen. Ich tue dies auch in
Vertretung von Herrn Oberbürgermeister Dr. Twenhöven, der mich gebeten hat,
Ihnen seine Grüße und guten Wünsche zu übermitteln.

Ich habe es in zweifacher Hinsicht gern übernommen, zu Ihnen zur Eröffnung
des diesjährigen Symposiums ein Grußwort zu sprechen.

Einmal als Mitglied des Rates der Stadt Münster, die als Gründungsmitglied der
Gesellschaft für Arterioskeroseforschung die inzwischen weltweit bekannten Ar-
beiten dieses Institutes, im übrigen des einzigen in Deutschland, mit ganz besonde-
rem Interesse verfolgt. Die Bedeutung der Arterioskleroseforschung — wobei man
sich in diesem Zusammenhang vor Augen halten sollte, daß die Arteriosklerose mit
einem Anteil von 50%, bei Personen ab 60 Jahren sogar 80—90% die am häufigsten verbreitete Krankheit ist — wird nicht zuletzt auch dadurch besonders hervor-
gehoben, daß zu diesem Symposium Wissenschaftler aus aller Welt in Münster in
den Räumen unserer Universität zusammengekommen sind, um in einer Reihe von
Veranstaltungen ihre Erfahrungen auszutauschen und neue Aspekte zu beleuch-
ten.

Wenn ich sage, in unserer Universität, so möchte ich damit die ganz besondere
Verbundenheit der Stadt Münster und ihrer Bürgerinnen und Bürger mit der Westfälischen Wilhelms-Universität, ihrer Medizinischen Fakultät und den Universitäts-
kliniken zum Ausdruck bringen.

Die Universität mit ihren vielen in Forschung und Lehre tätigen Mitarbeitern,
mit ihren Studenten und allen anderen Beschäftigten prägt ganz entscheidend Cha-
rakter und Erscheinungsbild unserer Stadt.

Durch die vielen von der Universität ausgerichteten Kongresse ist Münster als
Standort für Wissenschaft und Forschung weit über die Grenzen unseres Landes
hinaus bekannt. Deshalb an dieser Stelle ein ganz besonderer Dank der Stadt an
die Veranstalter dieses sechsten Internationalen Arteriosklerosesymposiums.

Die vielen jungen Studenten der Universität sind aber auch ausschlaggebend
dafür, daß Münster trotz seiner fast 1200-jährigen Geschichte sich dem Besucher
als eine junge Stadt darstellt.

Meine sehr verehrten Damen und Herren, wenn ich einleitend bemerkt habe,
daß ich es in zweifacher Hinsicht gern übernommen habe, Grußworte zu sprechen,
so selbstverständlich in erster Linie als Vertreter des Rates der Stadt Münster. Ich
bin aber auch deshalb gern zu Ihnen gekommen, weil mir aus meiner früheren
beruflichen Tätigkeit als Mitglied der Geschäftsführung der Landesversicherungsanstalt Westfalen, die ebenfalls Gründungsmitglied der Gesellschaft für Arterioskleroseforschung ist, die hervorragende Arbeit der Gesellschaft gut bekannt ist.

Münster, die Stadt des Westfälischen Friedens, wird im Jahre 1993 ihr 1200-
jähriges Bestehen feiern. In unserer Stadt finden Sie noch heute viele Zeugnisse
dieser langen Geschichte, z.B. unser altes Rathaus, den Dom, das Schloß, um
nur einige zu nennen. Daneben können Sie aber auch sehen, wie wir uns bemühen,
den Erkenntnissen und Erfordernissen sowie den Bedürfnissen unserer Bürgerinnen
nen und Bürger aus heutiger Sicht gerecht zu werden. Wenn es Ihr umfangreiches
Tagungsprogramm zuläßt, möchte ich Sie herzlich einladen, sich etwas von unserer
Stadt anzusehen. Ich glaube, Sie werden nicht enttäuscht sein.

In diesem Sinne wünsche ich Ihrem Symposium, das sicherlich nicht nur von
unmittelbar betroffenen Bürgerinnen und Bürgern unserer Stadt mit Interesse be-
gleitet wird, einen guten Erfolg und Ihnen allen einen angenehmen Aufenthalt in
Münster, das Sie jederzeit gern wieder als Besucher begrüßt.

M. Gotthardt

Auch ich begrüße Sie sehr herzlich zum 6. internationalen Arteriosklerose-
Symposion in Münster. Sie sind nach Münster gekommen, einem Mittelpunkt der
Arterioskleroseforschung und -behandlung, wie wir Münsteraner stolz sagen.

In Münster finden Sie in besonders vorbildlicher Weise eine Verzahnung von
kliniknaher Forschung mit stationärer und ambulanter Krankenversorgung, wie
dies nicht überall der Fall ist. Das Institut für Arterioskleroseforschung nimmt
innerhalb der Medizinischen Einrichtungen einen besonderen Stellenwert ein. Dies
zeigt sich auch daran, daß bei dem Umbau und der Reorganisation der alten Kliniken das Institut besonders berücksichtigt wird, auch wenn nicht alle Wünsche des
Instituts immer und sofort in Erfüllung gehen können. Dies gilt aber für das Institut wie für viele andere Bereiche unserer Medizinischen Einrichtungen.

Sie werden es einem Verwaltungsdirektor verzeihen, wenn er einige Zahlen
nennt. Die Medizinischen Einrichtungen Münster bestehen aus 29 Instituten und
35 Kliniken. Innerhalb der Medizinischen Einrichtungen haben im letzten Seme-
ster 4.817 Studenten Medizin und Zahnmedizin im ersten Studienfach studiert.
Im Jahre 1989 wurden hier ca. 45.000 stationäre Patienten in 1.560 Betten behandelt. Im ambulanten Bereich wurden ca. 441.000 Patienten versorgt. Die Aufgaben in Forschung, Lehre und Krankenversorgung werden von etwa 5.600 Mitarbeitern geleistet.

Es stellt sich die Frage, ob bei diesen Patientenzahlen noch Zeit für Forschung und Lehre bleibt. Die Antwort darauf ist eindeutig: es bleibt genügend Zeit. Wenn man berücksichtigt, daß im Jahre 1989 in den Medizinischen Einrichtungen Münster etwa 380 Drittmittelprojekte von fremden Geldgebern gefördert wurden, aus denen etwa 340 Mitarbeiter finanziert werden konnten, so zeigt dies eindeutig, welchen Stellenwert die Forschung in Münster hat. Auch die insgesamt eingeworbene Höhe von etwa 23 Millionen DM Drittmittel im Jahre 1989 spricht hier eine deutliche Sprache. Forschung ist in den Medizinischen Einrichtungen Münster ein wichtiger Faktor neben Krankenversorgung und Lehre, auch wenn dies an anderen Stellen nicht immer sofort so erkannt wird.

Mit Ihrer Tagung möchten Sie der Forschung neue Anstöße geben. Wir hoffen, daß daraus auch neue Anstöße für Versorgung und Verhütung von Krankheiten, insbesondere der Arteriosklerose, erwachsen.

In diesem Sinne wünsche ich Ihnen einen erfolgreichen Verlauf Ihrer Tagung und eine schöne Zeit in Münster.

Wilhelm Riehemann

Mit besonderer Freude begrüße ich Sie, meine Damen und Herren, und überbringe Ihnen die herzlichsten Grüße und alle guten Wünsche von Mitgliederversammlung, Kuratorium und Vorstand der Gesellschaft für Arterioskleroseforschung in Münster. Als Vorsitzender des Vorstandes der Trägergesellschaft bin ich hocherfreut, stolz und dankbar zugleich, daß Sie, verehrter Herr Professor Hauss, Ehrenvorsitzender unseres Instituts, nun schon zum sechsten Male dieses internationale Arteriosklerose-Symposium ausrichten.

Daß Ihrer Einladung, lieber Herr Professor Hauss, so viele Wissenschaftler aus dem In- und Ausland gefolgt sind, zeigt mir, welche Bedeutung diesem Symposium beigemessen wird.

Aber nicht nur die Wissenschaft, sondern auch wir – die Mitglieder des Vereins – sind gespannt auf die Ergebnisse Ihrer Beratungen, ja, wie uns die Arbeit des Instituts überhaupt brennend interessiert.

Warum das so ist? Warum interessieren sich Verwaltungen für Arterioskleroseforschung? Die Zahlen der deutschen Rentenversicherungsträger belegen unser Interesse. Bei der LVA Westfalen stehen die Herzkreislauferkrankungen mit gut einem Drittel an erster Stelle der Ursachen der Renten wegen Berufs- und Erwerbsunfähigkeit, bei den Männern sogar mit 36%.

106.000 Heilmaßnahmen wurden von allen Rentenversicherungsträgern in der Bundesrepublik 1988 wegen Krankheiten des Kreislaufsystems durchgeführt.

Also Ausgaben in Milliardenhöhe allein durch die Rentenversicherungsträger. Deshalb unser menschliches, wie unser wirtschaftliches Interesse an der Arterioskleroseforschung. Deshalb fördern wir – auch finanziell – die so bedeutsame

Arbeit unseres Instituts, weil nur durch engagierte Forschung weitere Aufschlüsse über die Ursachen und damit auch über die mögliche Verhinderung der Arteriosklerose zu erhalten sind.

Darum bin ich auch so froh und dankbar, daß unser Institut seit der letzten Mitgliederversammlung vor einigen Wochen nicht mehr nur den Zweck hat, die Erforschung der Entstehung, der Verhütung und der Behandlung der Arteriosklerose zu fördern, sondern daß das Institut nun auch die Aufgabe hat, der Prävention zu dienen.

Der Rektor der Universität Münster hat die Arterioskleroseforschung zur Schwerpunktforschung an unserer Universität erklärt. Dafür sind wir ihm sehr dankbar. Der Trägerverein hat expressis verbis nun die Prävention in den Aufgabenkatalog seines Instituts aufgenommen. Herr Professor Hauss hat in seinem neuesten Buch "Die Arteriosklerose" geschrieben, die Arteriosklerose sei heute "als die häufigste Seuche in den modernen Industriestaaten" zu bezeichnen.

Wissenschaft und Rentenversicherungsträger haben in einem beispiellosen Kampf über viele Jahrzehnte die Volksseuche Tuberkulose bekämpft und besiegt.

Es ist des Schweißes aller Edlen wert, den gleichen Kampf gegen die Arteriosklerose zu führen. Wir als Rentenversicherungsträger fühlen uns dazu aufgerufen.

In diesem Sinne wünsche ich dem 6. Arteriosklerose-Symposium einen guten Verlauf.

Werner H. Hauss

I welcome you to the Sixth Münster International Arteriosclerosis Symposium.

This time you have come to our country which — after a long and dark time — has recovered to a peaceful, free and reunited Germany.

Our institute, the university and the city of Münster are in the happy situation to celebrate a second cheerful event: Exactly 20 years ago the government of Nordrhine-Westfalia foundet on my initiative the Institute of Arteriosclerosis Research at the University of Münster to continue a long German scientific tradition older than a hundred years.

My co-workers and I are thankful to all people who helped to create this institute and especially to the scientists all over the world who educated the "baby" growing up. Many of you, my dear guests, have been engaged for which we thank you very much.

Especially, my dear friend Bob Wissler advised us from the beginning — and me even for years longer. He taught us to become active members in the international scientific medical community. My co-workers and I thank him heartily for his help. I asked him to have the kindness to speak about the history of our institute and as always he agreed to my request.

SESSION I:
ARTERIAL WALL AND BLOOD CELL INTERACTIONS IN THE PATHOGENESIS OF ARTERIOSCLEROSIS

1

The Biochemical Basis of Atherosclerosis: Roles for Cytokines

Peter Libby M.D.
Vascular Medicine and Atherosclerosis Unit
Brigham & Women's Hospital
and Harvard Medical School, Boston, Mass., USA

Clinical, epidemiological, and experimental evidence continues to accumulate linking disordered lipid metabolism with a development of atherosclerosis in humans and other animals. Over the last fiften years a great deal of information has become available regarding protein growth factors that can influence the proliferation of smooth muscle cells, a process thought crucial in the transition from the fatty to the fibrious complicated atheroma. Although a definite rôle for any given growth factor during the pathogenesis of atherosclerosis is uncertain, it is reasonable to adopt the working hypothesis that disordered growth control of proliferation involving such factors contributes to atherogensis. Despite remarkable advances in understanding the structure of apolipoproteins and their receptors and the metabolism of lipids in the organism and within cells and a burgeoning of structural information regarding protein growth factors, there is little information regarding the mechanisms that link these two biochemical factors implicated in the pathogenesis of arterial diseases. Our laboratory has been interested in the possibility that cytokines may provide a link between dyslipidemia and atherosclerosis. This brief review will outline some of the concepts regarding interrelations between cytokine gene expression and other factors postulated to contribute to atherogenesis. Current approaches should permit testing these concepts.

The cytokines are protein mediators of inflammation, immunity, and the host response to infectious agents. They include an ever-growing series of interleukins designated by number (Table 1). These factors, originally thought to provide signals among leukocytes, actually effect many other cell types including vascular endothelial and smooth muscle cells. Tumor necrosis factor α and lymphotoxin, also known as tumor necrosis factor β, share many of the properties of certain interleukins as well. The colony stimulating factors (CSFs) are hematopoietic growth factors and activators of certain leukocyte functions. The biological ac-

Table 1: Partial listing of cytokines possibly produced by cells in the atheroma

Cytokine:	Major Function:
Interleukin 1	See table 2
Interleukin 2	T lymphocyte activation
Interleukin 6	T & B lymphocyte activation
Interleukin 8	Granulocyte activation/adhesion inhibition
TNF α	Similar to IL-1, Macrophage activation
TNF β	Similar to TNF α
MCP-1/MCAF/JE	Macrophage chemotaxis and activation
M-CSF	Macrophage growth and activation
GM-CSF	Granulocyte/Monocyte growth and activation
Interferon β	Class I histocompatibility gene expression, smooth muscle cell growth inhibiton
Interferon γ	Class I and II histocompatibility gene expression, smooth muscle cell growth inhibition

tivities of the CSFs overlap with those of the interleukins, earning them a place within the cytokine family. The interferons constitute another subgroup of protein mediators that affect diverse functions of leukocytes and other cell types. Type 1 interferons (IFNs α and β) exhibit antiviral and other biological activities. These types of interferon are produced by leukocytes (interferon α) and fibroblasts and smooth muscle cells (interferon β). Interferon γ, also known as immune interferon, is produced only by activated T lymphocytes or natural killer (NK) cells. Interferon γ stimulates expression of histocompatibility antigens on the surface of many cell types and can activate macrophages, a property which may prove relevant to atherogenesis.

Over the last half dozen years results from a number of laboratories have established that many of the key functions of vascular cells of important in maintenance

Table 2: Some functions of Interleukin 1 on Vascular Cell Functions

Augments:	Supresses:
Leukocyte adhesion molecule expression	
Tissue factor procoagulant	Thrombomodulin expression
Plasminogen activator inhibitor expression	Plasminogen activator activity
Smooth muscle cell growth	Endothelial cell growth
Platelet-derived growth factor expression	
Acidic fibroblast growth factor expression	
Interleukin-1 gene expression	
M-CSF, GM-CSF, IL-8, MCP-1/JE expression	

of normal vascular homeostasis and the pathogenesis of vascular disease are subject to cytokine regulation *in vitro* (Table 2). For example, cytokines can modulate the properties of endothelial cells that render their surface able to maintain blood in a liquid state. Interleukin-1 or TNF can alter the balance of anticoagulant, antithrombotic, and fibrinolytic mechanisms of endothelial cells in an fashion that reduces hemocompatibility [1, 2, 3, 4].

Adhesive interactions between leukocytes and endothelium contribute importantly to normal leukocyte trafficking and the mobilization of host defenses and in the pathogenesis of certain diseases. Early in the response to atherogenic diets in many species, blood monocytes adhere to the endothelium of lesion-prone areas of arteries, enter the intima, and accumulate lipids [5, 6, 7, 8]. These lipid-laden macrophages make up an important component of the foam cell lesion characteristic of consumption of diets high in cholesterol and fat. The recent explosion in structural information concerning leukocyte adhesion molecules (LAMs) on endothelial and other cells has yielded greater understanding of the mechanisms of these adhesive interactions [9, 10]. One feature that emerges from recent studies of the expression of LAMs is their regulability by cytokines. Interleukin-1, tumor necrosis factor, and interferon γ can all modulate the expression of well characterized LAMs.

Cytokines can also influence the growth of endothelial and smooth muscle cells by either direct or indirect mechanisms. TNF and IL-1 tend to reduce the proliferation of endothelial cells *in vitro*. Interleukin-1 treatment stimulates proliferation of smooth muscle cells [11], perhaps by inducing autocrine growth factor production [12]. Interferon γ limits the proliferation of both endothelial and smooth muscle cells [13, 14, 15]. The induction of expression of endogenous growth factor or CSF genes by cytokines appears common. For example IL-1 or modified lipoproteins can modulate the expression of granulocyte-monocyte CSF (GM-CSF) in cultured human endothelial cells [16, 17]. Tumor necrosis factor and IL-1 can enhance platelet-derived growth factor gene expression in vascular endothelial and smooth muscle cells [12, 18].

Cytokines also regulate the production of lipid mediators by vascular wall cells. Interleukin-1 and TNF potently stimulate arachadonic acid metabolism in these cells. This pathway yields production of prostanoids such as prostacyclin or PGE_2 by vascular cells [19, 20]. Interleukin-1 can also elicit endothelial production of platelet activating factor [21].

Finally, a characteristic action of cytokines are target cells including those in the vessel wall is stimulation of expression of other cytokine genes. For example, IL-1 can stimulate expression of genes that encode both isoforms of this mediator [22, 23]. Likewise tumor recrosis factor can induce interleukin-1 gene expression in both vascular cell types [24, 25]. Interleukin-1 is a common trigger for expression of other interleukin genes in vascular cells including interleukin-6 [26, 27, 28], interleukin-8 [29, 30], and MCP1/MCAF/JE [31].

This overview of the manifold effects of cytokine such as IL-1 on vascular cells highlights why these molecules seem attractive candidates for mediating some of the changes in vascular functions associated with initiation and progression of the atheroslerotic plaque. How might cytokine gene expression be linked to factors implicated in the initiation of atherosclerosis, notably hyperlipoproteinemia? In monkeys fed diets that produce moderate levels of hypercholesterolemia extracts of affected arteries contain IL-1 messenger RNA. Chronic lesion in *Cynomologus* monkeys with moderate hypercholesterolemia contain endothelial cells, smooth muscle cells, and macrophages that exhibit IL-1 α and β mRNA as revealed by immunochemistry and *in situ* hybridization [32].

Recent studies in our laboratory have shown that rabbit aortae, 10 weeks after the initiation of diets supplemented with saturated fat and graded levels of cholesterol, do not contain augmented levels of RNA encoding IL-1 α or β or TNF mRNA, as estimated by polymerase chain reaction amplification of cDNA prepared by reverse transcription (Fleet et al., unpublished data). Interestingly, an intravenous injection of a classical cytokine inducer, bacterial endotoxin, elicited greater elevation of cytokine mRNA levels in animals fed diets containing 0.3 or 0.9% cholesterol in addition to saturated fat. We believe that this finding indicates that macrophage derived foam cells, and/or other cells types in the fatty lesions produced by ten weeks of this type of atherogeneic diet in rabbits, although they do not have spontaneous activation of cytokine gene expression, retain the ability respond to exogenous stimuli. Thus, foam cells *per se* may not be in an activated state in regard to cytokine gene expression. Our results cannot indicate whether individual vascular wall cells in the cholesterol-fed animal have altered sensitivity to endotoxin. However, the very accumulation of phagocytes within the lesion area appears to yield an augmentation in overall cytokine mRNA levels. Further studies will be required to determine whether corresponding increases in cytokine protein level or biological activity accompany the changes noted in RNA levels. Delineation of the contribution of various cell types to this exaggerated cytokine gene expression induced by endotoxin in the aortae of cholesterol-fed rabbits will also require additional study.

The identity of the proximate chemical messenger(s) linking the dietary changes to the altered metabolism of the arterial wall remain speculative. Work from a number of laboratories has suggested modified lipoproteins or their lipid or protein derivatives as mediators of the effects of hypercholesterolemia on arterial wall metabolism. Steinberg, Witztum and their colleagues have produced several lines of evidence that oxidized lipoproteins accumulate in atherosclerotic lesions and may play a rôle in monocyte chemotaxis and in other aspects of lesion formation [33]. Monoclonal antibody raised against oxidized lipoproteins has localized reactive material within experimental atherosclerotic lesions [34]. Fogelman, Berliner and colleagues have recently established that low densitiy lipoprotein subjected to "minimal" oxidative modification can induce cytokine production by endothelial cells [17, 35]. Fox and DiCorleto have argued that oxidized lipoproteins can alter growth factor production by cultured endothelial cells [36]. Hamilton and Chisolm have found that oxidized low density lipoprotein suppresses induced tumor necrosis factor-α mRNA expression in murine macrophages [37].

Thus, accumulating experimental evidence supports the concept that modified lipoprotein derivatives may provide a connection between the hypercholesterolemic state and evolution of the atherosclerotic plaque. Much work remains to establish a direct causal relationship between such lipoprotein derivativesand pathologic changes. The intiguing postulate that lipoprotein-induced modulation of cytokine and growth factor elaboration by vascular wall cells and infiltrating leukocytes also requires further investigation.

Acknowledgements

The author thanks his colleagues who contributed to the work in his laboratory related to the subject of this manuscript including Stephen K. Clinton, Hong Mei Li, James C. Fleet, and Helen Palmer. Dr. Libby is an Established Investigator of the American Heart Association. These studies were supported by a grant from the National Heart, Lung and Blood Institute, HL-34636.

References

[1] Bevilacqua, M.P., Pober, J.S., Majeau, G.R., Cotran, R.S., Gimbrone, Jr., M.A. (1984): Interleukin-1 (IL-1) induces biosynthesis and cell surface expression of procoagulant activity in human vascular endothelial cells. J. Exp. Med., 160: 618–623.
[2] Stern, D., Nawroth, P., Handley, D., Kisiel, W. (1985): An endothelial cell-dependent pathway of coagulation. Proc. Natl. Acad. Sci. USA 82: 2523–2527.
[3] Stern, D.M., Bank, I., Nawroth, P.P., Cassimeris, J., Kisiel, W., J.W. 2. Fenton, Dinarello, C., Chess, L., Jaffe, E.A. (1985): Self-regulation of procoagulant events on the endothelial cell surface. J. Exp. Med. 162: 1223–1235.
[4] Bevilacqua, M.P., Schleef, R., Gimbrone, Jr., M.A., Loskutoff, D.J. (1986): Regulation of the fibrinolytic system of cultured human vascular endothelium by IL-1. J. Clin. Invest. 78: 587–591.
[5] Poole, J.C.F., Florey, H.W. (1958): Changes in the endothelium of the aorta and the behavior of macrophages in experimental atheroma of rabbits. J. Path. Bact. 75: 245–253.
[6] Gerrity, R.G., Naito, H.K., Richardson, M., Schwartz, C.J. (1979): Dietary induced atherogenesis in swine: Morphology of the intima in prelesion stages. Am. J. Pathol. 95: 775–786.
[7] Faggiotto, A., Ross, R., Harker, L. (1984): Studies of hypercholesterolemia in the non-human primate. I. Changes that lead to fatty streak formation. Arteriosclerosis 4: 323–340.
[8] Rosenfeld, M.E., Tsukada, T., Gown, A.M., Ross, R. (1987): Fatty streak initiation in watanabe heritable hyperlipemic and comparably hypercholesterolemic fat-fed rabbits. Arteriosclerosis 7: 9–23.
[9] Bevilacqua, M.P., Stengelin, S., Gimbrone, M.A. Jr., Seed, B. (1989): Endothelial Leukocyte Adhesion Molecule 1: An inducible receptor for neutrophils related to complement regulatory proteins and lectins. Science 243: 1160–1165.

[10] Johnston, G.I., Cook, R.G., McEver, R.P. (1989): Cloning of GMP-140, a granule membrane protein of platelets and endothelium: sequence similarity to proteins involved in
cell adhesion and inflammation. Cell 56: 1033−1044.

[11] Libby, P., Warner, S.J.C., Friedman, G.B. (1988): Interleukin-1: a mitogen for human
vascular smooth muscle cells that induces the release of growth-inhibitory prostanoids.
J. Clin. Invest. 88: 487−498.

[12] Raines, E.W., Dower, S.K., Ross, R. (1989): Interleukin-1 mitogenic activity for fibroblasts and smooth muscle cells is due to PDGF-AA. Science 243: 393−396.

[13] Friesel, R., Komoriya, A., Maciag, T. (1987): Inhibition of endothelial cell proliferation
by gamma-interferon. J. Cell. Biol. 104: 689−96.

[14] Hansson, G.K., Jonasson, L., Holm, J., Clowes, M.K., Clowes, A. (1988): Gamma interferon regulates vascular smooth muscle proliferation and Ia expression in vivo and in
vitro. Cir. Research 712−719.

[15] Warner, S.J.C., Friedman, G.B., Libby, P. (1989): Immune interferon inhibits proliferation and induces 2'-5'-oligoadenylate synthetase gene expression in human vascular
smooth muscle cells. J. Clin. Invest. 83: 1174−1182.

[16] Bagby, G.C.J., Dinarello, C.A., Wallace, P., Wagner, C., Hefeneider, S., McCall, E. (1986):
Interleukin 1 stimulates granulocyte macrophage colony-stimulating activity release by
vascular endothelial cells. J. Clin. Invest. 78: 1316−1323.

[17] Rajavashisth, T.B., Andalibi, A., Territo, M.C., Berliner, J.A., Navab, M., Fogelman,
A.M., Lusis, A.J. (1990): Induction of endothelial cell expression of granulocyte and
macrophage colony-stimulating factors by modified low-density lipoproteins. Nature
344: 254−257.

[18] Hajjar, K.A., Hajjar, D.P., Silverstein, R.L., Nachman, R.L. (1987): Tumor necrosis
factor-mediated release of platelet-derived growth factor from cultured endothelial cells.
J. Exp. Med. 166: 235−245.

[19] Dejana, E., Breviario, F., Erroi, A., Bussolino, F., Mussoni, L., Gramse, M., Pintucci, G.,
Casali, B., Dinarello, C.A., Van Damme, J., Mantovani, A. (1987): Modulation of endothelial cell functions by different molecular species of interleukin 1. Blood 69: 695−699.

[20] Albrightson, C.R., Baenziger, N.L., Needleman, P. (1985): Exaggerated human vascular
cell prostaglandin biosynthesis mediated by monocytes: role of monokines and interleukin 1. J. Immunol. 135: 1872−1877.

[21] Bussolino, F., Breviario, F., Tetta, C., Aglietta, M., Mantovani, A., Dejana, E. (1986):
Interleukin 1 stimulates platelet-activating factor production in cultured human endothelial cells. J. Clin. Invest. 77: 2027−2033.

[22] Warner, S.J.C., Auger, K.R., Libby, P. (1987): Human interleukin 1 induces interleukin 1 gene expression in human vascular smooth muscle cells. J. Exp. Med. 165: 1316−
1331.

[23] Warner, S.J.C., Auger, K.R., Libby, P. (1987): Interleukin-1 induces interleukin-1. II.
Recombinant human interleukin-1 induces interleukin-1 production by adult human
vascular endothelial cells. J. Immunol. 139: 1911−1917.

[24] Libby, P., Ordovàs, J.M., Auger, K.R., Robbings, H., Birinyi, L.K., Dinarello, C.A.
(1986): Endotoxin and tumor necrosis factor induce interleukin-1 gene expression in
adult human vascular endothelial cells. Am. J. Path. 124: 179−186.

[25] Warner, S.J.C., Libby, P. (1989): Human vascular smooth muscle cells: Target for and
source of tumor necrosis factor. J. Immunol. 142: 100−109.

[26] Sironi, M., Breviario, F., Proserpio, P., Biondi, A., Vecchi, A., Van Damme, J., Dejana,
E., Mantovani, A. (1989): IL1 stimulates IL6 production in endothelial cells. J. Immunol.
142: 549−553.

[27] Loppnow, H., Libby, P. (1989): Adult human vascular endothelial cells express the IL6
gene differentially in response to LPS or IL1. Cell. Immunol. 122: 493−503.

[28] Loppnow, H., Libby, P. (1990): Proliferating or Interleukin 1-activated Human Vascular
Smooth Muscle Cells Secrete Copious Interleukin 6. J. Clin. Invest. 85: 731−738.

[29] Strieter, R.M., Kunkel, S.L., Showell, H.J., Remick, D.G., Phan, S.H., Ward, P.A. Marks,
R.M. (1989): Endothelial cell gene expression of a neutrophil chemotactic factor by
TNF-alpha, LPS, and IL-1 beta. Science 243: 1467−9.

[30] Sica, A., Matsushima, K., Van Damme, J., Wang, J.M., Polentarutti, N., Dejana, E., Colotta, F., Mantovani, A. (1990): IL-1 transcriptionally activates the neutrophil chemotactic factor/IL-8 gene in endothelial cells. Immunology 69: 548–553.

[31] Sica, A., Wang, J.M., Collota, F., Dejana, E., Mantovani, A., Oppenheim, J.J., Larsen, C.G., Zachariae, C.O., Matsushima, K. (1990): Monocyte chemotactic and activating factor gene expression induced in endothelial cells by IL-1 and tumor necrosis factor. J. Immunol. 144: 3034–3038.

[32] Williams, K., Sajuthi, D., Tulli, H., Huggins, E., Moyer, C. (1990): Vascular cells in atherosclerotic plaques of cynomolgous monkeys sythesize interleukin-1. FASEB J. 4: A 1154.

[33] Steinberg, D., Parthasarathy, S., Carew, T.E., Khoo, J.C., Witztum, J.L. (1989): Beyond cholesterol. Modifications of low-density lipoprotein that increase its atherogenicity. N. Engl. J. Med. 320: 915–924.

[34] Boyd, H.C., Gown, A.M., Wolfbauer, G., Chait, A. (1989): Direct evidence for a protein recognized by a monoclonal antibody against oxidatively modified LDL in atherosclerotic lesions from a Watanabe heritable hyperlipidemic rabbit. Am. J. Pathol. 135: 815–25.

[35] Berliner, J.A., Territo, M.C., Sevanian, A., Ramin, S., Kim, J.A., Bamshad, B., Esterson, M., Fogelman, A.M. (1990): Minimally modified low density lipoprotein stimulates monocyte endothelial interactions. J. Clin. Invest. 85: 1260–1266.

[36] Fox, P.L., DiCorleto, P.E. (1986): Modofied low density lipoproteins suppress production of a platelet-derived growth factor-like protein by cultured endothelial cells. Proc. Natl. Acad. Sci. USA 83: 4774–4778.

[37] Hamilton, T.A., Ma, G.P., Chisolm, G.M. (1990): Oxidized low density lipoprotein suppresses the expression of tumor necrosis factor-alpha mRNA in stimulated murine peritoneal macrophages. J. Immunol. 144: 2343–50.

The Role of T Lymphocyte Activation in Arteriosclerosis and Vascular Inflammation

Göran K. Hansson and Sten Stemme
Department of Clinical Chemistry,
Sahlgren's Hospital,
University of Göteborg, Sweden

Introduction

The atherosclerotic plaque is a site of inflammation, tissue repair and lipid accumulation. It is composed of three main cell types, smooth muscle cells, macrophages, and T lymphocytes [1]. Macrophages dominate the lipid-rich core region of the plaque, whereas smooth muscle cells are most frequent in the fibrous cap surrounding it [1]. T lymphocytes are present throughout the plaque and constitute approximately 10% of all cells [1-4].

Immunology active cells (T lymphocytes and macrophages) have a high capacity for production of cytokines that exert important regulatory functions on a variety of cell types. The presence of such cells in tissues does not, however, necessarily imply that cytokine production is taking place. Alternatively, the cells could be in a resting state with little or no production of bioactive signal substances.

We have characterized the T lymphocytes of the atherosclerotic plaque with regard to phenotype, activation state, and clonality, and also identified lymphokine-mediated effects on growth and differentiation of vascular cells by cell culture studies and animal experiments.

Plaque T cells are in a state of chronic activation

The T lymphocyte population of the atherosclerotic plaque is a mixture of CD4- and CD8-type cells [1, 2], the proportions of which may vary under different phases of the disease [4-5].

The activated T cell expresses cell surface proteins that differ from those expressed by resting T lymphocytes [6]. Furthermore, T lymphocytes that have once been activated can be distinguished from naive T lymphocytes on the basis of their cell surface proteins [7]. Immunohistochemical and flow cytometric analysis of T cells using monoclonal antibodies to such proteins provides detailed information on the functional state of the cells.

We have used this approach to characterize T cells of human atherosclerotic plaques. The tissue was obtained at endarterectomy, and samples were either snap-frozen and sectioned, or digested for cell isolation. In the former case, avidin-biotin enhanced immunohistochemical analysis was used to stain T cell activation markers. The isolated cells were labelled with fluorescent antibodies and analyzed by flow cytometry.

The immunohistochemical analysis revealed expression of receptors for the autocrine T-cell growth factor, interleukin-2 (IL2R), in the atherosclerotic plaques. Both scattered IL2R-positive cells and small clusters of positive cells were identified in the fluorescent microscope [3]. Staining of serial sections with the pan-T-cell antibody, CD3, clarified that IL2R expression was confined to areas with T cell infiltrates. This suggests that IL2R were expressed only by T cells. The overall frequency of IL2R positive T cells was, however, relatively low, or approximately 6% [3].

Autocrine growth occurs during the first phase of in vitro activation of T cells; this phase is followed by a late activation stage characterized by expression of integrin receptors [8]. We therefore analyzed expression of the integrin receptor, VLA-1, on CD3-positive T cells isolated from plaques. The flow cytometric analysis revealed a 25-fold higher proportion of VLA-1 positive T cells in the plaque when compared to peripheral blood from the same patient [2].

Plaque T cells are of polyclonal origin

The finding of T cell infiltrates in an inflammatory lesion such as the atherosclerotic plaque raises the question whether local, clonal proliferation of antigen-specific T cells may have occurred. Such a mechanism could be driven by a small number of antigens and result in an oligoclonal population of T cells. This appears to be the case in multiple sclerosis [10], whereas synovial T cells of rheumatoid arthritis patients appear to be polyclonal [11]. We have now evaluated the degree of clonality of the T cell population in the human atherosclerotic plaque.

For this purpose, we generated T cell cultures, each of which were derivated from one sigle progenitor T cell of the plaque (Fig. 1). The degree of monoclonality of such cultures is reflected in the organization of the genes for the T cell receptors (TCR) and can be determined by DNA hybridization. The rationale is the following.

The TCR genes are present in the genome of germline cells as gene segments dispersed along the chromosome. During T cell differentiation, these segments are rearranged in order to form a functional TCR gene [12]. The precise sequence of the rearranged gene is unique for each T lymphoblast and will remain unchanged throughout the life not only of the lymphoblast but also of the mature T lymphocyte and all daughter cells derived from it. Therefore, clonal proliferation during an immune response will result in a population of T cells with identical TCR genes. In contrast, a polyclonal T cell population will contain as many TCR gene patterns as there are cells.

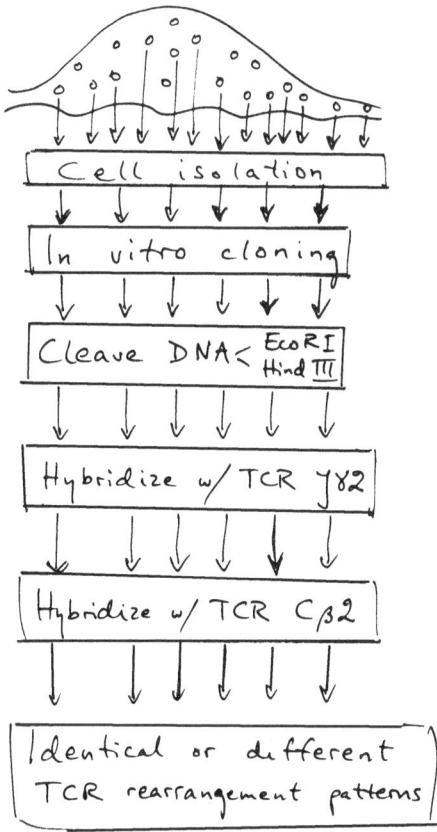

Figure 1: Schematic representation of the technique for isolation and TCR gene characterization of plaque T lymphocytes.

The rearranged TCR gene can be distinguished from the germline gene by DNA hybridization. Furthermore, each individual TCR rearrangement pattern is unique and can be distinguished from other TCR patterns by Southern blotting after cleavage of the gene with appropriate restriction enzymes. If individual T cells of a plaque can be analyzed with regard to TCR genes, it is possible to determine whether they represent individual members of one clone, or alternatively, a polyclonal cell population. We have been able to carry out such an analysis by first isolating plaque T cells, then expanding them in culture under clonal conditions to amplify the DNA of each cell sufficiently for analysis, i.e., to μg quantities or approx 5×10^6 cells (Fig. 1).

T cells were isolated from endarterectomy specimens and immediately cloned by the limiting dilution technique. Irradiated autologous peripheral mononuclear cells were used as feeder cells and both growth factor (interleukin-2) and a poly-

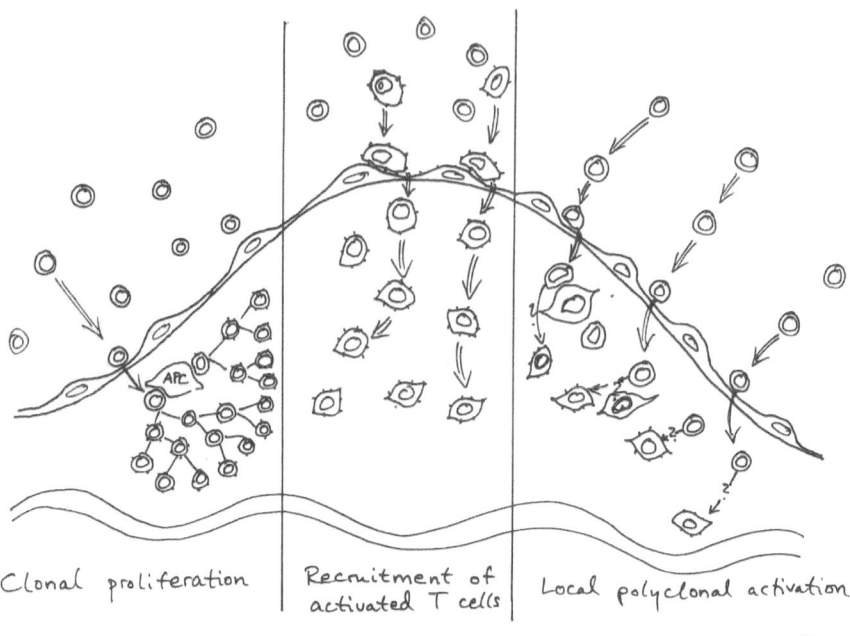

Figure 2: Three mechanisms that could explain the accumulation of T lymphocytes in the plaque.
Left, a local immune response induced by antigen-presenting cells (APC) which activate antigen-specific T cells to proliferate clonally.
Center, preferential recruitment of activated T cells accomplished by receptor interactions with cells at the plaque surface.
Right, polyclonal activation of T cells in plaque tissue.

clonal mitogen (CD3 antibody) were added to promote growth of the cultures. Cloning efficiencies were approx. 30% for plaque T cells under these conditions, and permitted expansion of 30–50 clones from each plaque.

DNA was isolated from each clone, cleaved with the restriction enzymes EcoRI and HindIII, separated by electrophoresis and blotted to nitrocellulose. The membranes were hybridized with gene probes specific for the TCR β and γ genes.

Analysis of the TCR γ gene using a probe for its J segment showed heterogeneity among the T cell preparations. Only 9, 5, 4 and 3 clones, respectively, from the four patients contained indistinguishable, rearranged TCR-γ genes [13]. When the DNA of these clones were reanalyzed using a probe for the constant segment of the TCR-β gene, all but two of the clones could be separated into different TCR gene patterns. The last pair was analyzed also after cleavage with another restriction enzyme, KpnI. TCR-γ gene hybridization revealed that also these two clones were different and thus not derived from the same progenitor T cell in the tissue.

In conclusion, the analysis indicated that the T cell population of the athe-rosclerotic plaque is polyclonal. This argues against a local immune response to one or a few antigenic epitopes as being a significant fenomenon in the mature atherosclerotic plaque. It cannot, however, be ruled out that such a response could take place earlier during the pathogenesis of the disease.

Our two findings that (i) the T cells of the plaque are in a state of chronic activation, and (ii) that they are polyclonal, suggest that there is a preferential recruitment of activated T cells into the atherosclerotic plaque (Fig. 2). The reason for this is unclear. One possibility is that the (endothelial or other) surface-forming cells of the plaque or in the vasa vasorum express receptors that bind to cell surface proteins that are specifically expressed on activated T lymphocytes. The mechanism and regulation of such cell-cell interactions are, however, not known. The further characterization of the interactions between immune and mesenchymal cells during pathological conditions should therefore be a fruitful research field in years to come.

Acknowledgment

This work was supported by the Swedish Medical Research Council (proj. 6816), the Swedish Heart-Lung Foundation, King Gustav V 80th Anniversary Foundation and the University of Göteborg.

References

[1] Jonasson, L., Holm, J., Skalli, O., Bondjers, G., Hannsson, G.K.: Arteriosclerosis 6: 131–138, 1986.
[2] Jonasson, L., Holm, J., Skalli, O., Gabbiani, G., Hansson, G.K.: J. Clin. Invest. 76: 125–131, 1985.
[3] Hansson, G.K., Holm, J., Jonasson, L.: Am. J. Pathol. 135: 169–175, 1989.
[4] Hansson, G.K., Jonasson, L., Seifert, P.S., Stelle, S.: Arteriosclerosis 9: 567–578, 1989.
[5] Emeson, E.E., Robertson, A.L.: Am. J. Pathol. 130: 369–376, 1988.
[6] Waldmann, T.A.: Science 232: 727–732, 1986.
[7] Thomas, M.L.: Ann. Rev. Immunol. 7: 339–370, 1989.
[8] Hemler, M.E., Glass, D., Coblyn, J.S., Jacobson, J.G.: J. Clin. Invest. 78: 696–702, 1986.
[9] Stemme, S., Holm, J., Hansson, G.K.: Submitted for publication, 1991.
[10] Hafler, D.A., Duby, A.D., Lee, S.J., Benjamin, D., Seidman, J.G., Weiner, H.L.: J. Exp. Med. 167: 1313–1322, 1988.
[11] Duby, A.D., Sinclair, A.K., Osborne-Lawrence, S.L., Zeldes, W., Kan, L., Fox, D.A.: Proc. Natl. Acad. Sci., USA 86: 6206–6210, 1989.
[12] Caccia, N., Mak, T.W.: Transpl. Proc. 12: 18–21, 1989.
[13] Stemme, S., Rymo, L., Hansson, G.K.: Lab. Invest., in press 1991.

Platelets and Atherosclerosis
– Experimental and Clinical Studies –
(Abstract)

Fujio Numano and Yukio Kishi
Dept. of Internal Medicine
Tokyo Medical and Dental University

Modern studies on atherogenesis have elucidated the important role platelets play not only in initiating thrombus formation, but in causing vascular injury which develops into atheromatous lesions. Our in vitro studies using animal models demonstrated that activated platelets release thromboxane A_2 and other vasoactive substances which induce edematous changes in the arterial wall. These changes result in acute plasmal infiltration into the arterial wall, including lipid particles. In vitro studies further indicate that activated platelets directly damage luminal endothelial cells. Cultured endothelial cells isolated from bovine aorta and preincubated with ^{3}H-adenine were subjected to collagen-activated or sonicated human platelets, and resulted in damage to the cells as estimated by ^{3}H-adenine release into the media. The release of ^{3}H-adenine depended on their dosage and on the incubation time with activated platelets. The content of intracellular ATP and cyclic AMP decreased in endothelial cells treated with activated platelets.

On the other hand, pretreatment of the endothelial cells with cAMP-promoting agents such as ZK36.374(10^{-6}M) IBMX (10^{-3}M), cilostazol (10^{-3}M) phthalazinol (10^{-2}M) protected the cells from activated platelet induced damage.

These experimental data suggest that antiplatelet therapy could be meaningful not only for the prevention of thrombotic episodes but also for the protection of the arterial wall from vascular injury and the atherosclerotic process. In fact, many antiplatelet agents clinically employed in Japan were reported to increase cAMP content in both endothelial cells and platelets. The results with patients treated with these agents have revealed their favorable clinical effects in parallel with decreased platelet aggregability and an increase in plasma cAMP levels. Even long term treatement with a small dose of aspirin (80 mg/day, cyclooxygenase inhibitor) revealed the increase in cAMP levels in the plasma of patients, so that this remedy is becoming one of the essential treatment for atherosclerotic disorders.

The Role of Type 1 Plasminogen Activator Inhibitor in the Regulation of the Fibrinolytic System of the Normal and Atherosclerotic Vessel Wall

Dietmar Seiffert and David J. Loskutoff
Committee on Vascular Biology
Research Institute of Scripps Clinic
La Jolla, California, USA

Introduction

It is generally assumed that vascular homeostasis results from the regulated interaction of the coagulation and fibrinolytic systems. These systems appear to be in dynamic equilibrium, and any imbalance in them leads to an increased risk of thrombosis or the tendency to develop a bleeding diathesis (Astrup, 1958). This balance is severely disturbed in the atherosclerotic vessel wall (Balkuv-Ulutin, 1986; Breddin, 1986). Thrombosis is most likely initiated upon plaque rupture, a process which undoubtedly exposes the flowing blood to the procoagulant activity present in the necrotic core of the vessel wall (for review, see Chandler, 1982). The fibrinolytic system (for review, see Bachmann, 1987) is responsible for the dissolution of fibrin deposits in the vasculature. Degradation of fibrin normally results from the action of plasmin, which circulates in plasma as an inactive proenzyme, plasminogen, and is activated by plasminogen activators (PAs) like urinary-type PA (u-PA) and tissue-type PA (t-PA). The presence of type 1 plasminogen activator inhibitor (PAI-1), the physiological inhibitor of both u-PA and t-PA (for review, see Loskutoff et al., 1989), in the plaque will prevent this system from being activated. This review will emphasize the role of PAI-1 in regulating the fibrinolytic system of the vessel wall. Particular attention will be paid to the interaction between PAI-1 and extracellular matrix (ECM) proteins including vitronectin (Vn) and the potential importance of this interaction for vascular disease.

Properties of PAI-1

Human PAI-1 is a single-chain glycoprotein of Mr 50,000, and is synthesized and secreted by a variety of cell types in culture (for reviews, see Sprengers and Kluft, 1987; Loskutoff et al., 1989). PAI-1 is also present in blood (Erickson et al.,

1986; Sprengers and Kluft, 1987; Kruithof et al., 1987) and platelets (Erickson et al., 1984; Booth et al., 1985; Kruithof et al., 1986; Sprengers et al., 1986; Preissner et al., 1989). Its primary structure has been elucidated by molecular cloning studies (for review, see Loskutoff et al., 1989). The pre-PAI-1 molecule is 402 amino acids in length, including a signal peptide of 23 amino acids. Removal of the signal peptide yields a mature secreted form of PAI-1 that is 379 amino acids in length and contains three potential N-linked glycosylation sites.

PAI-1 inhibits both t-PA and u-PA by forming sodium dodecyl sulfate (SDS)-stable 1:1 stoichiometric complexes with them (Wiman et al., 1984). Kinetic studies indicate that the dissociation constant for the interaction of human PAI-1 and t-PA is less then 1×10^{-13} mol/L (van Mourik et al., 1984; Colucci et al., 1986). The binding of PAI-1 to t-PA and u-PA is extremely rapid with second-order rate constants between $10^7 - 10^8 / M^{-1} s^{-1}$ (Coleman et al., 1986; Colucci et al., 1986; Hekman and Loskutoff, 1988b).

PAI-1 is present in the medium conditioned by a variety of cells primarily in an inactive (latent) form (Hekman and Loskutoff, 1985; Sprengers and Kluft, 1987). Latent PAI-1 can be converted into its active form by treatment with denaturants (e.g., SDS, guanidine hydrochloride, urea; Hekman and Loskutoff, 1985) and heat (Katagiri et al., 1988). Activation of latent PAI-1 with reagents that disrupt the secondary structure of proteins suggest that the activation process is associated with a conformational change in the molecule (Loskutoff et al., 1989). This hypothesis is consistent with the observation that active and latent PAI-1 migrate quite differently from each other when analyzed by gel filtration (Hekman and Loskutoff, 1985) and ultracentrifugation (Levin and Santell, 1987a). The demonstration that negatively charged phospholipids (Lambers et al., 1987) and Vn (Wun et al., 1989) activate latent PAI-1 raises the possibility that the conversion of latent PAI-1 into an active inhibitor in vivo may be of physiological significance. For example, platelets assume a net negative charge upon activation (Zwall, 1978), raising the possibility that latent PAI-1 may bind to and be activated on the platelet surface. There is, at present, little available data concerning this possibility. Although Vn is present in plasma at high concentrations (Conlan et al., 1988), it seems to convert latent PAI-1 into its active form only slowly (days) (Wun et al., 1989) compared to the rapid (minutes) clearance time for PAI-1 from the circulation (Colucci et al., 1985).

PAI-1 in cell extracts was shown to be present primarily in the active form (Levin and Santell, 1987b), and to spontaneously decay into the latent form in solution (Kooistra et al., 1986; Levin and Santell, 1987a; Hekman and Loskutoff, 1988a). These results suggest that PAI-1 is synthesized in the active form, but decays into the latent form following its release from cells. The binding of PAI-1 to ECM (Mimuro et al., 1987) and Vn (Declerk et al., 1988; Lindahl et al., 1989; Seiffert et al., 1989) appears to stabilize it against this rapid loss of activity (see below).

PAI-1 also rapidly loses its activity in the presence of oxidants, presumably by the oxidation of at least one critical methionine residues (Lawrence and Loskutoff, 1986). In analogy with the oxidative inactivation of alpha-1-proteinase inhibitor in inflammatory process (Travis and Salvesen, 1983; Weiss and Regiani, 1984), the oxidative inactivation of PAI-1 may be important for the regulation of the PA-system.

Regulation of PAI-1 Biosynthesis

PAI-1 ist a major biosynthetic product of endothelial cells, representing up to 10–15% of the proteins secreted by these cells into the serum-free conditioned medium, and its synthesis is highly regulated. Our laboratory has been studying the regulation of PAI-1 biosynthesis by molecules likely to be generated in, and released from platelets and leukocytes when they become activated in response to inflammatory processes, vascular injury, and thrombosis, all events implicated in the pathogenesis of atherosclerosis (Rokitansky, 1852; Duguid, 1946; Ross, 1986). In this regard, it is now clear that cytokines represent a group of molecules that may regulate PAI-1 synthesis by endothelium. For example, interleukin 1 stimulates the production of PAI-1 by cultured human umbilical vein endothelial cells (Bevilacqua et al., 1986a; Emeis and Kooistra, 1986; Gramse et al., 1986; Nachman et al., 1986; Schleef et al., 1988), causing a 4 to 8-fold increase in active PAI-1 in conditioned media (Bevilacqua et al., 1986a) and cell extracts (Schleef et al., 1988). Interleukin 1 may also suppress t-PA production (Bevilacqua et al., 1986a; Schleef et al., 1988) suggesting that the antifibrinolytic effects of this monokine occur at the level of both PAI-1 and t-PA. Tumor necrosis factor-alpha, a cytokine that mediates septic shock and the hemorrhagic necrosis of certain tumors, also stimulates PAI-1 synthesis in endothelial cells, again with concomitant decreases in t-PA production (Schleef et al., 1988). Tumor necrosis factor also induces tissue factor activity in endothelial cells (Bevilacqua et al., 1986b; Nawroth and Stern, 1986). The decreased fibrinolytic activity and increased procoagulant activity may therefore promote both the formation and maintenance of fibrin.

The induction of procoagulant activity by inflammatory mediators such as interleukin 1 and tumor necrosis factor alpha (Bevilacqua et al., 1986b; Nawroth and Stern, 1986), may lead to the increased generation of thrombin. The addition of thrombin to human umbilical vein endothelial cells caused an increase of PAI-1 activity in the medium (Gelehrter and Sznycer-Laszuk, 1986). Thrombin has also been shown to cleave and inactivate PAI-1 present in the ECM (Knudsen et al., 1987), and to stimulate the biosynthesis and release of t-PA from endothelial cells (Levin et al., 1984). The effects of thrombin on the fibrinolytic activity of these cells are therefore complex, and difficult to interpret.

A number of growth factors have been tested for their effects on PAI-1 synthesis. One of the most potent is transforming growth factor beta (TGF-beta), a polypeptide growth modulator present in platelets (for reviews see Sporn et al., 1987; Barnard et al., 1990) and released from platelet alpha-granules upon activation with physiological agonists (Assoian and Sporn, 1986). TGF-beta stimulates the synthesis of extracellular matrix proteins, including fibronectin and procollagen (Ignotz and Massague, 1986; Roberts et al., 1986). Picomolar concentrations of TGF-beta increased synthesis of PAI-1 in endothelial cells (Laiho et al., 1987; Saksela et al., 1987). These results thus raised the possibility that activated platelets may be able to suppress the fibrinolytic system of the vessel wall by releasing TGF-beta. This conclusion is supported by the observation that platelet releasates increased the rate of PAI-1 biosynthesis in endothelial cells, and that this increase could be blocked by pretreating the platelet releasates with antisera to TGF-beta (Slivka and Loskutoff, 1991). These results indicate that platelets can communicate with endothelial cells to modulate their fibrinolytic system, and suggest that platelet-rich thrombi may have high local concentrations of PAI-1, both as a direct consequence of its release from platelet alpha-granules, and because its production by surrounding endothelial cells is stimulated by platelet-derived TGF-beta. Neither epidermal growth factor, platelet-derived growth factor, or endothelial cell growth factor stimulated PAI-1 synthesis in bovine endothelial cells (Mimuro and Loskutoff, 1987b). Interestingly, platelet-derived growth factor and TGF-beta have recently been shown to increase PAI-1 synthesis in smooth muscle cells (McFall and Reilly, 1990). This latter observation suggests that these growth factors may promote fibrin deposition in the vessel wall at sites of endothelial injury.

Endotoxin or lipopolysaccharide (LPS), a component of the cell wall of gram-negative bacteria (Morrison and Ulevitch, 1978), elevates PAI-1 activity in plasma of patients with gram-negative septicaemia (Colucci et al., 1985). Other investigators have noted increased PAI-1 activity in the plasma of rats injected with LPS (Emeis and Kooistra, 1986), and in LPS-treated cultured endothelial cells of both human (Emeis and Kooistra, 1986; Dubor et al., 1986) and bovine (Crutchley and Conanan, 1986; Podor et al., 1988) origin. The elevated PAI-1 level may predispose these individuals to develop thrombotic disease, and indeed, disseminated intravascular coagulation is one of the major clinical manifestations of gram-negative septicaemia.

Finally, a variety of observations indicate that hormones may regulate PAI-1 biosynthesis. For example, steroids have been noted to stimulate PAI-1 synthesis in several cell culture systems (Loskutoff et al., 1986; Coleman et al., 1982; Busso et al., 1987). Despite these findings, no effect of steroids on PAI-1 activity has been demonstrated in vivo. A positive correlation has also been demonstrated between PAI-1 and plasma insulin levels (Juhan-Vague et al., 1987; Vague et al., 1986). Insulin caused a two-fold increase in PAI-1 production by primary cultures of human hepatocytes (Kooistra et al., 1989), while no effect of insulin could be detected in human umbilical vein endothelial cells (Alessi et al., 1988). These observations suggest that hepatic synthesis may contribute to the elevated concentrations of PAI-1 found in the plasma of hyperinsulinemic subjects (Juhan-Vague et al., 1987; Vague et al., 1986).

Presence of PAI-1 in the ECM and its Interaction with VN

PAI-1 has been detected in ECM from a number of cultured cells, including bovine smooth muscle cells (Knudsen et al., 1987), and bovine (Mimuro et al., 1987a) and human (Levin and Santell, 1987b; Schleef et al., 1990) endothelial cells. The generality of these findings are the basis of speculation that PAI-1 also may be present in ECM in vivo. In this instance, ECM-proteins may serve to localize and concentrate PAI-1 in the subendothelium. The ECM associated PAI-1 binds to and inhibits both t-PA (Knudsen et al., 1987; Levin and Santell, 1987b; Mimuro et al., 1987a) and u-PA (Knudsen et al., 1987; Laiho et al., 1987), indicating that PAI-1 in the ECM is active. The resulting PAI-1/t-PA complexes have a relatively low affinity for ECM and thus rapidly dissociate from it (Mimuro and Loskutoff, 1989b; Schleef et al., 1990). As mentioned previously, this behavior is in marked contrast to PAI-1 in the conditioned medium which is mostly found in the latent form. The PAI-1 in the ECM is biologically stable over a 24-hour period (Mimuro et al., 1987a) whereas PAI-1 in the conditioned medium decays into the latent form with a half-life of approximately 2–3 hours.

The association between PAI-1 and ECM is of relatively high affinity since bound PAI-1 cannot be eluted from ECM by treatment with high concentrations of sodium chloride, heparin sulfate, or sugars (Mimuro et al., 1987a; Knudsen et al., 1987). However, as mentioned above, PAI-1 can be eluted from ECM with PA's and can also be specifically removed with low-pH buffer and high concentrations of arginine (Mimuro et al., 1987a; Knudsen et al., 1987). ECM depleted of endogenous PAI-1 by these treatments can still bind exogenously added PAI-1 indicating that these agents do not act by destroying the PAI-1 binding protein(s) in ECM. Latent PAI-1 binds to ECM only weakly compared to the active form (Mimuro and Loskutoff, 1989b) and is not activated as a consequence of this interaction (Mimuro et al., 1987a; Mimuro and Loskutoff, 1989b). Thus, the ECM does not appear to contain an activator of latent PAI-1.

ECM-associated PAI-1 is distributed as a rather homogeneous carpet under the cells, and this pattern is interrupted by striae of negative staining at focal contacts (Pollanen et al., 1987). It should be noted that u-PA also was detected under the cells but in discrete cellular contact sites (Pollanen et al., 1987; Pollanen et al., 1988). Thus, the localization of PAI-1 is in distinct contrast to that of u-PA.

Recent studies identified Vn as the primary PAI-1 binding protein in ECM (Mimuro and Loskutoff, 1989b; Seiffert et al., 1990). However, the relatively uniform pattern of PAI-1 associated with the culture substrate surface suggests that this inhibitor may be binding to Vn derived from the serum present in the culture medium rather then from Vn synthesized by the cells themselves. This

conclusion is supported by the observation that three cell lines, including bovine
and human endothelial cells (Seiffert et al., 1990), and human smooth muscle
cells (unpublished observation) each shown previously to contain PAI-1 in their
ECM, did not actually synthetisize detectable amounts of Vn. Moreover, the same
partially proteolyzed fragments of Vn detected in ECM were also present in the
serum used to culture these cells (Seiffert et al., 1990). Taken together, these
results indicate that PAI-1 is bound to Vn derived from the culture medium. The
interaction of PAI-1 and Vn is relatively specific, since no PAI-1 was detected in
ECM when endothelial cells were plated on culture dishes coated with fibronectin,
type IV collagen, or laminin, and direct binding studies using ^{35}S-labeled PAI-1
failed to detect significant interactions between these ECM-proteins and PAI-1
(Seiffert et al., 1990).

When plasma (Wiman et al., 1988) or serum (Erickson et al., 1986) was fractionated by gel filtration chromatography, the majority of active PAI-1 was
recovered in fractions that migrated with an apparent molecular weight in excess
of Mr 250,000, whereas latent PAI-1 migrated with the expected Mr of 50,000.
Thus, plasma contains PAI-1 binding protein(s) with molecular weight of 150,000—
200,000, and these protein(s) bind active PAI-1 but not the latent form (Wiman
et al., 1988). One of these proteins was purified from bovine (Mimuro and Loskutoff, 1989a) and human (Declerk et al., 1988; Wiman et al., 1988) plasma and
shown to be Vn. Solution-phase Vn (Declerk et al., 1988; Lindahl et al., 1989)
and solid-phase Vn (Seiffert et al., 1989) appear to increase the biological half-life
of PAI-1 by approximately 2—3 fold. It has been reported that PAI-1 bound to
Vn is less sensitive to oxidants (Lindahl et al., 1989) suggesting that Vn may
protect PAI-1 from oxidative inactivation. These results thus raise the possibility
that Vn may locally protect PAI-1 from oxidants liberated by activated inflammatory cells (Weiss and Regiani, 1984). PAI-1 bound to Vn appears to be a better
thrombin-inhibitor than free PAI-1 (Ehrlich et al., 1990) suggesting that Vn may
modulate the substrate specificity of PAI-1 in some settings. However, the majority
of PAI-1 in plasma circulates in complex with Vn and no PAI-1/thrombin complexes have been reported in plasma.

Kinetic studies indicate that the dissociation constant for the interaction of
activated PAI-1 and immobilized Vn is in the order of 10^{-10} mol/L (Salonen
et al., 1989; Seiffert et al., 1989). A second low-affinity interaction (1.9×10^{-7}
mol/L) was also noted and presumably involves the binding of the various inactive
forms of PAI-1 (e.g., latent, oxidized, proteolytically modified, or complexed
with PAs) with Vn (Salonen et al., 1989).

PAI-1 and Atherosclerosis

Recent studies employing in situ hybridization provide evidence that PAI-1 is synthesized in human atherosclerotic plaques (Gordon et al., 1989). Endothelial cells expressing PAI-1 were a consistent feature of these lesions. In addition, mesenchymal-appearing cells were shown to be strongly positive for PAI-1 mRNA. In the development of these lesions, the presence of both PAI-1 and tissue factor, which is extensively expressed within atheromatous plaques (Wilcox et al., 1989) may promote local thrombus formation. These thrombi may subsequently be incorporated into the atherosclerotic plaques (for review, see Woolf, 1981). Interestingly, Vn also was detected in both intimal thickenings and fibrous plaques of atherosclerotic lesions (Guettier et al., 1989; Niculescu et al., 1989). Rupture of the plaque would expose the blood to tissue factor procoagulant activity, initiating clot formation and thrombosis. Vn may serve to locally concentrate and stabilize the PAI-1, thus impairing the otherwise normal clearance of these thrombi by the fibrinolytic system. The recurrence of such episodes would promote the growth and development of the plaques, leading ultimately to severe stenosis and thrombotic occlusion of the vessel (Woolf, 1981).

Deficient fibrinolysis due to increased plasma PAI-1 activity has been noted in obese subjects (Vague et al., 1986), and in non-insulin dependent diabetes (Auwerx et al., 1988), hyperinsulinemia (Juhan-Vague et al., 1987), and hypertriglyceridemia (Juhan-Vague et al., 1987; Hamsten et al., 1985). These conditions are recognized risk factors for the development of atherosclerosis. In addition, evidence for increased PAI-1 levels in patients with coronary artery disease has been obtained. For example, Paramo et al. (1985) found elevated PAI-1 level in patients with angiographically documented coronary artery disease. However, similar studies by Oseroff et al. (1989) could demonstrate no such relationship. This discrepancy may, in part, reflect differences in the patient populations chosen for these studies and the exclusion of subjects with other risk factors codistributing with PAI-1 (Oseroff et al., 1989). Hamsten et al. (1985) demonstrated elevated levels of PAI-1 in young survivors of myocardial infarction, raising the possibility that PAI-1 may be a risk factor for the development of coronary artery disease.

While the identity of the stimulus for PAI-1 synthesis in atherosclerotic lesions is unknown, it is likely that many of the agents described above (see section entitled, "Regulation of PAI-1 biosynthesis") are involved. For example the release of TGF-beta from platelets, or TGF-beta together with interleukin 1 or tumor necrosis factor alpha from activated monocytes, may activate PAI-1 synthesis in atherosclerotic lesions. Similarly, the release of platelet derived growth factor from activated platelets, which may act as a mitogenic stimulus for smooth muscle cells (Ross, 1986), may also stimulate PAI-1 biosynthesis in these cells (McFall and Reilly, 1990). In conclusion, localized increases in PAI-1 activity, resulting either from increased synthesis in response to the action of mediators of inflammatory or repair processes on cells of the vessel wall, and/or from the concentration and stabilization of PAI-1 by Vn in atherosclerotic plaques, may compromise normal fibrinolysis and contribute to the development of thrombotic occlusion of atherosclerotic vessels. However, although a positive correlation between locally and systemically increased PAI-1 activity and vascular disease can be found, a causal role of PAI-1 remains to be proven.

Acknowledgements

This work was supported by grant HL 31950 to DJL from the National Institute of Health and a research fellowship to DS from the American Heart Association, California Affiliate, with funds contributed by the Orange County Chapter.

References

[1] Alessi, M.C., Juhan-Vague, I., Kooistra, T., Declerck, P.J., and Collen, D.: Insulin stimulates the synthesis of plasminogen activator inhibitor 1 by the human hepatocellular cell line hep G2. Thromb. Haemostas. 1988; 60: 491–494.

[2] Assoian, R.K., Sporn, M.B.: Type-beta transforming growth factor in human platelets: Release during platelet degranulation and action on vascular smooth muscle cells. J. Cell. Bio. 1986; 102: 1217–1223.

[3] Astrup, T.: The haemostatic balance. Thromb. Diath. Haem. 1958; 2: 347.

[4] Auwerx, J., Bouillon, R., Collen, D.: Geboers. Tissue-type plasminogen activator inhibitor activity in diabetes mellitus. Arteriosclerosis 1988; 8: 68.

[5] Bachmann, F., Fibrinolysis. In: Thrombosis and Haemostasis. Ed. Verstraete, M., Vermylen, J., Lijnen, H.R., Arnout, J. Leuven University Press, Leuven, 1987.

[6] Balkuv-Ulutin: Fibrinolytic system in atherosclerosis. Sem. Thromb. Haemost. 1986; 12: 91–101.

[7] Barnard, J.A., Lyons, R.M., Moses, H.L.: The cell biology of transforming growth factor beta. Biochem. Biophys. Acta 1990; 1032: 79–87.

[8] Bevilacqua, M.P., Schleef, R.R., Gimbrone, M.A. Jr., Loskutoff, D.J.: Regulation of the fibrinolytic system of cultured human vascular endothelium by interleukin 1. J. Clin. Invest. 1986a; 78: 587–591.

[9] Bevilacqua, M.P., Pober, J.S., Majeau, G.R. Fiers, W., Cotran, R.S., Gimbrone, M.A. Jr.: Recombinant tumor necrosis factor induces procoagulant activity in cultured human vascular endothelium: Characterization and comparison with the actions of interleukin 1. Proc. Natl. Acad. Sci. USA 1986b; 83: 4533–4537.

[10] Booth, N.A., Anderson, J.A., Bennett, B.: Platelet release protein which inhibits plasminogen activators. J. Clin. Pathol. 1985; 38: 825–830.

[11] Breddin, K.: Detection of prethrombotic states in patients with atherosclerotic lessions. Sem. Thromb. Haemost. 1986; 12: 110–123.

[12] Busso, N., Belin, D., Failly-Crepin, C., Vassalli, J.D.: Glucocorticoid modulation of plasminogen activators and of one of their inhibitors in the human mammary carcinoma cell line MDA-MB-231. Can. Res. 1987; 47: 364–370.

[13] Chandler, A.B.: Thrombotic processes in coronary disease. In: Hemostasis and Thrombosis: Basic principles and clinical practice. Ed. Colman, R.W., Hirsh, J., Marder, V.J., Salzman, E.W. J.B. Lippincott Company, Philadelphia-Toronto, 1982.

[14] Coleman, P.L., Barouski-Miller, P.A., Gelehrter, T.D.: The dexamethsaone-induced inhibitor of fibrinolytic activity in hepatoma cells – a cellular product which specifically inhibits plasminogen activation. J. Biol. Chem. 1982; 257: 4260–4264.

[15] Coleman, P.L., Patel, P.D., Cwikel, B.J., Rafferty, U.M., Sznycer-Laszuk, R., Gelehrter, T.D.: Characterization of the dexamethasone-induced inhibitor of plasminogen activator in HTC hepatoma cells. J. Biol. Chem. 1986; 261: 4352–4357.

[16] Colucci, M., Paramo, J.A., Collen, D.: Generation in plasma of a fast-acting inhibitor of plasminogen activator in response to endotoxin stimulation. J. Clin. Invest. 1985; 75: 818–824.

[17] Colucci, M., Paramo, J.A., Collen, D.: Inhibition of one-chain and two-chain forms of human tissue-type plasminogen activator by the fast-acting inhibitor of plasminogen activator in vitro and in vivo. J. Lab. Clin. Med. 1986; 108: 53–59.

[18] Conlan, M.G., Tomasini, B.R., Schultz, R.L., Mosher, D.J.: Plasma vitronectin polymorphism in normal subjects and patients with disseminated intravascular coagulation. Blood 1988; 72: 185–190.

[19] Crutchley, D.J., Conanan, L.B.: Endotoxin induction of an inhibitor of plasminogen activator in bovine pulmonary artery endothelial cells. J. Biol. Chem. 1986; 261: 154–159.

[20] Declerk, P.J., De Mol, M., Alessi, M.C., Baudner, S., Paques, E.P., Preissner, K.T., Mueller-Berghaus, G., Collen, D.: Purification and characterization of a plasminogen activator inhibitor 1 binding protein from human plasma. J. Biol. Chem. 1988; 263: 15454–15461.

[21] Dubor, F., Dosne, A.M., Chedid, L.A.: Effect of polymyxin B and colimycin on induction of plasminogen antiactivator by lipopolysaccharide in human endothelial cell culture. Infect. Immun. 1986; 52: 725–729.

[22] Duguid, J.B.: Thrombosis as a risk factor in the pathogenesis of aortic atherosclerosis. J. Path. Bact. 1948; 60: 925.

[23] Ehrlich, H.J., Klein Gebbink, R., Keijer, J., Linders, M., Preissner, K.T., Pannekoek, H.: Alteration of serpin specifity by a protein cofactor. J. Biol. Chem. 1990; 265: 13029–13035.

[24] Emeis, J.J., Kooistra, T.: Interleukin 1 and lipopolysaccharide induce an inhibitor of tissue-type plasminogen activator in vivo and in cultured endothelial cells. J. Exp. Med. 1986; 163: 1260–1266.

[25] Erickson, L.A., Ginsberg, M.H., Loskutoff, D.J.: Detection and partial characterization of an inhibitor of plasminogen activator in human platelets. J. Clin. Invest. 1984; 74: 1465–1472.

[26] Erickson, L.A., Hekman, C.M., Loskutoff, D.J.: The primary plasminogen-activator inhibitors in endothelial cells, platelets, serum, and plasma are immunologically related. Proc. Natl., Acad. Sci. USA 1985; 82: 8710–8714.

[27] Gelehrter, T.D., Sznycer-Laszuk, R.: Thrombin induction of plasminogen activator-inhibitor in cultured human endothelial cells. J. Clin. Invest. 1986; 77: 165–169.

[28] Gordon, D., Augustine, A.J., Smith, K.M., Schwartz, S.M., Wilcox, J.N.: Localization of cells expressing tPA, PAI-1, and urokinase by in situ hybridization in human atherosclerotic plaques and in the normal rhesus monkey. Atherogenesis 1989; 1: 419.

[29] Gramse, M., Breviario, F., Pintucci, G., Millet, I., Dejana, E., Van Damme, J., Donati, B.M., Mussoni, L.M.: Enhancement by interleukin-1 (IL-1) of plasminogen activator inhibitor (PAI) activity in cultured human endothelial cells. Biochem. Biophys. Res. Commun. 1986; 139: 720–727.

[30] Guettier, C., Hinglais, N., Bruneval, P., Kazatchkine, M., Bariety, J., Camilleri, J.P.: Immunohistochemical localization of S protein/vitronectin in human atherosclerotic versus arteriosclerotic arteries. Virchows Archiv. A. Pathol. Anat. 1989; 414: 309–313.

[31] Hamsten, A., Wiman, B., deFaire, U., Blomback, M.: Increased plasma levels of a rapid inhibitor of tissue plasminogen activator in young survivors of myocardial infarction. N. Engl. J. Med. 1985; 313: 1557–1563.

[32] Hekman, C.J., and Loskutoff, D.J.: Endothelial cells produce a latent inhibitor of plasminogen activators that can be activated by denaturants. J. Biol. Chem. 1985; 260: 11581–11587.

[33] Hekman, C.M., and Loskutoff, D.J.: Bovine plasminogen activator inhibitor 1: Specificity determinations and comparison of the active, latent and guanidine-activated forms. Biochemistry 1988a; 27: 2911–2918.

[34] Hekman, C.M., and Loskutoff, D.J.: Kinetic analysis of the interactions between plasminogen activator inhibitor 1 and both urokinase and tissue plasminogen activator. Archives of Biochem. and Biophys. 1988b; 262: 199–210.

[35] Ignotz, R., Massague, J.: Transforming growth factor-beta stimulates the expression of fibronectin and collagen and their incorporation into the extracellular matrix. J. Biol. Chem. 1986; 261: 4337–4345.

[36] Juhan-Vague, I., Vague, P., Alessi, M.C., Badier, C., Valadier, J., Aillaud, M.F. Atlan, C.: Relationship between plasma insulin, triglyceride, body mass index, and plasminogen activator inhibitor 1. Diabetes Metab. 1987; 13: 331.

[37] Katagiri, K., Okada, K., Hattori, H., Yano, M.: Bovine endothelial cell plasminogen activator inhibitor. Purification and heat activation. Eur. J. Bioch. 1988; 176: 81–87.

[38] Knudsen, B.S., Hapel, P.C., Nachman, R.L.: Plasminogen activator inhibitor is associated with the extracellular matrix of cultured bovine smooth muscle cells. J. Clin. Invest. 1987; 80: 1082–1089.

[39] Kooistra, T., Sprengers, E.D., van Hinsbergh, V.W.M.: Rapid inactivation of the plasminogen-activator inhibitor upon secretion from cultured human endothelial cells. Biochem. J. 1986; 239: 497–503.

[40] Kooistra, T., Bosma, P.J., Tons, H.A.M., van den Berg, A.P., Meyer, P., Princen, H.M.B.: Plasminogen activator inhibitor 1: Biosynthesis and mRNA level are increased by insulin in cultured human hepatocytes. Thromb. Haemost. 1989; 62: 723–728.

[41] Kruithof, E.K.O., Tran-Thang, C., Bachmann, F.W.: Studies on the release of a plasminogen activator inhibitor by human platelets. Thromb. Haemost. 1986; 55: 201–205.

[42] Kruithof, E.K.O., Nicolosa, G., Bachmann, F.W.: Plasminogen activator inhibitor 1: Development of a radioimmunoassay and observations on its plasma concentration during venous occlusion and after platelet aggregation. Blood 1987; 70: 1645–1653.

[43] Laiho, M., Saksela, O., Keski-Oja, J.: Transforming growth factor-beta induction of type 1 plasminogen activator inhibitor. J. Biol. Chem. 1987; 262: 17467–17474.

[44] Lambers, J.W.J., Cammenga, M., Konig, B., Pannekoek, H., van Mourik, J.A.: Activation of human endothelial type plasminogen activator inhibitor (PAI-1) by negatively charged phospholipids. J. Biol. Chem. 1987; 262: 17492–17496.

[45] Lawrence, D., and Loskutoff, D.J.: Inactivation of plasminogen activator inhibitor by oxidants. Biochemistry 1986; 21: 6351–6355.

[46] Levin, E.G., Marzec, U., Anderson, J., and Harker, L.A.: Thrombin stimulates tissue plasminogen activator release from cultured human endothelial cells. J. Clin. Invest. 1984; 74: 1988–1995.

[47] Levin, E.G., Santell, L.: Conversion of the active to latent plasminogen activator inhibitor from human endothelial cells. Blood 1987a; 70: 1090–1098.

[48] Levin, E.G., Santell, L.: Association of plasminogen activator inhibitor (PAI-1) with the growth substratum and membrane of human endothelial cells. J. Cell. Biol. 1987b; 105: 2543–2549.

[49] Lindahl, T., Wiman, B.: Purification of high and low molecular weight plasminogen activator inhibitor 1 from fibrosarcoma cell-line HT 1080 conditioned medium. Biochim. Biophys. Acta. 1989; 994: 253–257.

[50] Loskutoff, D.J., Roegner, K., Erickson, L.A., Schleef, R.R., Huttenlocher, A., Coleman, P.L., Gelehrter, T.D.: The dexamethasone-induced inhibitor of plasminogen activator in hepatoma cells is antigenically-related to an inhibitor produced by bovine aortic endothelial cells. Thromb. Haemost. 1986; 55: 8–11.

[51] Loskutoff, D.J. Sawdey, M., and Mimuro, J.: Type 1 plasminogen activator inhibitor. In: B. Coller (Ed.) Progress in Hemostas Thromb., 9: 97–115, 1989.

[52] McFall, B.C., and Reilly, C.F.: TGF beta and PDGF induce plasminogen activator inhibitor release from vascular smooth muscle cells. FASEB J. 1990; 4: 3631.

[53] Mimuro, J., Schleef, R.R., and Loskutoff, D.J.: The extracellular matrix of cultured bovine aortic endothelial cells contains functionally active type 1 plasminogen activator inhibitor. Blood 1987a; 70: 721–728.

[54] Mimuro, J., Loskutoff, D.J.: Effect of transforming growth factor-beta on the fibrinolytic system of cultured bovine aortic endothelial cells (BAEs). Thromb. Haemost. 1987b; 58: 1647.

[55] Mimuro, J., and Loskutoff, D.J.: Binding of type 1 plasminogen activator inhibitor to the extracellular matrix of cultured bovine endothelial cells. J. Biol. Chem. 1989a; 264: 5058–5063.

[56] Mimuro, J., and Loskutoff, D.J.: Purification of a protein from bovine plasma that binds to type 1 plasminogen activator inhibitor and prevents its interaction with extracellular matrix. Evidence that the protein is vitronectin. J. Biol. Chem. 1989b; 264: 936–939.

[57] Morrison, D.C., Ulevitch, R.J.: The effects of bacterial endotoxins on host mediation systems. Am. J. Path. 1978; 93: 527–617.

[58] Nachman, R.L., Hajjar, K.A., Silverstein, R.L., Dinarello, C.A.: Interleukin 1 induces endothelial cell synthesis of plasminogen activator inhibitor. J. Exp. Med. 1986; 163: 1595–1600.

[59] Nawroth, P.P., Stern, D.M.: Modulation of endothelial cell hemostatic properties by tumor necrosis factor. J. Exp. Med. 1986; 163: 740–745.

[60] Niculescu, F., Rus, H.G., Porutiu, D., Ghiurca, V., Vlaicu, R.: Immunoelectron-microscopic localization of S-protein/vitronectin in human atherosclerotic wall. Atherosclerosis 1989; 78: 197–203.

[61] Oseroff, A., Krishnamurti, C., Hassett, A., Tang, D., and Alving B.: Plasminogen activator and plasminogen activator inhibitor activities in men with coronary artery disease. J. Lab. Clin. Med. 1989; 113: 88–93.

[62] Paramo, J.A., Colucci, M., Collen, D.: Plasminogen activator inhibitor in the blood of patients with coronary artery disease. Br. Med. J. 1985; 291: 573–574.

[63] Podor, T., Sawdey, M., Mathison, J., Tobias, P., Ulevitch, R., Loskutoff, D.J.: Serum-derived lipopolysaccharide (LPS) binding factors enhance the LPS-mediated induction of type 1 plasminogen activator inhibitor in endothelial cells. Fibrinolysis 1988; 2 (supp 1): 149.

[64] Pollanen, J., Saksela, O., Salonen, E.M., Andreasen, P.A., Nielsen, L., Dano, K., Vaheri, A.: Distinct localizations of urokinase-type plasminogen activator and its type 1 inhibitor under cultured human fibroblast and sarcoma cells. J. Cell. Biol. 1987; 104: 1085–1096.

[65] Pollanen, J., Hedman, K., Nielsen, L.S., Dano, K., Vaheri, A.: Ultrastructural localization of plasma membrane-associated urokinase-type plasminogen activator at focal contacts. J. Cell. Biol. 1988; 106: 87–95.

[66] Preissner, K.T., Holzhuter, S., Justus, C., Muller-Berghaus, G.: Identification and partial characterization of platelet vitronectin: Evidence for complex formation with platelet-derived plasminogen activator inhibitor-1. Blood 1989; 74: 1989–1996.

[67] Roberts, A.B., Sporn, M.B., Assoian, R.K., Smith, J.M., Roche, N.S., Wakefield, L.M., Heine, U.I., Liotta, L.A., Falanga, V., Kehrl, J.H., and Fauci A.S.: Transforming growth factor type-beta: Rapid induction of fibrosis and angiogenesis in vivo and stimulation of collagen formation in vitro. Proc. Natl. Acad. Sci. USA 1986; 83: 4167–4171.

[68] Rokitansky, C.V.: A manual of pathologic anatomy. The Sydenham Society 1852; p. 271.

[69] Ross, R.: The pathogenesis of artherosclerosis: an update. N. Engl. J. Med. 1986; 314: 488–500.

[70] Saksela, O., Moscatelli, D., and Rifkin, D.B.: The opposing effects of basic fibroblast growth factor and transforming growth factor beta on the regulation of plasminogen activator activity in capillary endothelial cells. J. Cell. Biol. 1987; 105: 957–963.

[71] Salonen, E.M., Vaheri, A., Pollanen, J., Stephens, R., Andreasen, P., Mayer, M., Dano, K., Gailit, J., Ruoshlahti, E.: Interaction of plasminogen activator inhibitor (PAI-1) with vitronectin. J. Biol. Chem. 1989; 264: 6339–6343.

[72] Schleef, R.R., Bevilacqua, M.P., Sawdey, M., Gimbrone, M.A., Jr., and Loskutoff, D.J.: Cytokine-activation of vascular endothelium: Effects on tissue-type plasminogen activator and type 1 plasminogen activator inhibitor. J. Biol. Chem. 1988; 263: 5797–5803.

[73] Schleef, R.R., Podor, T.J., Dunne, E., Mimuro, J., and Loskutoff, D.J.: The majority of type 1 plasminogen activator inhibitor associated with cultured human endothelial cells is located under the cells and is accessible to solution-phase tissue-type plasminogen activator. J. Cell. Biol. 1990; 110: 155–163.

[74] Seiffert, D., Mimuro, J., Loskutoff, D.J.: Analysis of the interaction between type 1 plasminogen activator inhibitor and its binding protein vitronectin. Fibrinolysis 1989a; 3 (suppl. 1), 39.

[75] Seiffert, D., Wagner, N.N., and Loskutoff, D.J.: Serum-derived vitronectin influences the pericellular distribution of type 1 plasminogen activator inhibitor. J. Cell. Biol. 1990b; 111: 1283–1291.

[76] Slivka, S.R., and Loskutoff, D.J.: Platelets stimulate endothelial cells to synthesize type 1 plasminogen activator inhibitor. Blood 1991; 77: 1013–1019.

[77] Sporn, M.B., Robert, A.B., Wakefield, L.M., de Crombrugghe, B.: Some recent advances in the chemistry and biology of transforming growth factor beta. J. Cell. Biol. 1987; 105: 1039–1045.

[78] Sprengers, E.D., Akkerman, J.W.N., Jansen, B.G.: Blood platelet plasminogen activator inhibitor: Two different pools of endothelial cell type. Thromb. Haemost. 1986; 55: 325–329.

[79] Sprengers, E.D., Kluft, C.: Plasminogen activator inhibitors. Blood 1987; 69: 381–387.

[80] Travis, J., Salvesen, G.S.: Human plasma protein inhibitors. Ann. Rev. Biochem. 1983; 52: 655–709.

[81] Vague, P., Juhan-Vague, I., Aillaud, M.F., Badier, C., Viard, R., Alessi, M.C., Collen, D.: Correlation between blood fibrinolytic activity, plasminogen activator inhibitor level, plasma insulin level and relative body weight in normal and obese subjects. Metabolism 1986; 35: 250.

[82] van Mourik, J.A., Lawrence, D.A., Loskutoff, D.J.: Purification of an inhibitor of plasminogen activator (antiactivator) synthesized by endothelial cells. J. Biol. Chem. 1984; 259: 14914–14921.

[83] Weiss, S.J., Regiani, S.: Neutrophils degrade subendothelial matrices in the presence of alpha-1-proteinase inhibitor. J. Clin. Invest. 1984; 73: 1297–1303.

[84] Wilcox, J.N., Smith, K.M., Schwartz, S.M., and Gordon, D.: Localization of tissue factor in the normal vessel wall and in the atherosclerotic plaque. Prov. Natl. Acad. Sci. USA 1989; 86: 2839–2843.

[85] Wiman, B., Chmielewska, J., Ranby, M.: Inactivation of tissue plasminogen activator in plasma. J. Biol. Chem. 1984; 259: 3644–3647.

[86] Wiman, B., Almquist, A., Sigurdardottir, O., Lindahl, T.: Plasminogen activator inhibitor 1 (PAI) is bound to vitronectin in plasma. FEBs Letters 1988; 242: 125–128.

[87] Woolf, N.: Thrombosis and atherosclerosis. In: Haemostasis and thrombosis. Ed. Bloom AL, Thomas, D.P. Churchill Livingstone, Edinburgh 1981; p. 527–552.

[88] Wun, T.C., Palmier, M.O., Siegel, N.R., Smith, C.E.: Affinity purification of active plasminogen activator inhibitor-1 (PAI-1) using immobilized anhydrourokinase. J. Biol. Chem. 1989; 264: 7862–7868.

[89] Zwall, R.F.A.: Membrane and lipid involvement in blood coagulation. Biochim. Biophys. Acta 1978; 515: 163–205.

5

The Cell Populations and other Components of the Atheromatous Lesions in Young People
– A Preliminary Report –

Robert W. Wissler, Akio Komatsu, Clifford Ko, Yoshiaki Kusumi, Dragoslava Vesselinovitch
Department of Pathology and the PDAY Center at
The University of Chicago
Chicago, IL, USA

Introduction

Atherosclerosis is a chronic disease process which develops over a period of many years in most individuals who are at risk in the more highly developed industrialized countries of the world. In general there is a much better understanding of the advanced lesions which lead to clinical disease as compared to knowledge about the factors influencing developing plaques in young people at the cellular and chemical artery wall level. In the USA a fourteen-center cooperative research program is aimed at learning more about how several risk factors lead to progression of the atherosclerotic plaque by utilizing pathobiological methods which can be applied to autopsy samples of arteries and other tissues. This program [1–3], which is called the Pathobiological Determinants of Atherosclerosis in Youth (PDAY), has now collected carefully standardized artery samples from over 1500 young people. These anatomically standardized samples of aortas and coronary arteries are obtained at nine forensic collection centers and come from autopsies of individuals aged 15 through 34 who are free of chronic disease and who have succumbed suddenly and unexpectedly, usually of traumatic causes. These nine collection centers are following a very detailed protocol and manual of procedures in order to insure that the artery samples and the other samples utilized for risk factor assessment from these autopsy cases meet the requested criteria and that they are preserved, processed, and distributed to the various study centers under as near ideal conditions as possible. As is shown in Figure 1, the sampling of the aorta and the left anterior descending coronary artery (LAD) for the core studies and for special studies is performed in a carefully planned way so that "lesion prone" and "lesion resistant" areas, as previously determined

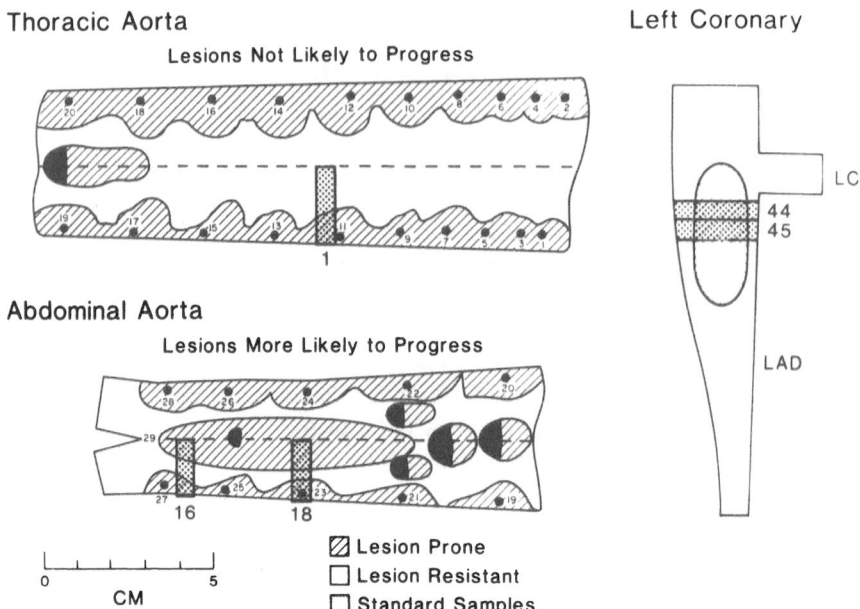

Thoracic Aorta   Left Coronary

Lesions Not Likely to Progress

Abdominal Aorta

Lesions More Likely to Progress

0   5
         CM

▨ Lesion Prone
☐ Lesion Resistant
☐ Standard Samples

Figure 1: This figure illustrates in diagrammatic form some of the strengths and advantages of the core sampling strategy which PDAY is employing on all of its cases. As can be seen, these samples make it possible to study and to evaluate quantitatively the thoracic aorta core sample area (# 1) as compared to the standard abdominal aorta areas (# 16 and # 18). It also makes it possible to evaluate similarly the left anterior descending coronary artery (LAD) standard samples (# 44 and # 45) and to compare "lesion prone" and "lesion resistant" areas in each of these standard samples. The arteries are oriented and marked so that under the microscope it is relatively easy to distinguish "lesion prone" and "lesion resistant" areas and to match up the sections stained for lipid with the sections stained for connective tissue components. These are less than a millimeter from each other because of the way samples are prepared for microscopic examination. (As modified from Wissler, R.W. et al. [1])

by Cornhill et al. [4], can be compared in each microscopic section that is studied. Furthermore, these core samples are processed and prepared for micromorphometry in a way that makes it possible to study the localization of lipid by means of oil red-O (ORO) staining in a section that is very close to a paraffin imbedded section which is stained for smooth muscle cells, specific mononuclear inflammatory cells, selected apolipoproteins, and connective tissue elements [5].

The risk factors are measured by means of methods carefully worked out and verified by the PDAY group at the Louisiana State University Medical Center in New Orleans [6]. They are able to generate quantitative data reflecting the individual's use of cigarettes, his or her blood lipids, the presence of chronic hypertension, as well as previously undetected diabetes and pre-diabetes. Furthermore, quantitative evaluation of the gross extent and severity of atherosclerosis in both the aorta and the coronary arteries are carried out both at the LSU center and at

PDAY MATERIALS AND DATA FLOW

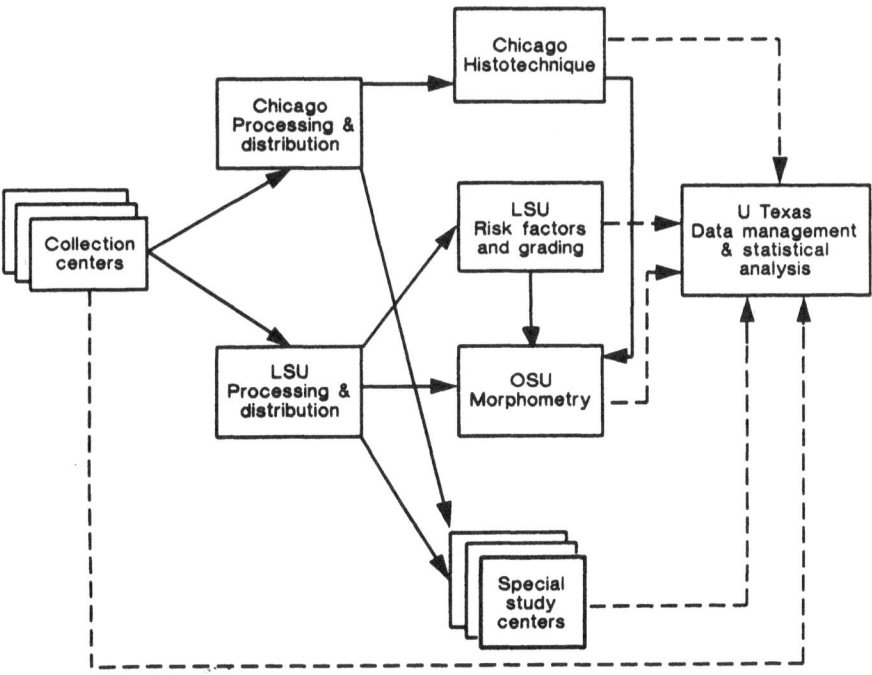

Figure 2: This diagram indicates how the collection centers interact with the various core centers in preserving and transmitting samples for processing, for risk factor measurements, for statistical evaluation of data, or gross and microscopic morphometry, and for use in the various special studies which are being carried out at a number of centers. This system, which was demonstrated to be workable during a "Phase 1 feasibility trial" involving samples, data, and information generation and utilization on more than 200 cases, has now been used successfully in more than 1500 cases. (This diagram was developed by Dr. Henry C. McGill, Jr. [3])

the computer assisted morphometry center at the Ohio State University. Many other special studies are in progress at other centers and these have been delineated in a recent publication [2]. Figure 2 diagrams the general flow of samples, data, and the ways in which the centers relate to each other to produce some of the early results of this study relating risk factors to the quantitatively determined gross involvement of the aorta. Some of these have recently been published [6], thus far limited to data collected in black and white males. The main purpose of this report is to present some of the preliminary cellular pathobiological and immunohistochemical results which are being produced by the special study center at the University of Chicago.

The Methods of Quantitating the Cell Populations in the "Lesion Prone" and
"Lesion Resistant" Areas of the Coronary Artery and the Aorta

In order to identify and to make it possible to quantitate the two major cell populations in the developing atherosclerotic plaques in the "lesion prone" and "lesion resistant" areas (Fig. 1) immunohistochemical approaches were utilized. In preliminary studies it became evident that the Vector ABC approach using peroxidase as the indicator on adjacent sections of the core samples of aorta and LAD coronary artery would give reproducible and consistently high quality results [7]. The antibodies employed were obtained through the kindness of Professor Allan Gown at the University of Washington. These antibodies have been extensively utilized for a number of studies of human lesions at that institution [8, 9]. The cell quantitation techniques developed by us have made it possible to identify and count the cells in both the superficial and the deeper portions of the thickened intima and to obtain reproducible quantitative data [10]. The quantitative values were obtained by counting the cells under standard conditions in twelve areas bounded by two of the pre-selected squares in an eyepiece reticule and then eliminating the two most deviating counts in order to arrive at a final total number in the ten remaining squares [10].

The micromorphometry system employed in these special studies was developed in this laboratory a few years ago with the assistance of Drs. Schaffner, Glagov, and Wied at this institution and with the advice and guidance of Dr. Gene Bond from the Bowman-Gray School of Medicine [11, 12]. This computer assisted digitizer with its very skillfully programmed software developed in Dr. Wied's laboratory, and the carefully oriented and high quality microscopic slides which are produced by our laboratory, have made it possible to measure many lesion and other artery wall components in these core artery samples. We are able to express the micromorphometric results in a quantitative mode which permits comparison from one case to another or from one part of the arterial tree to another with special emphasis, in this report, on comparing standard samples from the thoracic and abdominal aorta and comparing the "lesion prone" and "lesion resistant" areas of each sample which we studied.

Summary of Cellular and Related Quantitative Data

A preliminary report of a few of the overall results which have been published recently [2] and which were presented both nationally [10] and internationally [2, 13] indicate that the smooth muscle cell population in both the "lesion prone" and "lesion resistant" areas as well as the numbers of monocyte derived macrophages can be quantitated. The results as recently presented [2, 10, 13] are shown in Table 1. They indicate that the monocyte derived macrophage population is substantially higher in the "lesion prone" areas of the thoracic aorta where lesions

Table 1: Macrophage (Mϕ) populations, quantitatively enumerated as a percentage of the total number of cells in the dorsal (lesion prone) parts of the core samples of the aorta based on immunohistochemical identification on a standardized reticule counting system developed and utilized by Dr. Akio Komatsu in a study of 50 randomly distributed PDAY cases.
* Only 47 samples were available.

	Number of Cases with less than 15% Mϕ	Number of Cases with more than 15% Mϕ
Thoracic aorta sample # 1	20	30
Midabdominal aorta sample # 18	27	23
Lower abdominal aorta sample # 16*	34	13

generally progress slowly or do not progress at all as compared to the "lesion prone" areas of the lower abdominal aorta where lesions generally progress most rapidly. Furthermore the results indicate that the smooth muscle cell population remains rather constant in all of the "lesion prone" areas where quantitative results were obtained and that the monocyte derived macrophages tend to be greater in the superficial parts of the lesions than in the deeper portions. There is also a definite trend for the monocyte derived macrophage population to be greater in the "lesion prone" areas of all three of the aortic samples and in the LAD coronary artery "lesion prone" areas as compared to the "lesion resistant" areas of these so-called core samples.

Additional cell population data from additional cases are now being rapidly developed by one of us (AK). These should make it possible to obtain quantitative data on a sufficient number of cases of white males so that significant correlations can be made with the quintiles of age, as well as with the results of the measurements of the various risk factors which are being quantitated independently at the LSU PDAY center in New Orleans.

The additional variables which have been studied on all of these cases include computer assisted results of the specifically immunohistochemically stained extent of apo B, apo E, and Lp(a) deposition as visualized in adjacent sections from paraffin embedded fixed samples of these same core areas. These data, some of which also have been recently reported [10], indicate that apo B and apo E reveal similar patterns of quantitative localization, but even more recently Dr. Kusumi and I have found that Lp(a) is present to a much lesser extent (Table 2) and tends to be localized on the fibrous elements of the plaque and especially on the lumenal surface of the intima [14]. The results also indicate that abundant apo B can be demonstrated in the "lesion resistant" areas of these samples under conditions in which oil red O stained slides taken from an adjacent section of the same sample reveal no evidence of deposited stainable lipid. This is a phenomenon which we and others have observed previously [15, 16]. It can be interpreted in a number of

Table 2: The morphometric data from ten special study PDAY cases für the percentage of intima involved by immunohistochemical labeling of Apo B and Apo Lp(a) in aortic samples number 1 (thoracic) and number 16 (lower abdominal) standardized "lesion prone" areas.
* Averages were compared using paired Student's t-test

F PDAY Case #	Graph Case #	#1 Sample Lesion Prone		#16 Sample Lesion Prone	
		Apo B	Lp(a)	Apo B	Lp(a)
57289	1	51.61	23.97	36.66	07.36
41868	2	59.13	26.20	81.54	13.74
38127	3	16.54	13.78	00.00	03.34
37430	4	53.71	43.24	42.52	11.25
32630	5	58.22	08.29	54.13	14.99
70102	6	62.72	10.87	63.97	00.00
47809	7	32.53	02.45	68.55	09.73
55057	8	71.64	07.21	73.96	04.29
21714	9	26.06	00.48	59.26	00.00
44323	10	24.42	09.15	14.34	02.30
Average		45.66	14.56	49.49	06.70
SE		±5.71	±3.91	±7.88	±1.66
			$P < 0.001$*		$P < 0.001$*

ways. We believe that it indicates that low density lipoproteins are making their way into the intima of the artery and that the apo B retains its antigenicity under conditions in which little if any stainable lipid, including cholesterol esters and triglycerides, is retained to accumulate.

The overall results thus far would seem to indicate that increased numbers of monocyte derived macrophages are more likely to be present in those developing atheromatous lesions which are least likely to progress and that the numerical population is best correlated with protective mechanisms which may inhibit progression of the plaque.

The results thus far also indicate that most of the "intermediate" aortic lesions can be classified as *fatty plaques* because they are definitely raised when viewed grossly, with very sharp and discrete edges and with little gross or microscopic evidence of increased overlying collagen. They are usually characterized micro-scopically on high resolution fat stains by abundant intracellular lipid deposits mostly in cells that are clearly identifiable as modified smooth muscle cells (Plate I). As the lesions progress and before there is evidence of definite central necrosis of the developing plaque it is common to find increasing quantities of extracellular lipid (Plate II). This type of "fatty plaque" with abundant extracellu-lar lipid is found more frequently on the lower abdominal aorta (Table 3) where it is known that lesions are more likely to progress to fibrous plaques. This observa-tion is similar to results being reported by others which appear to establish a de-finite relationship between progression of the plaque and an increase in quantities of extracellular lipid [17].

Table 3: The average percent of the intima involved by extracellular lipid as determined by micromorphometric measurement of the "lesion prone" (dorsal) areas of the three standard core samples of the aortas of the same 50 cases as studied for cell population (see Table 1).

	Extracellular lipid (% of intima)
Thoracic aorta sample # 1	2.9
Midabdominal aorta sample # 18	3.2
Lower abdominal aorta sample # 16	7.0

The Effects of Circulating Immune Complexes on the Microarchitecture of the Developing Plaque

The special studies now being carried out at the University of Chicago PDAY Center also include an investigation of the role that circulating immune complexes may play in the accelerated progression of atherosclerosis and the effects which this immunological phenomenon has on the microarchitecture, the light microscopic features, and the reversibility of the atherosclerotic process. These investigations stem in part from a longstanding interest which investigators in this laboratory have had in the effects of experimental serum sickness [18] and its role in producing a polyarteritis in muscular arteries [19]. This interest was reawakened recently when it became apparent that the atherosclerosis developing in cynomolgus monkeys which have been previously reported to have a high incidence of immune complex disease manifested in their renal glomeruli [20] was marked by a very high proportion of concentric and transmural atheroarteritic lesions [12, 21]. In a number of studies it has become apparent that this type of atheroarteritis is definitely different from the experimental atherosclerosis which develops in the rhesus monkey fed a high fat, high cholesterol diet [22, 23]. Furthermore it is apparent that the cynomolgus arterial lumens tend to increase very little when intervention is carried out by means of a low fat, low cholesterol diet plus a bile acid sequestrant which in turn produces remarkably favorable regression of lesions and increased lumen size in the rhesus monkey [21, 23, 24]. Similar results indicate that it is difficult to demonstrate lumen enlargement in cynomolgus monkeys when intervention has led to removal of lipid from the lesions [25]. A plausible explanation of these paradoxical results is that when the arterial media of these muscular arteries is involved concentrically and transmurally then removal of lipid results in concentric scarring of the arterial media. This leads to a lack of the effective lumen enlargement which occurs so consistently when the lesions are eccentric and largely intimal.

Recently, we have reported preliminary results from our extension of these studies to the coronary arteries of the young people in the PDAY study [26]. Although the results are not definitive they appear to indicate that concentric lesions which have evidence of extensive medial involvement by stainable lipid deposition and by a substantial increase in monocyte derived macrophages in the media are also the cases where immune complex concentrations, as measured by enzyme-linked immunosorbent assays (ELISA) and by polyethylene glycol (PEG) precipitation, are frequently at a very high level in the circulation. The results also indicate that the values obtained by the two methods usually agree remarkably well. These studies are now being extended to additional cases and to an expanded study of the quantitation of immune complexes not only in the serum but also in the lesions of the coronary arteries.

If the results continue to support the role of circulating immune complexes in the development of concentric atheroarteritic lesions it would appear that at least some of the paradoxical cases of accelerated atherosclerosis in the absence of the three most commonly involved risk factors (namely: hyperlipidemia, cigarette smoking and hypertension) may involve circulating immune complexes as a main risk factor. In our current formulation we think that this pathogenetic mechanism and its resulting effects on the microarchitecture of lesions may be similar to mechanisms involved in the development of the similar atheroarteritis frequently described and illustrated in studies of young women with lupus erythematosus who succumb to ischemic heart disease [27] and in transplant arteritis [28, 29].

Summary

These investigations at the University of Chicago represent only a small proportion of the special studies which are being conducted in the PDAY research program [2]. It is clear from the early results obtained thus far that much can be learned from a well organized study of small standardized samples of arteries from a large number of forensic autopsies performed on young people who die suddenly and unexpectedly from traumatic causes. When the results are quantitated and carefully correlated with a number of other observations, including the quantitation of classical risk factors and the generic features of age, sex, and race, then many meaningful new relationships are discovered. As the numbers of cases available increase and as the results are interrelated from the various study centers it is likely that many additional new correlations will be found at the chemical and pathobiological level which will help us understand the factors supporting progression of this very common pathological process which is by far the leading cause of death in the USA. As the study continues, we are confident that the results will define some of the mechanisms by which risk factors operate in the artery wall of young people in our environment and that a number of new pathobiological determinants of progression of atherosclerosis in youth will be discovered.

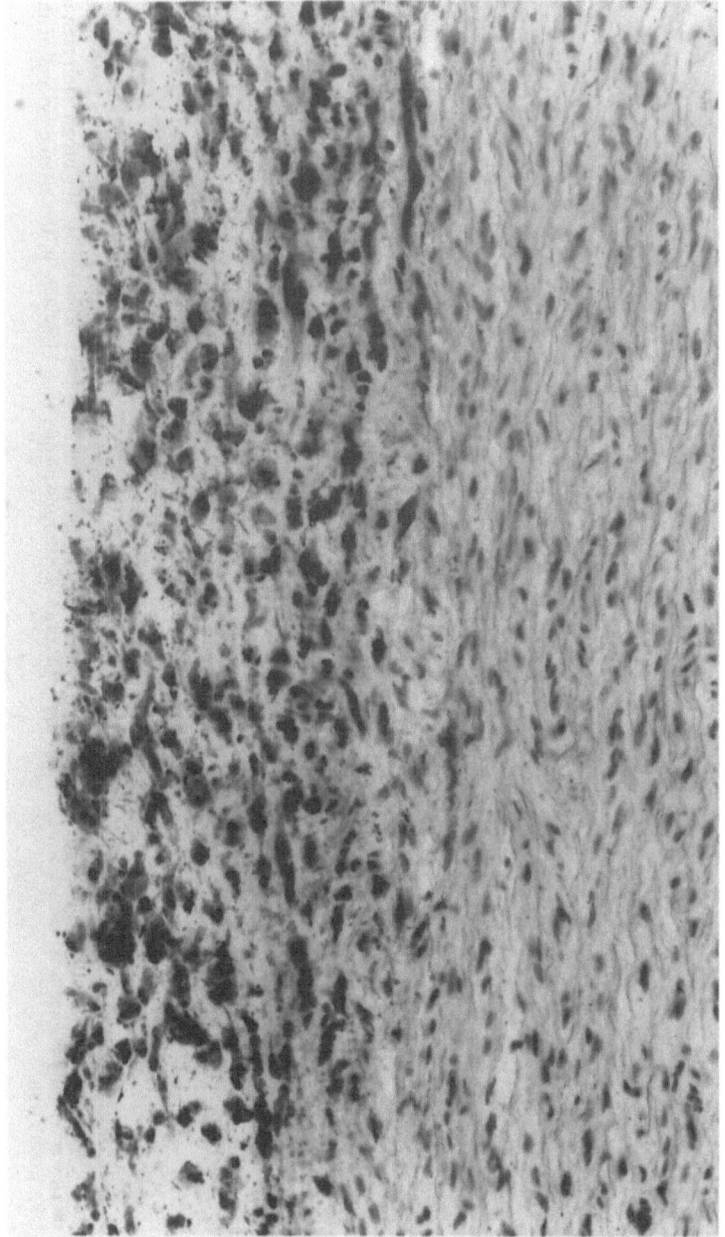

Plate I: This is a photomicrograph of a typical fatty plaque from the lower abdominal aorta of a 19 yr. old white male. It was, by actual measurement, about half the thickness of the underlying media. Note the relative paucity of monocyte derived foam cells. The majority of the cells are elongated and enlarged lipid containing smooth muscle cells which on adjacent sections are clearly positive for alpha actin using the HHF 35 antibody. Cells which are positive when the slide is prepared with HAM 56 primary antibody to macrophages are found only in small numbers in most instances.

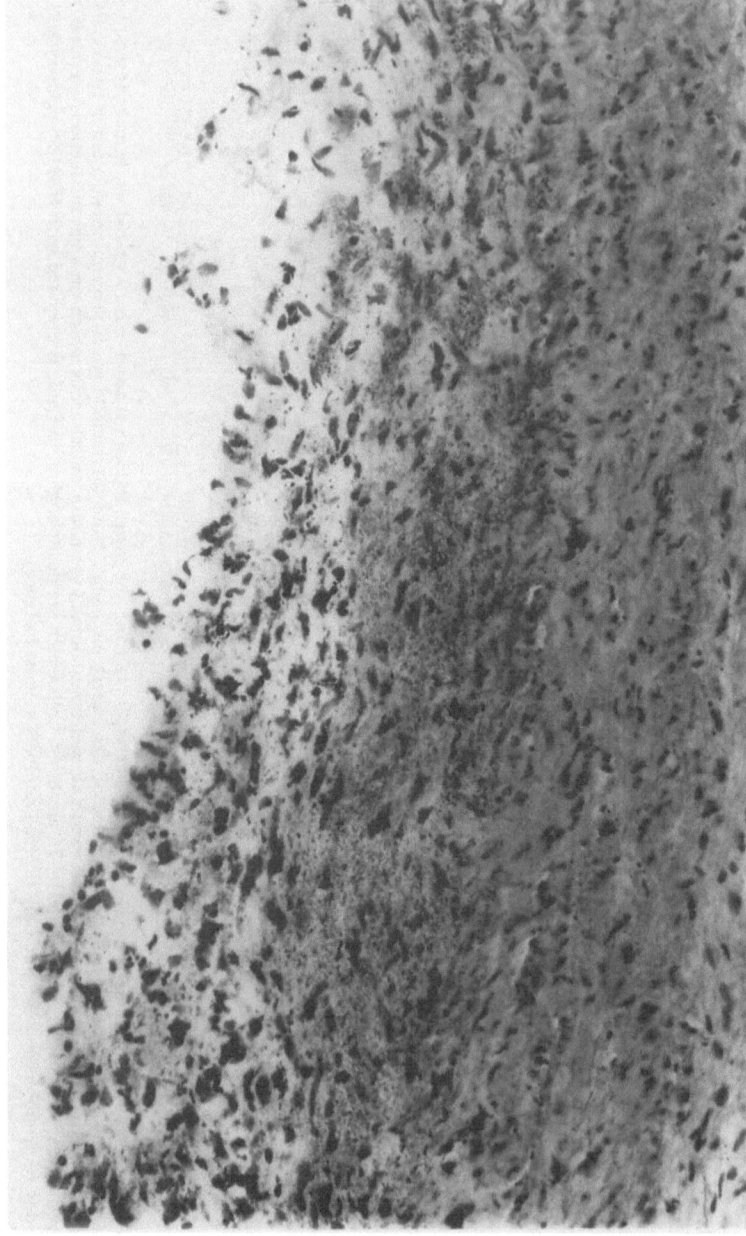

Plate II: In this fatty plaque from the abdominal aorta of a 26 yr. old black male, note the evidence of extracellular lipid in between the numerous lipid filled smooth muscle cells. This appears to be the most noticable correlate with the progression seen in the lower abdominal aorta where lesions are more likely to go on to fibrous plaque than elsewhere in the arterial system of the USA population.

Acknowledgement

This research was conducted as part of the Pathobiological Determinants of Atherosclerosis in Youth (PDAY) research program. Participating centers and principal investigators are the University of Alabama, Birmingham, AL, Steffen Gay, MD [HL-33733], and Edward J. Miller, PhD [HL-33728]; Albany Medical College, Albany, NY, Assaad Daoud, MD [HL-33765]; Baylor College of Medicine, Houston, TX, Louis C. Smith, PhD [HL-33750]; University of Chicago, Chicago, IL, Robert W. Wissler, PhD, MD, Program Director [HL-33740]; University of Illinois, Chicago, IL, Abel L. Robertson, Jr., MD, PhD [HL-33758]; Louisiana State University Medical Center, New Orleans, LA, Jack P. Strong, MD, Margaret C. Oalmann, DrPH [HL-33746]; University of Maryland, Baltimore, MD, Wolfgang J. Mergner, MD, PhD [HL-33752]; Medical College of Georgia, Augusta, GA, A. Bleakley Chandler, MD, Raghunatha N. Rao, MD [HL-33772]; University of Nebraska Medical Center, Omaha, NE, Bruce M. McManus, MD, PhD [HL-33778]; The Ohio State University, Columbus, OH, J. Fredrick Cornhill, D. Phil [HL-33760]; Southwest Foundation for Biomedical Research, San Antonio, TX, James E. Hixson, PhD [HL-33913]; The University of Texas Health Science Center, San Antonio, TX, C. Alex McMahan, PhD, Henry C. McGill, Jr., MD [HL-33749]; Vanderbilt University, Nashville, TN, Renu Virmani, MD [HL-33770]; and West Virginia University Health Science Center, Morgantown, WV, Singanallur N. Jagannathan, PhD [HL-33749].

References

[1] Wissler, R.W., Vesselinovitch, D., Komatsu, A., and Bridenstine, R.T.: The arterial wall and atherosclerosis in youth. In: Biology of the arterial wall. Rome, CIC Edizioni Internazionali, 1988; 265–274.

[2] Wissler, R.W., Vesselinovitch, D., and Komatsu, A.: The contribution of studies of atherosclerotic lesions in young people to future research. Ann. NY. Acad. Sci. 1990; 598: 418–434.

[3] Wissler, R.W.: USA multicenter study of the pathobiology of atherosclerosis in youth. Ann. NY. Acad. Sci. 1991; 623: 26–39.

[4] Cornhill, J.F., Herderick, E.E., and Stary, H.C.: Topography of human aortic sudanophilic lesions. In: Beynen, A.C., Kritchevsky, D., Pollak, O.I., eds. Monographs on atherosclerosis. Basel: S. Karger, 1990; 15: 13–19.

[5] Vesselinovitch, D., Getz, G.S., Hughes, R.H., and Wissler, R.W.: Atherosclerosis in the rhesus monkey fed three food fats. Atherosclerosis 1974; 20: 303–321.

[6] PDAY Research Group: Relationship of atherosclerosis in young men to serum lipoprotein cholesterol concentrations and smoking. JAMA 1990; 264: 3018–3024.

[7] Yomantas, S., Elner, V.M., Schaffner, T., and Wissler, R.W.: Immunohistochemical localization of apolipoprotein B in human atherosclerotic lesions. Arch. Pathol. Lab. Med. 1984; 108: 374–378.

[8] Gown, A.M., Vogel, A.M.: Monoclonal antibodies to intermediate filament proteins of human cells: Unique and cross-reacting antibodies. J. Cell. Biol. 1982; 95: 414–424.

[9] Gown, A.M., Tsukada, T., Ross, R.: Human atherosclerosis. II. Immunocytochemical analysis of the cellular composition of human atherosclerotic lesions. Am. J. Pathol. 1986; 125: 191–207.

[10] Komatsu, A., Wissler, R.W., and Vesselinovitch, D.: Cell populations in atheromatous lesions in young people. Arteriosclerosis. 1989; 9: 709a.

[11] Wissler, R.W., Vesselinovitch, D., Schaffner, T.J., and Glagov, S.: Quantitating rhesus monkey atherosclerosis progression and regression with time. In: Gotto, A.M., Jr., Smith, L.C., and Allen, B., eds. Atherosclerosis V (Proc. Vth. Int. Symp.). New York: Springer-Verlag, 1980; 757–761.

[12] Vesselinovitch, D., and Wissler, R.W.: Quantitation of certain qualitative differences in the atherosclerotic process. In: Schettler, G., Gotto, A.M., Middelhoff, G., Habenicht, A.S., and Jurutka, K.R., eds. Atherosclerosis VI (Proc. VIth. Int. Symp.). Berlin: Springer-Verlag, 1983; 174–179.

[13] Wissler, R.W.: Morphological characteristics of the developing atherosclerotic plaque: animal studies and studies of lesions from young people. In: International Workshop on Atherosclerosis. New York, Raven Press, 1991; Athero. Rev. 23: 91–103.

[14] Kusumi, Y., and Wissler, R.W.: Aortic Lp(a) deposition in young people. FASEB 1991; FASEB J. 5: A 1254.

[15] Kao, V.C., and Wissler, R.W.: A study of the immunohistochemical localization of serum lipoproteins and other plasma proteins in human atherosclerotic lesions. Exp. Mol. Pathol. 1965; 4: 465–479.

[16] Hoff, H.F., Gaubatz, J.W., and Gotto, A.M., Jr.: Apo B concentration in the normal human aorta. Biochem. Biophys. Res. Comm. 1978; 85: 1424–1430.

[17] Bocan, T.M.A., Schifani, T.A., and Guyton, J.R.: Ultrastructure of the human aortic fibrolipid lesion: formation of the atherosclerotic lipid-rich core. Am. J. Pathol. 1986; 123: 413–424.

[18] Hopps, H.C., and Wissler, R.W.: The experimental production of generalized arteritis and periarteritis (periarteritis nodosa). J. Lab. Clin. Med. 1946; 31: 939–957.

[19] Rich, A.R., and Gregory, J.E.: The experimental demonstration that periarteritis nodosa is a manifestation of hypersensitivity. Bull Johns Hopkins Hosp. 1943; 72: 65–88.

[20] Poskitt, T.R., Fortwengler, Jr., H.P., Bobrow, J.C., and Roth, G.J.: Naturally occurring immune-complex glomerulonephritis in monkey (Macaca irus). I. Light, immunofluorescence, and electron microscopic studies. Am. J. Pathol. 1974; 76: 145–164.

[21] Vesselinovitch, D., and Wissler, R.W.: Correlation of types of induced lesions with regression of coronary atherosclerosis in two species of macaques. In: Noseda, G., Fragiacomo, C., Fumagalli, R., and Paoletti, R., eds. Lipoproteins and coronary atherosclerosis. Amsterdam: Elsevier, 1982; 401–406.

[22] Wissler, R.W., and Vesselinovitch, D.: Atherosclerosis – Relationship to coronary blood flow. Am. J. Cardiol. 1983; 52: 2A-7A.

[23] Wissler, R.W., Vesselinovitch, D., Davis, H.R., Lambert, P.H., and Bekermeier, M.: A new way to look at atherosclerosis involvement of the artery wall and the functional effects. Ann. NY Acad. Sci. 1985; 454: 9–22.

[24] Wissler, R.W., and Vesselinovitch, D.: The time course of atherosclerotic lesion regression in macaque monkeys. In: Descovitch, G.C., Gaddi, A., Magri, G.L., and Lenzi, S. Atherosclerosis & Cardiovascular Desease: 7th International Meeting. Dordrecht: Kluwer, 1990; 391–400.

[25] Hollander, W., Kirkpatrick, B., Paddock, J., Colombo, M., Nagraj, S., and Prusty, S.: Studies on the progression and regression of coronary and peripheral atherosclerosis in the cynomolgus monkey. I. Effects of dipyridamole and aspirin. Exp. Mol. Pathol. 1979; 30: 55–73.

[26] Wissler, R.W., Vesselinovitch, D., and Ko, C.: The effects of circulating immune complexes on atherosclerotic lesions in experimental animals and in younger and older humans. Transplant. Proc. 1989; 21: 3707–3708.

[27] Bulkley, B.H., and Roberts, W.C.: The heart in systemic lupus erythematosus and the changes induced in it by corticosteroid therapy. Am. J. Med. 1975; 58: 243–264.

[28] Uys, C.J., Rose, A.G., and Barnard, C.N.: The pathology of human cardiac transplantation. S. Afr. Med. J. 1979; 56: 887–896.

[29] Alonso, D.R., Starek, P.K., and Minick, R.C.: Studies on the pathogenesis of athero-arteriosclerosis induced in rabbit cardiac allografts by the synergy of graft rejection and hyperchoesterolemia. Am. J. Pathol. 1977; 87: 415–442.

Differentiation and Role of Macrophages in the Early Human Atherosclerotic Plaque

A. Roessner[1], E. Vollmer[1], E. Jaeger[2],
J. Rauterberg[2], W. Böcker[1]
[1] Gerhard-Domagk-Institut für Pathologie
[2] Institut für Arterioskleroseforschung
der Westfälischen Wilhelms-Universtität Münster

Introduction

New Morphological investigations on the pathogenesis of atherosclerosis have refocused the attention on the role of monocytes and macrophages, especially in the early phases of the disease. This is somewhat opposed to the recent concentration on smooth muscle cells. Various factors have prompted the reorientation: Macrophages were found to be essentially involved in the intimal lipoprotein metabolism (Brown and Goldstein, 1983; 1986). They are incorporating cholesterol-binding lipoproteins that enter the intima, but if they have taken up more than they can possibly digest, the excess cholesterol will be stored as drop-like cytoplasmic deposits. Recent experimental data suggested that the majority of foam cells observed in the atherosclerotic plaque, must be of this origin. Foam cell transformation of smooth muscle cells was found to be rather less common (Schwartz et al., 1985). Although the functional importance of macrophages in lipoprotein metabolism has been verified in vitro, our knowledge about their behaviour especially in the human atherosclerotic plaque is still fairly vague, as most of the morphological studies conducted in this field, have been based on experimental models.

Monoclonal antibodies revealed a distinct heterogeneity of human aortic intimal cells (Orekhov et al., 1986). Further phenotypic characterization of macrophages and their differential identification from other cell types of the human atherosclerotic plaque is facilitated by application of this technique (Radzun, 1985; Zwadlo et al., 1985, 1986). The present study was aimed at a more detailed characterization of the macrophage-derived foam cells of the atherosclerotic plaque. We performed immunohistological investigations with appropriate antibodies for differentiating the respective cell types of the mononuclear phagocyte system.

Materials and Methods

Our investigations were performed on samples excised from the human ascending aorta of patients undergoing coronary bypass surgery. Since the employed antibodies were also applicable to formol-fixed tissue, the samples were fixed in 4% formol and carefully embedded in paraffin, a procedure that ensures better morphological preservation than the usual work-up in frozen section.

Immunohistochemical studies were performed with single and double indirect peroxidase and alkaline phosphatase methods, using the substrate 3.3 diaminobenzidine tetrahydrochloride (DAB) or $3'9'$ ethylcarbazole (AEC) and naphthol salts as coupling reagent with hexazotic neofuchsin (Sigma/Munich and Merck/Darmstadt). Endogenous peroxidase was suppressed by $NaNO_3$, endogenous alkaline phosphatase by levamisole. For secondary and tertiary antibodies we used products of Sigma/Munich, Dakopatts/Hamburg, and Dianova/Hamburg. Nuclear counterstaining was performed with acid hemalum. For negative controls we omitted the primary antibody, or incubated normal serum of the respective species. For positive controls we used the remaining slides of each set.

Light microscopical controls were stained with hematoxilin eosin. Antibodies for demonstration of monocytes (27-E-10, Zwadlo et al., 1986) and macrophages (25-F-9, Zwadlo et al., 1985) and the antibody against apolipoprotein E were kindly supplied by Prof. Dr. C. Sorg, Institute of Experimental Dermatology of Münster University. The antibody against the inflammatory differentiation antigen (4-D-10) was supplied by Dr. Goerdt from the same institute. The polyclonal antibodies against human apolipoproteins A_1, A_2, and B are commercially available from Boehringer/Mannheim. The monoclonal antibody against muscle specific alpha actin (HHF 35, Tsukada et al., 1987) was purchased from Dakopatts/Hamburg.

Demonstration and differentiation of macrophages in fatty streaks

Conventional light microscopy in HE staining demonstrates typical foam cells in incipient fatty streaks that are characterized by a lucent cytoplasm and darkly staining nuclei. Their cytologic nature, however, cannot be inferred from the mere histologic picture. Immunohistological studies, using antibodies against alpha-1-antichymotrypsin known as a marker for cells of the mononuclear macrophage system, identified the majority of such foam cells as members of the macrophage population. Since that antibody is known to be non-specific, we have applied specific monoclonal antibodies to cells of the mononnuclear phagocyte system.

Vessels with incipient fatty streaks showed isolated subendothelial blood monocytes with positive staining with antibody 27-E-10, directed against blood monocytes (Fig. 1). Foam cells would never stain with this antibody. Developing fatty streaks were characterized by a considerable infiltration of macrophages changing to foam cells which displayed negative staining to antibody 27-E-10 against blood monocytes, but strong positive staining to antibody 25-F-9 against mature tissue macrophages. Subendothelial clusters of foamy macrophages were early manifestations. During the progression of lipid streaks we observed extended subendothelial clusters of foam cells thickening the intima. The clusters were identified as mature tissue macrophages by their positive reaction to antibody 25-F-9, too (Fig. 2). Only some isolated smooth muscle cells were observed within lipid streaks. These results permit the conclusion that blood monocytes should be able to pervade the endothelial layer, then stay in the intima, and to be transformed into mature tissue macrophages, from which the majority of foam cells are derived. These foam cells supply the structural characteristics of fatty streaks; the specific antibodies applied in our study allow for appropriate discrimination of infiltrating macrophage populations in the arterial intima (Roessner et al., 1987).

Endothelial pervasion of macrophages

The next question would be how macrophages are managing to enter and pervade the vascular endothelium. According to recent investigations, a certain phenotypic modulation of the endothelial cells may be involved in that process (Munro and Cotran, 1988). There is an increasing experimental evidence for the diversity of endothelial cells which may be comparable to that of cells belonging to the mononuclear phagocyte system proper. It has been possible to raise specific monoclonal antibodies against different subtypes of endothelial cells (Goerdt et al., 1987). We were using an antibody (4-D-10) reacting with a certain differentiation antigen which is expressed exclusively by endothelial cells in tissues undergoing inflammatory changes.*)

Investigations on endothelial cell cultures have clearly shown that the inflammatory differentiation antigen that reacts with antibody 4-D-10 can be induced on endothelial cells by various inflammatory stimuli such as endotoxines, phorbol esters, and tumor necrosis factor. If stimulation is discontinued, antigen expression will decrease again. So the antibody can be used to discriminate endothelial cells in inflammatory tissue. According to current opinion, there is increasing evidence for the possibly inflammatory basis of atherosclerosis. The similarities between the two processes were recently stressed (Joris and Majno, 1977). We therefore wanted to find out whether an expression of the inflammatory differentiation antigen could also be found in the endothelial cells covering early atherosclerotic plaques. Staining of fatty streaks in fibrous/fatty lesions showed distinct

---

*) The antibody 4-D-10 was kindly supplied by Dr. Goerdt, Institute of Experimental Dermatology of Münster University.

positivity for antibody 4-D-10 against the inflammatory differentiation antigen (Fig. 3). In endothelial cells covering unaltered aortic walls the inflammatory differentiation antigen was not detected.

Localization by immunoelectron microscopy reveals the exclusive expression of that antigen in the outer plasma membrane of endothelial cells, but not in their cytoplasmic organelles (Fig. 4). Monocytic adherence of endothelial cells is known to increase along with the expression of the inflammatory activation antigen in a highly significant fashion (Goerdt et al., 1987; Bevilaqua et al., 1985; Pober et al., 1986). Our results have shown that endothelial cells will express inflammatory differentiation antigens in their outer cytoplasmic membrane even above early atherosclerotic plaques (Fig. 4), thereby obviously facilitating the entering of blood monocytes through the endothelium into the underlying intima of the vessel.

Macrophages and lipoprotein metabolism

According to the theory of Brown and Goldstein (1983), macrophages are functioning as scavenger cells in lipoprotein metabolism, and their major role in atherogenesis seems to be in the clearance of lipids from the very area where a lesion is forming. Further in vitro studies have shown that macrophages play a major role in lipoprotein metabolism, incorporating various lipoproteins (LDL and β-VLDL) by receptormediated endocytosis (Brown and Goldstein, 1983; Goldstein et al., 1980). The internalized lipoproteins are transported to lysosomes, and hydrolysed cholesterol is released into the cytoplasm, then re-esterified, and stored as cholesteryl droplets in the cytoplasmic compartment. The cholesteryl esters in the cytoplasm are continually undergoing hydrolysation and reesterification. If the extracellular medium contains cholesterol acceptors such as HDL, cellular unesterified cholesterol is released from these cells. Along with increasing cholesterol accumulation, macrophages also synthesize and secrete increasing amounts of Apolipoprotein E which associates with cholesterol-enriched HDL to form the HDL complex.

The HDLc particles target the secreted cholesterol to hepatocytes (Mahley, 1981), thereby mediating the "reverse cholesterol transport" to the liver. These are, however, the results of in vitro studies, so far. In our morphologic investigations we tried to trace some of the possible steps in this metabolic pathway within the atherosclerotic plaque.

The main lipoprotein component of LDL is Apolipoprotein B. Staining for that substance with antibodies shows in the early atherosclerotic plaque, distinct and predominantly extracellular deposits, and so we may safely infer that LDL is present in these areas (Vollmer et al., 1990a). The LDL observed in the arterial intima is most likely incorporated by macrophages. The cholesterol esters are deposited in cytoplasmic lipid vacuoles which ultimately appear as foam cells, and can be demonstrated by conventional electron microscopy. According to ultrastructural findings, the number of lipid vacuoles increases, and the typical foam cells develop, forming the cytologic basis of fatty streaks. Eventually, these macrophage-derived foam cells may become necrotic to form the so-called "atheroma" (Fagiotto et al., 1984). It was also suggested that lipid-laden macrophages may also re-enter the vessel lumina.

On the other hand, macrophages are also able in vitro to resecrete cholesterol via the reverse cholesterol transport. Until now the exact mechanism of cholesterol secretion by macrophages, and the origin of plasma HDL with regard to the reverse cholesterol transport have been rather unclear. Observations by Schmitz et al. (1985), using biochemical and electron microscopical techniques, led to the assumption that HDL are binding to specific receptors on the surface of macrophages. Subsequently, bound HDL particles are internalized and transported in endosomes. These endosomes are not fusing with the lysosome compartment, but taking up cytoplasmic cholesterol, and are ultimately re-secreted. In our morphologic studies we wanted to find out whether macrophages in the atherosclerotic plaque would be equally capable of secreting Apo E, and if so, whether the reverse cholesterol transport could be of importance in the atherosclerotic plaque. Staining of fatty streaks with antibodies against Apo E shows distinct positivity in the cytoplasm of foam cells which obviously contain Apo E (Fig. 5). Comparable results were also observed by Murase et al. (1986). To confirm the macrophage nature of these foam cells which contain or probably secrete Apo E, we performed an immunohistological double labelling: Apo E was stained red, using the alkaline phosphatase method, while the peroxidase method using antibody 25-F-9 identified these cells as mature tissue macrophages. The cytoplasm of foam cells appeared in a mixed, brown-reddish color, signalling these cells as macrophages carrying or probably actively secreting Apo E (Vollmer et al., 1991b). Preliminary electron microscopic studies on the atherosclerotic plaque for demonstrating Apo E have shown that the reaction product is localized on the granular endoplasmic reticulum and the Golgi apparatus of macrophages, i.e. their secretory apparatus. So we may infer that macrophages in the atherosclerotic plaque are indeed able to secrete Apo E.

As emphasized in the reverse cholesterol transport, Apo E is associating with re-secreted cholesterol and HDL present in the surrounding medium to produce the HDLc particle, which is then targeted to liver cells. The question is whether HDL can also be demonstrated morphologically in the arterial intima, signalling their potential role as cholesterol acceptors. Staining with antibodies against Apo A_1, the main component of HDL, reveals the mainly extracellular localization of Apo A_1 in the arterial intima undergoing early atherosclerotic change. It can be assumed that HDL is present in corresponding localization. In addition, immunohistological double-labelling for Apo A_1 and 25-F-9 for demonstrating macrophages revealed that numerous foam cells characterized as macrophages in brownish color by 25-F-9, are also containing cytoplasmic Apo A_1. We may infer that HDL are incorporated at least temporarily by these macrophages, forming the HDLc complex. However, an in-depth study of the intracytoplasmic metabolism that leads to potential formation of the HDLc complex, is not feasibly by these light microscopic findings, and will require further immunoelectron microscopic studies of the Apolipoprotein metabolism in the macrophages of the atherosclerotic plaque, which are currently in progress (Vollmer et al., 1991a).

In conclusion, our morphologic data demonstrating the secretion of Apo E by macrophage-derived foam cells, and the occurrence of HDL in the extracellular spaces of the arterial intima and also in the cytoplasm of foam cells, suggests that the so-called reverse cholesterol transport to the liver may also play a significant role in the development of the atherosclerotic plaque.

The role of macrophages in the synthesis of collagen by smooth muscle cells

Increased biosynthesis and deposition of proteins in the extracellular matrix, especially of collagens, are contributing essentially to the atherosclerotic transformation of the arterial wall. The potential role of macrophages in the synthesis of collagen types principally effected by smooth muscle cells, is still insufficiently explained. Those smooth muscle cells are readily identified in the proliferating fibrous plaque by immunohistology after staining with antibodies against muscle-specific alpha actin (Tsukada et al., 1987). The substances synthesized by smooth muscle cells can also be discriminated on histologic section by appropriate antibody staining.

Studies of Voss et al. (1986) have shown that incipient fibrous plaques will manifest collagens in their intercellular matrix, preferably type I, but also type III collagen. With the aid of in situ hybridization, it is now possible to detect and distinguish mRNAs of the different collagen types within collagen-synthesizing smooth muscle cells (Jaeger, 1990).

Thus, cells with active collagen biosyntheses were identified and localized in frozen sections of human atheroclerotic arteries, using 25-S-labelled RNA probes complementary to the messenger RNA for type I and type III collagen, respectively. Increased messenger RNA was observed in particular in the smooth muscle cells of fibrous plaques. Immunohistochemical identification of parallel sections for smooth muscle cells and macrophages revealed regular coexistence or vicinity of mRNA-containing smooth muscle cells, and mature tissue macrophages or immigrating blood monocytes in the intima of atherosclerotic vessels. From these results the connection between the infiltration by macrophages and the activation of collagen synthesis in smooth muscle cells is evident, and may support the idea of cells from the mononuclear macrophage system playing an important role in the activation of collagen synthesis in smooth muscle cells of atherosclerotic vessels.

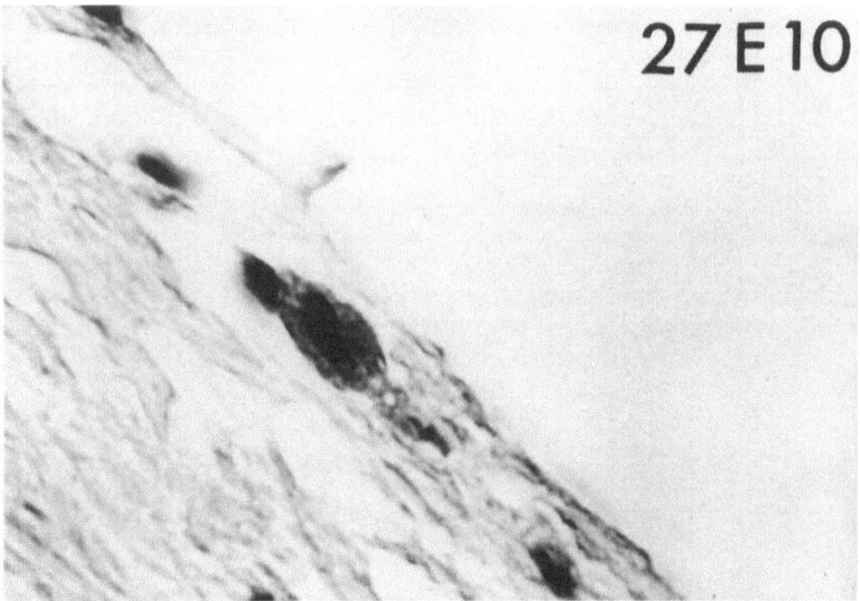

Fig. 1: Incipient fatty streak of human aorta stained with monoclonal antibody 27-E-10 directed exclusively against blood monocytes: single positive monocytes are observed in the subendothelial space. (x 550)

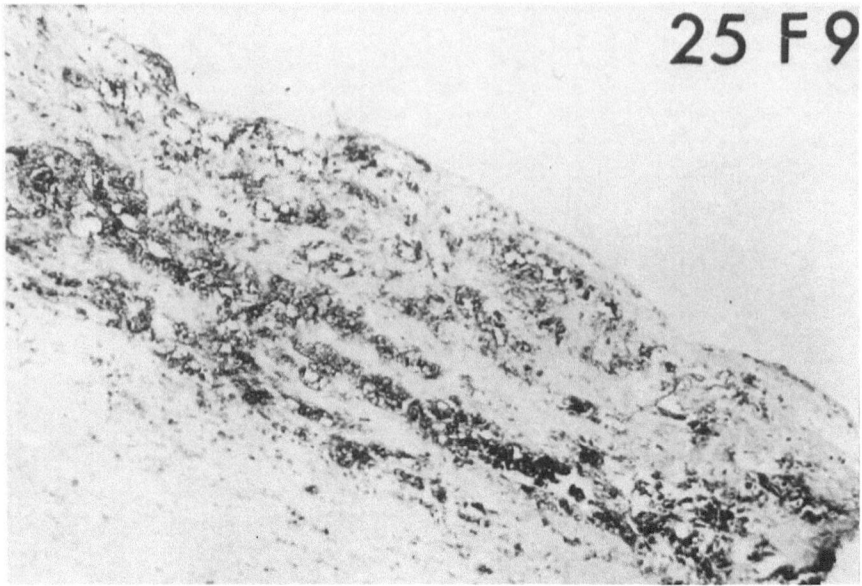

Fig. 2: Low power micrograph of fully developed fatty streak in the human aorta, stained with 25-F-9 against mature tissue macrophages, and showing abundant clusters of macrophage derived foam cells. (x 136)

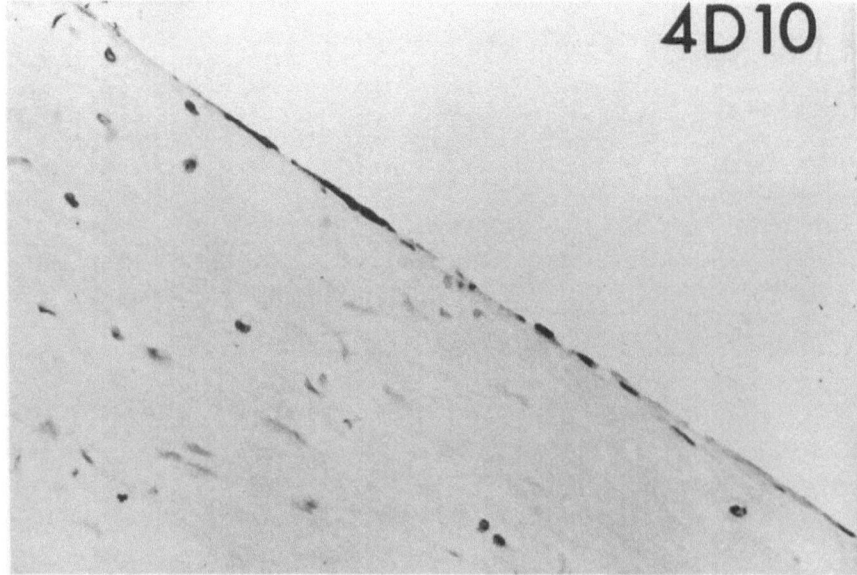

Fig. 3: Fibrous-fatty plaque of the human aorta, stained with antibody 4-D-10 against an inflammatory differentiation antigen, revealing strong positivity in the endothelial cells. (x 136)

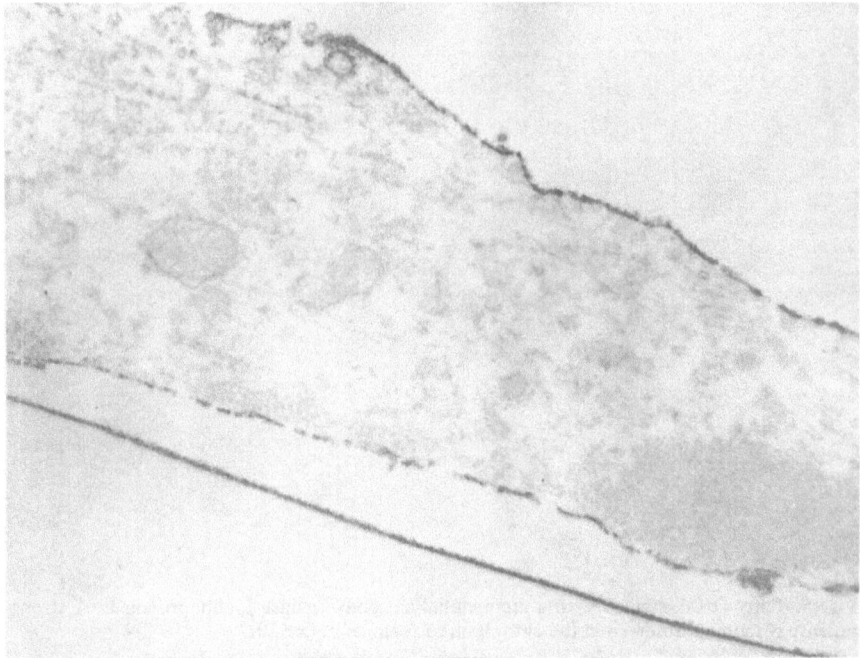

Fig. 4: Immunoelectron microscopic demonstration of the inflammatory differentiation antigen using the monoclonal antibody 4-D-10 in immune peroxidase technique. The reaction product es revealed exclusively on the outer cytoplasmic membrane where the antigen is obviously present. (x 9300)

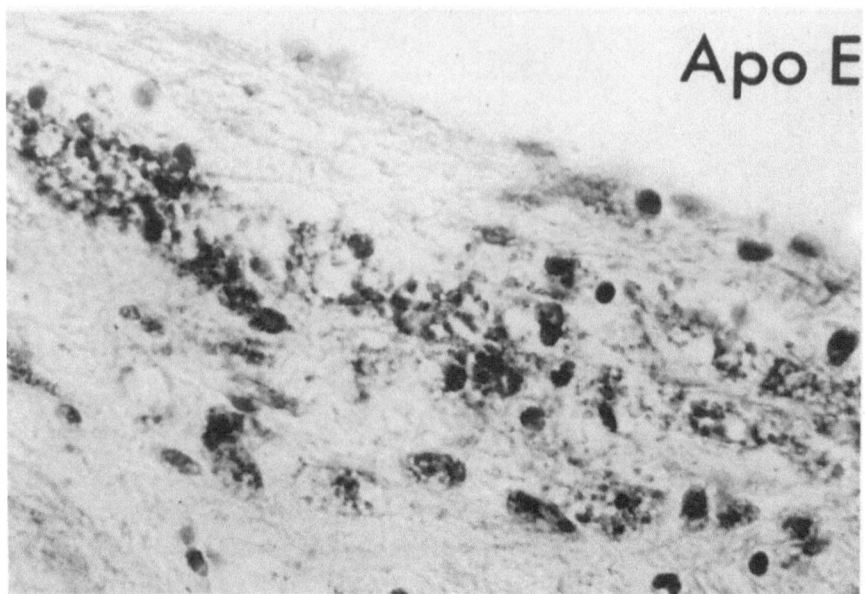

Fig. 5: Fatty streak stained with a monoclonal antibody against apolipoprotein E. A strong positive reaction is observed in the cytoplasm of foam cells. (x 550)

Conclusion

In its early stages, arteriosclerosis is in fact an intimal disease. Monocytes migrate from the vascular lumen through the endothelium into the arterial intima. Obviously, a certain phenotypic modulation of endothelial intimal cells, expressing an inflammatory differentiation antigen with increased monocytic adherence, plays an important role in this process. According to immunohistologic observations with differentiating antibodies, the immigrating monocytes are undergoing a transformation to tissue macrophages in the arterial intima. These macrophages are actively involved in lipoprotein metabolism ingesting cholesterol-carrying lipoproteins that have penetrated into the intima through the endothelium, thereby acting as scavenger cells. If these have incorporated more cholesterol than they are able to excrete under the conditions prevailing in the atherosclerotic plaque, macrophages are transformed to foam cells. So far, little is known about the fate of the intimal macrophages. One theory, however, suggests that some of them may pass through the endothelium and begin to recirculate after transformation into foam cells. On the other hand, our immunohistological results have shown that macrophages secrete Apo E, and that in the presence of HDL in the arterial intima, the so-called reverse cholesterol transport towards the liver may play a significant role in the pathogenesis of the atherosclerotic plaque.

On the other hand, the function of macrophages may also be a negative one. In the progression of an atherosclerotic lesion, the metabolically transforming macrophage seems to be able by activating the collagen synthesis of smooth muscle cells, to enhance and advance the atherosclerotic process itself.

References

[1] Bevilacqua, M.P., Pober, J.S., Wheeler, M.E., Cotran, R.S., Gimbrone, M.A., Jr. (1985): Interleukin-1 activation of vascular endothelium: Effects on procoagulant activity and leukocyte adhesion. Am. J. Pathol. 121: 394–400.
[2] Brown, M.S., Goldstein, J.L. (1983): Lipoprotein metabolism in the macrophage: Implications for cholesterol deposition in atherosclerosis. Annu. Rev. Biochem. 52: 223–261.
[3] Brown, M.S., Goldstein, J.L. (1986): A receptor-mediated pathway for cholesterol homeostasis. Science 232: 34–47.
[4] Fagiotto, A., Ross, R., Harker, L. (1984a): Studies of hypercholesterolemia in the nonhuman primate. I. Changes that lead to fatty streak formation. Arteriosclerosis 4: 323–340.
[5] Fagiotto, A., Ross, R. (1984b): Studies of hypercholesterolemia in the nonhuman primate. II. Fatty streak conversion to fibrous plaque. Arteriosclerosis 4: 341–356.
[6] Goerdt, S., Zwadlo, G., Schlegel, R., Hagemeier, H.H., Sorg, C. (1987): Characterization and expression kinetics of an endothelial cell activation antigen present in vivo only in acute inflammatory tissue. Exp. Cell. Biol. 55: 117–126.
[7] Goldstein, J.L., Ho, Y.K., Brown, M.S., Innerarity, T.L., Mahley, R.W. (1980): Cholesteryl ester accumulation in macrophages resulting from receptor-mediated uptake and degradation of hypercholesterolemic canine β-very low density liporpoteins. J. Biol. Chem. 255: 1839–1848.

[8] Goldstein, J.L., Brown, M.S. (1978): Familial hypercholesterolemia: Pathogenesis of a receptor disease. Johns Hopkins Med. J. 143: 8–43.

[9] Jaeger, E. (1990): Arterielle Kollagen-Expression bei Bluthochdruck und Arteriosklerose. Dissertation, Med. Fakultät Münster (Pharmazeutische Chemie).

[10] Joris, I., Majko, G. (1977): Atherosclerosis and inflammation. Adv. Exp. Med. Biol. 104: 227–225.

[11] Mahley, R.W. (1981): Cellular and molecular lipoprotein metabolism in atherosclerosis. Hum. Pathol. 16: 3–5.

[12] Munro, J.M., Cotran, R.S. (1988): The pathegenesis of atherosclerosis: Atherogenesis and inflammation. Lab. Invest. 58: 249–261.

[13] Murase, T., Oka, T., Yamada, N., Mori, N., Ishibashi, S., Takaku, F., Mori, W. (1986): Immunohistochemical localization of apolipoprotein E in atherosclerotic lesions of the aorta and coronary arteries. Atherosclerosis 60: 1–6.

[14] Orekhov, A.N., Kalantarov, G.F., Andreeva, E.R., Prokazova, N.V., Trakht, J.N. Bergelson, L.D., Smirnov, V.N. (1986): Monoclonal antibody reveals heterogeneity in human aortic intima: Detection of ganglioside antigen associated with subpopulation of intimal cells. Am. J. Pathol. 122: 279–385.

[15] Pober, J.S., Bevilacqua, M.P., Mendrick, D.L., Lapierre, L.A., Fiers, W., Gimbrone, M.A., Jr. (1986): Two distinct monokines, IL-1 and TNF, each independently induce biosynthesis and transient expression of the same antigen on the surface of cultured vascular endothelial cells. J. Immunol. 136: 1680–1687.

[16] Radzun, H.J. (1985): Immunhistochemie des menschlichen mononukleärphagozytischen Systems. Gustav Fischer Verlag, Stuttgart-New York.

[17] Roessner, A., Herrera, A., Höning, H.J., Vollmer, E., Zwadlo, G., Schürmann, R. Sorg, G., Grundmann, E. (1987): Identification of macrophages and smooth muscle cells with monoclonal antibodies in the human atherosclerotic plaque. Virchows Archiv. A. 412: 169–174.

[18] Schmitz, G., Robenek, H., Lohmann, U., Assmann, G. (1985): Interaction of high density lipoproteins with cholesteryl esterladen macrophages: Biochemical and morphological characterization of cell surface receptor binding, endocytosis and resecretion of high density lipoproteins by macrophages. EMBO J. 4: 613–622.

[19] Schwartz, C.J., Sprague, E.A., Kelley, J.L., Valente, A.J., Suenram, C.A. (1985): Aortic intimal monocyte recruitment in the normo- and hypercholesterolemic baboon (Papio cynocephalus). Virchow Archiv. A. 405: 175–191.

[20] Tsukada, T., Tippens, D., Gordon, D., Ross, R., Gown, A.M. (1987): HH F 35, a muscle-actin specific monoclonal antibody. I. Immunocytchemical and biochemical characterization. Am. J. Pathol. 126: 51–60.

[21] Vollmer, E., Brust, J., Roessner, A., Bosse, A., Kaesberg, B., Harrach, B., Robenek, H., Böcker, W. (1991a): Distribution patterns of apolipoproteins A_1, A_2, and B in the wall of atherosclerotic vessels. Virchows Archiv A (in press).

[22] Vollmer, E., Roessner, A., Bosse, A., Böcker, W., Kaesberg, B., Robenek, H., Sorg, C., Winde, G. (1991b): Immunohistochemical double labelling of macrophages, smooth muscle cells and apolipoprotein E in the atherosclerotic plaque. Path. Res. Pract. 187: 184–188.

[23] Voss, B., Rauterberg, J. (1986): Localization of collagen types I, III, IV and V, fibronectin, and laminin in human arteries by the indirect immunofluorescence method. Path. Res. Pract. 181: 568–575.

[24] Zwadlo, G., Bröcker, E.B., v. Bassewitz, D.B., Feige, U., Sorg, C. (1985): A monoclonal antibody to a differentiation antigen present on mature human macrophages and absent from monocytes. J. Immunol. 134: 1487–1492.

[25] Zwadlo, G., Schlegel, R., Sorg, C. (1986): A monoclonal antibody to a subset of human monocytes found only in the peripheral blood and inflammatory tissues. J. Immunol. 137: 512–518.

Atherogenic Factors of Blood:
Desialylated LDL and Anti-LDL Autoantibodies

Alexander N. Orekhov, Ph. D., *Vladimir V. Tertov*, Ph. D.
Institute of Experimental Cardiology,
USSR Cardiology Research Center, Moscow, Russia

This review is devoted to our recent finding that the plasma or serum of blood from patients suffering from coronary heart disease (CHD) with angiographically assessed coronary atherosclerosis has atherogenic properties. It has been established that atherogenicity of the serum is associated with low density lipoprotein (LDL) which differ from the LDL of healthy subjects. It was found out that atherogenic serum of patients contains anti-LDL autoantibodies which sharply increase LDL atherogenicity. And finally, some clinical applications based on the discovery of atherogenicity factors in the blood of CHD-patients are presented in this review.

Atherogenic Factors of Blood Plasma

The deposition of lipids and lipid overload represent the most prominent manifestation of atherosclerosis at the arterial cell level. It is quite possible that cellular pathology of atherosclerosis starts exactly from the accumulation of intracellular lipids. In this connection elucidation of their source becomes a high-priority problem. Indeed, where do lipids accumulating in the arterial cells come from? and what are the mechanisms of cellular lipidosis? It is commonly accepted idea that lipids accumulating in the arterial cells penetrate inside the vessel wall from the bloodstream. We have attempted to demonstrate that addition of blood plasma (or serum) of atherosclerotic patients to cultured cells can really cause the accumulation of intracellular fat. For this purpose, we obtained a culture of human aortic cells [1–4].

Cultured Human Arterial Cells

Cells were isolated from subendothelial part of human aortic intima, i.e. from the part of aorta which is localized between the endothelial lining and the media. The intima of adult human aorta is a well marked formation. The thickness of a normal intima varies from 50 to 120 μm [5]. Sometimes such a thickened intima is called a diffuse intimal thickening to underline its essential difference from a very thin intima of animal and adolscent aorta [5]. Unaffected intima of adult human aorta contains 10–12 lines of subendothelial cells.

To prepare primary culture, the cells are isolated by collagenase and elastase from the subendothelial layer of uninvolved intima [1–4]. The concentration of enzymes and the procedure for cell isolation were chosen so that cell viability could be retained. The viability of isolated cells amounted to 80–90% [1, 3]. Isolated cells are seeded in culture and spread within 3–4 days [1–4]. Our experiments were usually carried out on the fifth to seventh day.

By formal signs the cells cultured from the intima can be classified as the cells of smooth muscle origin. These cells are stained with antibodies to smooth muscle myosin [1–3]. For further identification of cultured cells we have used monoclonal antibody HHF-35 which interacts specifically with muscle alfa-actin and can reveal smooth muscle cells [6]. According to our calculations, primary culture of subendothelial cells contains about 90% of smooth muscle cells interacting with the HHF-35. Besides, cells cultured from subendothelial part of uninvolved intima have ultrastructural features of smooth muscle cells, namely: the basal membrane and filament bundles with dense bodies [2, 3]. The culture on which our experiments are performed is represented by mixed population of typical and modified smooth muscle cells revealed in human aorta earlier [5].

Discovery of Blood Plasma Atherogenicity

Having a primary culture of human aortic subendothelial cells, i.e. exactly those cells which accumulate lipids in atherosclerosis, we imitated cell lipidosis by addition to cultured cells of CHD-patients' blood serum. Incubation of smooth muscle cells cultured from normal human aortic intima with blood serum of CHD-patients with angiographically documented coronary atherosclerosis leads to the accumulation of intracellular cholesterol [7, 8]. The accumulation increases with the amount of serum added to culture. The sera taken from different patients caused different degree of intracellular cholesterol accumulation while the sera of healthy donors failed to induce the accumulation of cholesterol even if they have been used in high concentration. Cultivation of cells in the presence of patients' sera leads to the emergence of intracellular lipid inclusions while in the presence of healthy donors' sera no inclusions are formed [8]. It should be pointed out that the presence of lipid inclusions is the most characteristic feature of atherosclerotic changes in vascular cells [5].

The ability of patients' serum to induce the accumulation of intracellular cholesterol was termed atherogenicity. Later it was demonstrated that the deposition of intracellular cholesterol caused by the patients' sera is accompanied with the stimulation of cell proliferation enhanced synthesis of total protein, collagen, sulfated glycosaminoglycans and hyaluronic acid [9]. Thus, patients' sera possess a broad atherogenic potential which is realized in unaffected intima at the cellular level in the form of major cellular manifestations of atherosclerosis, namely: lipidosis, fibrosis and enhanced proliferation.

Most sera of healthy subjects free from any signs of coronary heart disease have no atherogenic properties [7]. On the other hand, some sera of healthy subjects bring about the accumulation of intracellular cholesterol, however, the degree of accumulation is much lower as compared to that caused by the sera of CHD-patients. Sometimes nonatherogenic sera are found among the sera of CHD-patients, but they are usually few. We have found that only 20–25% of healthy subjects devoid of any signs of CHD have atherogenic serum while nearly 90% of CHD-patients have atherogenic sera [7].

Atherogenicity of Lipoprotein

We decided to find out whether atherogenic properties of the serum are associated with lipoproteins. For this purpose the total lipoprotein fraction was isolated as well as LDL, very low density lipoprotein (VLDL), two high density lipoprotein fractions (HDL2 and HDL3). Both the total lipoprotein fraction and LDL obtained from an atherogenic plasma caused the accumulation of intracellular cholesterol in cultured cells, i.e. manifested atherogenic properties in culture [8–10]. The addition to cultured cells of LDL obtained from nonatherogenic plasma of healthy donors failed to induce the cholesterol accumulation [8–10]. It is necessary to point out that LDL of patients and healthy donors were added in equal concentrations both in terms of protein or cholesterol content, consequently, the atherogenic properties of patients' LDL are due to the qualitative difference from LDL of healthy subjects.

The accumulation of cholesterol caused by atherogenic LDL is accompanied with other atherosclerotic manifestations at the cellular level. If the cells are incubated with atherogenic LDL for three days with subsequent removal of lipoprotein from culture a high level of cholesterol, enhanced proliferative activity and increased rate of matrix synthesis are retained for at least seven following days [9]. These data indicate that LDL obtained from the plasma of CHD-patients bring about stable atherogenic alterations in the cells.

The LDL fraction is the only lipoprotein fraction possessing atherogenic properties. We failed to reveal atherogenicity in VLD, HDL2 and HDL3 obtained from an atherogenic blood plasma of CHD-patients [8, 10]. We also found no atherogenicity in any lipoprotein fraction of healthy donors' blood plasma.

Thus, we have established that blood plasma of atherosclerotic patients contains at least one component causing the accumulation of lipids in arterial cells, i.e. atherogenic LDL. This LDL is modified lipoprotein since nanatherogenic LDL of most healthy donors taken in the same concentration fails to induce the accumulation of lipids.

Desialylated LDL

Having revealed modified atherogenic LDL in the blood of atherosclerotic patients, we have attempted to find out possible differences between them and nonatherogenic LDL of healthy donors. LDLs were isolated from atherogenic patients' plasma and nonatherogenic plasma of healthy donors. The percentage of protein and major classes of lipids (phospholipids, triglycerides, free cholesterol and cholesteryl esters) in atherogenic and nonatherogenic lipoprotein preparations were the same [11]. The major protein in both types of LDL preparation was represented by apo-B. On the other hand, the sialic acid content in the LDL isolated from patients' blood was significantly lower than that of healthy donors' LDL [11, 12]. This was the only difference between the atherogenic LDL of patients and nonatherogenic LDL of healthy subjects that we could find.

We supposed that atherogenic properties of LDL circulating in the blood of atherosclerotic patients are explained exactly by a low sialic acid content. To test this hypothesis nonatherogenic LDL isolated from the blood of healthy donors was partially desialylated by incubating the lipoprotein with sialidase (neuraminidase). The addition to cultured cells of LDL treated with neuraminidase caused a more that two-fold increase of total intracellular cholesterol [11, 12]. Thus, initially nonatherogenic LDL of healthy donors can be turned atherogenic by partial desialylation. There exists a correlation between the degree of desialylation in vitro and lipoprotein atherogenicity: the higher the degree of LDL desialylation the more cholesterol is accumulated in cultured cells [12].

LDL preparations obtained from different patients had a different sialic acid content. We have found a negative correlation between the sialic acid content of LDL and their atherogenicity [11]. Thus, sialic acid contained in the LDL particle plays an essential role in the manifestation of lipoprotein atherogenic properties at the cellular level. We have assumed that the chemical nature of the modification of atherogenic LDL circulating in the blood of patients consists exactly in low sialic acid content in the lipoprotein particle.

Sialic acid is a terminal saccharide of N-linked biantennary carbohydrate chains of apolipoprotein B [13]. Terminal sialic acid is linked to galactose. During lipoprotein desialylation, that is following the loss of sialic acid, galactose becomes a terminal saccharide. We decided to make use of it to isolate desialylated lipoprotein from an LDL preparation. To isolate desialylated LDL we have used lectin, Ricin Agglutinin (RCA120), which has a high affinity to the terminal galactose. Using affinity chromatography on the basis of RCA120 immobilized on agarose, we have separated LDL with a normal sialic acid content and desialylated LDL from total LDL preparation isolated from atherogenic blood plasma of CHD-patients [14]. Thus, we have found both desialylated LDL and LDL with a normal sialic acid level in the blood of atherosclerotic patients.

Table 1 shows the data characterizing the two LDL subfractions separated by RCA120-agarose afinity chromatography. In the LDL preparations obtained from

Table 1: Characteristics of sialic acid rich LDL and sialic acid poor LDL subfractions separated by RCA120-agarose affinity chromatography

	Sialic acid rich LDL	Sialic acid poor LDL
Portion in total LDL preparation, %	40–80	20–60
Sialic acid, μg/mg protein	32± 3	14±1*
Cholesteryl esters, μg/10 mg protein	22±1	15±1*
Free cholesterol, μg/10 mg protein	8±1	4±1*
Triglycerides, μg/10 mg protein	5±1	2±1*
Lipid/protein ratio	3.6	2.1
Cellular cholesterol accumulation, % over control	6±7	215±18*

* significant difference between subfractions (p < 0.05).

patients, the subfraction of disealylated LDL account up to 60% of all circulating LDLs. Both subfractions naturally differed in the content of sialic acid. Besides, desialylated LDL subfraction was characterized by significantly lower levels of cholesteryl esters, free cholesterol and triglycerides. Desialylated LDL had a smaller lipid/protein ratio as compared with normal LDL. But, in our opinion, the major difference between these two subfractions is that normal LDL subfraction was nonatherogenic, i.e. failed to induce the accumulation of lipids in cultured cells while desialylated LDL was atherogenic and cause a 3-fold rise in intracellular cholesterol level. Thus, not all LDL, but only the subfraction of desialylated LDL represent an atherogenic component of blood plasma.

Figure 1: Agarose gel electrophoresis of normal and desialylated LDL.
Aliquots (2 mg of protein) of normally sialylated (1) and partially sialylated (2) LDL separated separated by affinity chromatography with RCA120 were subjected to 0.5% agarose gel electrophoresis and stained with fat red 7B according to Yla-Herttuala et al. [23].

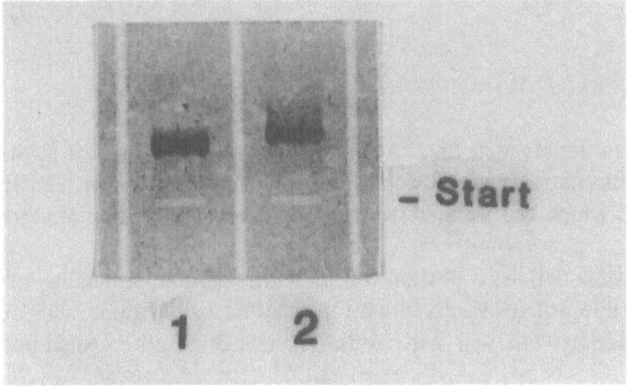

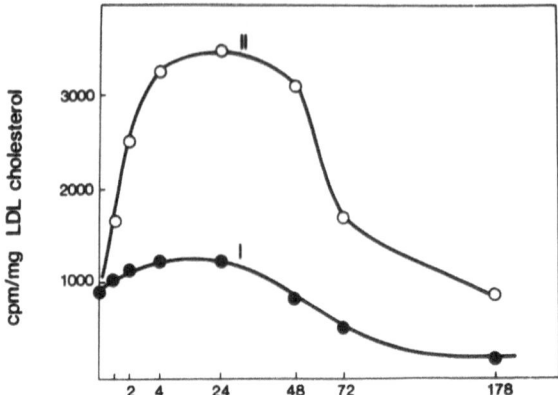

Figure 2: Specific radioactivity of [^{125}I]-labeled native LDL and desialylated LDL isolated from patient.

It has been established using gel electrophoresis that desialylated LDL has a smaller size as compared with normal lipoprotein, density of this desialylated LDL exceeds that of normal lipoprotein [15]. Desialylated LDL has a higher electrophoretic mobility, i.e. a higher negative charge (Fig. 1). It has been revealed using correlative photometry that desialylated LDL aggregate easily [16].

We have demonstrated that desialylated LDL are senescent lipoproteins which are older than normal LDL. Metabolic precursor of LDL, intermediate density lipoprotein, was isolated from the blood of a patient, labeled with [^{125}I] and reinjected to the circulation of the same patient. At certain time intervals, his blood was drawn and used to isolate normal and desialylated LDL. In all cases, specific radioactivity of desialylated LDL turned out to be higher than specific radioactivity of normal LDL (Fig. 2). Since lipoprotein radioactivity was determined by the initial radioactivity of the precursor, the obtained data allow to conclude that desialylated LDL is older lipoprotein which circulate in the bloodstream for a longer period of time as compared with normal LDL.

Discovery of Anti-LDL Autoantibodies

In addition to desialylated LDL, we have found one more factor in the blood of atherosclerotic patients which conditions its atherogenic potential. This is a non-lipid factor which was isolated from a lipoprotein-free portion of atherogenic blood serum.

If a lipoprotein-deficient portion of patients' plasma remaining after the removal of all lipoproteins is mixed with initially nonatherogenic LDL obtained from healthy donors, this will lead to the emergence of atherogenic properties in LDL [8].

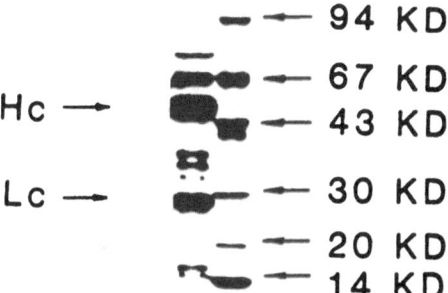

Figure 3: SDS-polyacrilamide gel electrophoresis of eluate obtained from LDL-agarose after atherogenic serum passing.

Twenty micrograms of eluate protein were subjected to SDS-PAGE (10% gel) in the presence of standard proteins (right column) and stained with Coomassie brilliant blue according to Stalenhoef et al. [24]. Hc and Lc: heavy and light immunoglobulin chains, respectively.

Using LDL immobilized on agarose, we have found out that non-lipid atherogenicity factor contained in the plasma directly interacts with LDL [8]. The substance interacting with LDL was retained on LDL-agarose and subjected to SDS gel electrophoresis. The major proteins sorbed on LDL are represented by light and heavy immunoglobulin chains (Fig. 3).

We assumed that a non-lipid factor interacting with LDL is represented by antibodies against LDL. Immunoglobulins were removed from an atherogenic serum of patients by passing the serum through a sorbent with antibodies against human immunoglobulins G (IgG), IgM and IgA. The elimination of IgG led to a sharp decrease of serum atherogenicity, a significant but less marked fall in serum atherogenicity was also observed after the removal of IgM but the removal of IgA practically did not affect the atherogenic properties of the serum [17]. Consequently, the atherogenicity of a non-lipid portion of the serum is associated mostly with IgG and to a less extent with IgM.

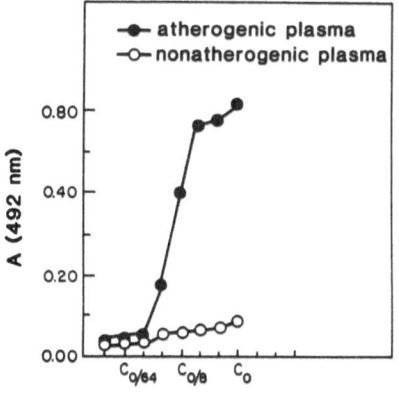

Figure 4: Discovery of anti-LdL IgG by ELISA technique.

To substantiate the hypothesis about the relationship of atherogenicity to autoantibodies we attempted to find in the serum IgG interacting with LDL. Using ELISA technique, the presence of IgG interacting with LDL was demonstrated in atherogenic sera of CHD-patients (Fig. 4). Nonatherogenic sera of healthy donors contained no anti-LDL-IgG.

To test the specificity of isolated anti-LDL IgG we carried out immunoblotting with electrophoretically separated serum proteins. Affinity purified anti-LDL bound only to the apolipoprotein B band but to not other serum proteins [18].

We established that the formation of an LDL-anti-LDL complex is accompanied with C1q complement component binding [18]. Besides F(ab')2 fragments of anti-LDL IgG interact with LDL [18]. We think that taken together these data proved that CHD-patients blood contains autoantibodies against LDL.

The constant of anti-LDL affinity to atherogenic LDL obtained from patients' blood was much high as compared with the affinity constant to nonatherogenic LDL derived from healthy donors' blood [18]. Taking into account this fact one may assume that autoantibodies in the blood are produced exactly against modified desialylated LDL. The antibodies had the highest affinity to LDL desialylated in vitro with neuraminidase [18]. We have investigated several more types of LDL modification in vitro. Autoantibodies had a roughly similar affinity to native LDL as well as Lp[a] and LDL modified by oxidation, glycosylation and acetylation but interacted with higher affinity with LDL treated by malon dialdehyde [18].

These data allow to conclude that we have found autoantibodies against modified desialylated LDL in the blood of atherosclerotic patients. Apparently, these antibodies are produced in response to the emergence of desialylated LDL in the bloodstream.

As was mentioned above, LDL obtained from the blood of healthy donors failed to bring about the accumulation of intracellular cholesterol. Simultaneous addition to culture of nonatherogenic LDL and autoantibodies led to a significant rise of cholesterol in the cells [18]. Atherogenic LDL obtained from the blood of patients had atherogenicity of their own. Addition of anti-LDL antibodies sharply increased atherogenic properties of LDL derived from patients [18].

Thus, we have established two atherogenicity factors in the plasma or serum of CHD-patiens. In the first place, these are modified desialylated LDL which is atherogenic in itself. Secondly, these are antibodies against modified LDL capable of increasing the atherogenicity of modified LDL and converted initially nonatherogenic lipoprotein into atherogenic.

Clinical Applications

Having established the origin of atherogenic blood properties, we are developing a simple method for the evaluation of patients' serum atherogenicity. It is based on the measurement of cholesterol or apo-B content in circulating immune complexes. We evaluated the significance of this index for the diagnosis of atherosclerosis. The second practical application is development of new approach to the therapy of atherosclerosis. We developed a sorbent on the basis of autologous LDL and used it for removal anti-LDL from patients' blood using extracorporeal circulation technique.

Diagnostic Value of Immune Cholesterol

Having established two factors of blood plasma atherogenicity, i.e. modified LDL and anti-LDL antibodies, we assumed that the blood of CHD-patients contains circulating immune complexes containing LDL. Circulating immune complexes were eliminated from an atherogenic serum by precipitation with polyethylenglycol (PEG) 6000. Removal of immune complexes led to a dramatic decrease in atherogenic properties of the serum [17, 19]. The isolated immune complexes proved to be atherogenic – their addition to cell culture brought about a substantial accumulation of intracellular cholesterol [17, 19]. Thus, atherogenic properties of the serum are related mostly with the presence of circulating immune complexes containing LDL.

We have developed a simple method for measuring the content of lipoprotein in circulating immune complexes. Basically, this method can be described as follows. The blood serum is mixed with PEG to the final concentration of 2.5% then, after incubation, the circulating immune complexes are sedimented by centrifugation and the apoB or cholesterol level is measured in the sediment [17, 19].

We have attempted to find out whether there is a relationship between the atherogenic properties of the serum which are manifested in culture and the cholesterol content of immune complexes. The atherogenicity was assessed by the accumulation of cholesterol in the cells cultured in the presence of the examined serum. A direct correlation was found between the cholesterol content in the serum immune complexes and the accumulation of intracellular cholesterol after the addition of this serum to cultured cells [17].

The cholesterol content in immune complexes (immune cholesterol) is associated with the presence of coronary atherosclerosis. Table 2 shows the correlation between presence of coronary atherosclerosis and immune cholesterol as well as other lipid and lipoprotein parameters. Only immune cholesterol and apoB/apoA-1 ration contributed strongly to the discrimination between patients with coronary atherosclerosis and those without stenoses. Sensitivity, specificity and accuracy of coronary atherosclerosis diagnosis were assessed for each parameter examined (Table 3). LDL-cholesterol and total cholesterol turned out highly sensitive, however, they were less specific as compared with immune cholesterol. HDL-cholesterol and apoB/apoA-1 ratio were less accurate markers, too. Triglycerides, apoA-1, apoB and Lp[a] appeared to be poor markers that provided only 50% discrimination or even less.

Table 2: Correlation between serum parameters and coronary
atherosclerosis

Parameter	P
CIC cholesterol	0.0001*
Total cholesterol	0.0575
Triglycerides	0.4852
LDL cholesterol	0.0591
HDL cholesterol	0.2146
apo B	0.0518
apoA-1	0.3342
apoB/apoA-1	0.0162*

The data presented are P values. * $p < 0.05$.

Table 3: Diagnostic value of serum parameters

Parameter	Cut off value	Sensitivity, %	Specificity, %	Accuracy, %
CIC cholesterol	15 μg/ml	81	70	78
Total cholesterol	200 mg/dL	74	33	69
Triglycerides	200 mg/dL	21	74	31
LDL cholesterol	125 mg/dL	87	11	68
HDL cholesterol	35 mg/dL	63	67	64
apo B	161 mg/dL	30	92	44
apo A-1	91 mg/dL	43	77	50
apo B/apo A-1	1.48	56	69	58
Lp[a]	30 μg/dL	41	37	40

It can be concluded that immune cholesterol level is the most reliable marker
of coronary atherosclerosis as compared to other chmical parameters used in
clinical practice.

Anti-LDL Apheresis

On the basis of our data indicating that the plasma atherogenisity can be substantially decreased by removing autoantibodies against LDL we decided to
develop a procedure using immobilized lipoproteins involved in the system of
extracorporeal circulation.

To obtaine a sorbent for anti-LDL removal we use autologous LDL, i.e. lipoprotein of the patient himself. The patient's blood plasma separated from the
blood cells was passed through a column containing this sorbent, then combined
with previously separated blood cells and returned to the patient circulation. The
procedure for elimination of anti-LDL was performed 2 hours.

Table 4: Repeated coronary angiography

	Patient				Total
	I	II	III	IV	
Total number of stenosis	5	3	4	3	15
New stenosis	0	0	0	0	0
Progression	3	1	2	1	7
Regression	1	1	0	2	4
Unchanged	1	1	2	0	4

After the anti-LDL elimination procedure the atherogenicity of blood plasma was dramatically reduced and the next day it practically fully disappeared [20]. Over the following days it gradually increased but did not achieved the initial level. Within a week the procedure was repeated, and again after the procedure atherogenicity disappeared. This time it could not be found within several days after the procedure and then it increased but slower than after the first session. If the procedure is repeated regularly (ones in two to three weeks) than atherogenicity of the patient's serum is retained at the relatively low level [20].

We have carried out a pilot study to find out the possibility of plasma atherogenicity elimination with the help of our procedure over a long period of time and to establish the effect of its chronic application on clinical and angiographic characteristics of atherosclerotic patients.

There were four patients participating in the trial. Their characteristics were shown elsewhere [20]. We performed the procedure of anti-LDL elimination on each patient for 2 years (ones in two weeks). We have not observed any serious complications of the treatment. All patients reported subjective improvement [20]. In three patients within the first several months of treatment the frequency of angina pectoris subsided, increased the patient's capacity of walking without pain. Patients reduces the doses of antianginal drugs. Tolerance of physical exercise, as judged by bycicle ergometer and holter monitoring, improved.

The second angiograms have been assessed after 20–25 months of treatment (Lyakishev, details will be published). There were no new stenoses, 50% stenosis have progressed, 25% — regressed and 25% — unchanged (Table 4). This situation is much better that the one observed in the normal course of coronary atherosclerosis [21, 22]. However, we understand that the number of our observations is to small to draw serious conclusions on the utility of this procedure. We hope that further investigations would allow us to arrive at a definite conclusion.

References

[1] Orekhov, A.N., Andreeva, E.R., Krushinsky, A.V., Smirnov, V.N.: Primary cultures of enzyme-isolated cells from normal and atherosclerotic human aorta. Med. Biol. 1984, 62: 255–259.

[2] Orekhov, A.N., Tertov, V.V., Novikov, I.D., Krushinsky, A.V., Andreeva, E.R. Lankin, V.Z., Smirnov, V.N.: Lipids in cells of atherosclerotic and uninvolved human aorta. I. Lipid composition of aortic tissue and enzyme isolated and cultured cells. Exp. Mol. Pathol. 1985, 42: 117–137.

[3] Orekhov, A.N., Krushinsky, A.V., Andreeva, E.R., Repin, V.S., Smirnov, V.N.: Adult human aortic cells in primary culture: heterogeneity in shape. Heart Vessels 1986, 2: 193–201.

[4] Smirnov, V.N., Orekhov, A.N.: Smooth muscle cells from adult human aorta. Cell Culture Techniques in Heart and Vessel Research. H.M. Piper (ed). Springer-Verlag, Berlin, 1990. pp 271–289.

[5] Geer, J.C., Haust, M.D.: Smooth muscle cells in atherosclerosis. Karger, Basel, 1972.

[6] Gown, A.M., Tsukada, T., Ross, R.: Human atherosclerosis. II. Immunocytochemical analysis of the cellular composition of human atherosclerotic lesions. Am. J. Pathol. 1986, 125: 191–207.

[7] Chazov, E.I., Tertov, V.V., Orekhov, A.N., Lyakishev, A.A., Perova, N.V., Kurdanov, Kh.A., Khashimov, Kh.A., Novikov, I.D., Smirnov, V.N.: Atherogenicity of blood serum from patients with coronary heart disease. Lancet 1986, 2: 595–598.

[8] Orekhov, A.N., Tertov, V.V., Pokrovsky, S.N., Adamova, I.Yu., Martsenyuk, O.N., Lyakishev, A.A., Smirnov, V.N.: Blood serum atherogenicity associated with coronary atherosclerosis. Evidence for nonlipid factor providing atherogenicity of low-density lipoproteins and an approach to its elimination. Circ. Res. 1988, 62: 421–429.

[9] Orekhov, A.N., Tertov, V.V., Kudryashov, S.A., Smirnov, V.N.: Triggerlike stimulation of cholesterol accumulation and DNA and extracellular matrix synthesis induced by atherogenic serum or low density lipoprotein in cultured cells. Circ. Res. 1990, 66: 311–320.

[10] Tertov, V.V., Orekhov, A.N., Martsenyuk, O.N., Perova, N.V., Smirnov, V.N.: Low density lipoproteins isolated from the blood of patients with coronary heart disease induce the accumulation of lipids in human aortic cells. Exp. Mol. Pathol. 1989, 50: 337–347.

[11] Orekhov, A.N., Tertov, V.V., Mukhin, D.N.: Desialylated low density lipoprotein – naturally occuring modified lipoprotein with atherogenic potency. Atherosclerosis 1990, 86: 153–161.

[12] Orekhov, A.N., Tertov, V.V., Mukhin, D.N., Mikhailenko, I.A.: Modification of low density lipoprotein by desialylation causes lipid accumulation in cultured cells. Discovery of desialylated lipoprotein with altered cellular metabolism in the blood of atherosclerotic patients. Biochem. Biophys. Res. Commun. 1989, 162: 206–211.

[13] Taniguchi, T., Ishikava, Y., Tsunemitsu, M., Fukuzaki, H.: The structure of the asparagine-linked sugar chains of human apolipoprotein B-100. Ach. Biochem. Biophys. 1989, 1989: 197–205.

[14] Tertov, V.V., Sobenin, I.A., Tonevitsky, A.G., Orekhov, A.N., Smirnov, V.N.: Isolation of atherogenic modified (desialylated) low density lipoprotein from blood of atherosclerotic patients: separation from native lipoprotein by affinity chromatography. Biochem. Biophys. Res. Commun. 1990, 167: 1122–1127.

[15] Jaakkola, O., Solakivi, T., Tertov, V.V., Orekhov, A.N., Miettinen, T., Nikkari, T.: Properties and cellular metabolism of low density lipoprotein subfractions. Arteriosclerosis 1990, 10: 858a.

[16] Tertov, V.V., Sobenin, I.A., Gabbasov, Z.A., Popov, E.G., Orekhov, A.N.: Lipoprotein aggregation as an essential condition of intracellular lipid accumulation caused by modified low density lipoproteins. Biochem. Biophys. Res. Commun. 1989, 163: 489–494.

[17] Tertov, V.V., Orekhov, A.N., Sayadyan, Kh.S., Serebrennikov, S.G., Kacharava, A.G., Lyakishev, A.A., Smirnov, V.N.: Correlation between cholesterol content in circulating immune complexes and atherogenic properties of CHD patients' serum manifested in cell culture. Atherosclerosis 1990, 81: 183–189.

[18] Orekhov, A.N., Tertov, V.V., Kabakov, A.E., Adamova, I.Yu., Pokrovsky, S.N., Smirnov, V.N.: Autoantibodies against modified low density lipoprotein – nonlipid factor of blood plasma that stimulates foam cell formation. Arteriosclerosis Thromb. 1991, 11: 316–326.

[19] Tertov, V.V., Orekhov, A.N., Kacharava, A.G., Sobenin, I.A., Perova, N.V., Smirnov, V.N.: Low density lipoprotein-containing circulating immune complexes and coronary atherosclerosis. Exp. Mol. Pathol. 1990, 52: 300–308.

[20] Chazov, E.I., Orekhov, A.N., Tertov, V.V., Pokrovsky, S.N., Adamova, I.Yu., Lyakishev, A.A., Gratsianski, N.W., Nechaev, A.S., Perova, N.V., Khashimov, Kh.A., Kurdanov, Kh.A., Kukharchuk, V.V., Smirnov, V.N.: Atherogenicity of blood plasma from patients with coronary atherosclerosis and its correction. Atherosclerosis Rev. 1988, 17: 9–20.

[21] Waters, D.D., Lesperance, J.: Regression of coronary atherosclerosis. Angiographic perspective. Drug. 1988, 36: 37–42.

[22] Hennerici, M., Rautenberg, W., Trockel, U., Kladetzky, R.G.: Spontaneous progression and regression of small carotid atheroma. Lancet. 1985, 1: 1415–1419.

[23] Yla-Herttuala, S., Jaakkola, O., Ehnholm, C., Tikkanen, M.J., Solakivi, T., Sarkioja, T., Nikkari, T.: Characterization of two lipoproteins containing apolipoproteins B and E from lession-free human aortic intima. J. Lipid. Res. 1988, 29: 563–572.

[24] Stalenhoef, A.F.H., Mallay, M.J., Kane, J.P., Havel, R.J.: Metabolism of apolipoproteins B-48 and B-100 of triglyceride-rich lipoproteins in normal and lipoprotein lipase-deficient humans. Proc. Natl. Acad. Sci. USA 1984, 81: 1839–1843.

Role of Lipoprotein Receptors on Macrophages in Atherogenesis

Horst Robenek, Gerd Schmitz
Institute for Arteriosclerosis Research, Dept. of Cell Biology and
Ultrastructure Research, University of Münster, Germany

Introduction

Lipoprotein receptors play a major role in the homeostasis of plasma lipo-proteins [1]. They are integrated constituents of cell membranes and bind certain lipoproteins which are then internalized by the cells [2, 3]. Insofar as lipoprotein receptors effect the concentration of lipoproteins in the plasma and may play a role in lipoprotein accumulation in arterial walls, they have both direct and in-direct influence on the progression of atherosclerosis [4, 5].

Foam cells derived from macrophages are the predominant constituents of atheromatous plaques [6–8]. Therefore, we have been studying the mechanisms of cholesterol influx and accumulation in macrophages in culture [9–12]. We could show that the uptake of lipoprotein-bound cholesterol in macrophages is mediated predominantly by receptor-mediated endocytosis [13]. Beside chemically modified low density lipoproteins (LDL), β-very low density lipoproteins (β-VLDL) are ingested by macrophages and catabolized in lysosomes [14].

The regulation of cholesterol homeostasis in macrophages is different from that of LDL-receptor cells such as fibroblasts. In the LDL-receptor cells, the activity of the receptor and the ratelimiting step of intracellular cholesterol synthesis are strictly controlled. Therefore, these cells do not need potent cholesterol acceptors for the secretion of surplus cholesterol. High density lipoproteins (HDL) stimulate the removal of cholesterol from macrophages in culture [15]. They have, there-fore, been implicated in the transport of cholesterol from peripheral tissues to the liver for disposal, a process called reverse cholesterol transport [16–18]. The cur-rent concept of reverse cholesterol transport from peripheral cells back to the liver is based on the assumption that HDL absorb unesterified cholesterol and incorporate apolipoprotein E. We have made a detailed study of the mechanisms of choleste-rol transfer from macrophages to HDL particles using biochemical and morpho-logical methods [19–21].

In this paper the mechanisms of cholesterol influx and efflux in macrophages and the receptors involved are described.

Results

1. Mechanisms of cholesterol influx in macrophages and foam cell formation

Distribution and dynamics of scavenger receptors

The mechanisms of foam cell formation by macrophages have been investigated in numerous studies [8]. The identification of a macrophage receptor mediating the endocytosis of chemically modified LDL raised the possibility that this AcLDL (acetylated LDL) or scavenger receptor plays a key part in the cholesterol influx and foam cell formation. The modifications of LDL that convert it into a ligand for the scavenger receptor include acetylation and oxydation. Recently two types of bovine macrophage scavenger receptors have been described [22, 23]. The scavenger receptor type I has three principal extracellular domains that could participate in ligand binding: Two fibrous coiled-coil-domains and the 110-amino-acid cysteine-rich C-terminal domain VI. Receptor type II is identical to the type I receptor, except that the cysteine-rich domain is replaced by a six-residue C terminus.

We have studied the distribution and dynamics of scavenger receptors in mouse peritoneal macrophages with the aid of AcLDL coupled to colloidal gold particles (Fig. 1A). Under normal culture conditions, mouse peritoneal macrophages are spread out and flat (Fig. 2A). Platinum/carbon surface replicas show the central region of the macrophage surface to be covered by numerous pleomorphic ridges and fingerlike extrusions having the appearance of microvilli. By contrast, the surface of the cell periphery is smooth, with very few or no microvilli. The borders of the cells are clearly outlined by numerous peripheral processes of variable length. After incubation of the mouse peritoneal macrophages with gold labelled AcLDL for 1 h at 4 °C, AcLDL was present on the cell surface, as can be discerned from the presence of gold label.

Exposure of macrophages to AcLDL gold complexes yielded preferential binding of gold label in the intermediate zone of the plasma membrane surface (Fig. 2B). The gold particles were more or less randomly distributed. When the cells incubated with gold labelled AcLDL for 1 h at 4 °C were warmed up to a temperature of 37 °C, within 2 min, the first signs of a rearrangement of AcLDL binding sites appeared. After 4 min the proportion of gold complexes present in larger aggregates increased considerably and after 8 min. almost all the gold particles were clustered in coated pits. After 12 to 15 min. the AcLDL gold complexes had almost completely disappeared from the cell surface.

Receptor-mediated endocytosis of AcLDL

Continuous exposure of mouse peritoneal macrophages to unlabelled AcLDL for 12 h at 37 °C resulted in the formation of numerous large multivesicular organelles with diameters of about 0.5 to 1.5 μm. Approximately 4 to 16 of these so-called 'foamy organelles' were observed per section of the cell (Fig. 4). Trimetaphosphatase and acid phosphatase reaction products in these organelles indicate that they represent the lysosomal compartments of the cells. When the macrophages were incubated further for 6 h at 37 °C in a lipoprotein-free culture medium, a substantial portion of the cytoplasm was occupied by lipid droplets. Approximately 6 to 15 lipid droplets were present per section of a cell. Their diameters ranged from 0.3 to 1.5 μm. In thin sections of macrophages warmed up to 37 °C in the presence of AcLDL gold complexes for 4 min., gold particles are found in coated pits and coated vesicles (Fig. 3), and after 15 min. in large vacuoles that often exhibit the characteristics of lysosomes (Fig. 4). This series of events is characteristic for receptor-mediated endocytosis. The following conclusions can be drawn from these results:

1. AcLDL receptors are distributed diffusely on a particular region of the cell surface of cultured mouse peritoneal macrophages.

2. The binding of AcLDL molecules to the receptors induces longrange clustering of the occupied receptors into coated pits. These two results show that both the distribution and dynamics of AcLDL and LDL receptors differ markedly, because LDL receptors in contrast to receptors for AcLDL, are always confined to presumptive coated pit regions, even prior to ligand binding, and do not migrate appreciably in the plane of the membrane.

3. AcLDL is removed rapidly from the plasma membrane and is delivered via coated vesicles to lysosomes for degradation.

Significant differences between peritoneal mouse macrophages and normal human monocyte-derived macrophages as well as macrophages from Tangier patients were observed when the cells were loaded with lipid by incubation with AcLDL. Control and Tangier-macrophages under normal culture conditions contain numerous mitochondria and cisternae of rough endoplasmic reticulum, abundant ribosomes and several vacuoles of variable size. Only occasionally single multivesicular bodies, lysosomes or lipid droplets are observed. The Golgi apparatus is well developed, although it is more extensive in the Tangier-macrophage than in the control cells (cp. Fig. 2A).

After exposure to AcLDL for 24 h at 37 °C control macrophages accumulated abundant small lipid droplets which occupied a substantial portion of the cytoplasm (Fig. 5A). In Tangier-macrophages, cytoplasmic lipid droplets were much less numerous after this treatment. Instead the cytoplasm was filled with two types of vacuoles referred to as type-I and type-II-vacuoles which were not observed in control macrophages (Fig. 5B). To determine whether the two vacuole types of Tangier cells were forms of lysosomes, immunogold cytochemistry was carried out to localize the lysosomal marker enzyme cathepsin D. This was done by postembedding immunoelectron microscopy with monospecific antibodies to cathepsin D. Both type-I- and type-II-vacuoles were found to be intensively and specifically labelled with this technique indicating that both forms of vacuoles represent lysosomes (Fig. 6A). In control macrophages the size of the lysosomal compartment was much smaller than that of Tangier-macrophages, and the individual lysosomes were less intensively stained with the cathepsin D antibody (Fig. 6B). Whether the two distinct morphological forms of the vacuoles in Tangier-macrophages reflect different stages in maturation of a single type of lysosomes or are separate type of lysosomes engaged in different types of degradative activity is uncertain. However, the fact that such a marked accumulation of lysosomes is seen, indicates that a block in the normal mechanism of transfer of cholesterol from the lysosomal compartment to storage as lipid droplets must exist in the Tangier-macrophages.

Accompanying the massive production of lysosomes in Tangier-macrophages there is a marked hyperplasia of the Golgi apparatus (Fig. 7A). As well as becoming widely distributed throughout the cell, the Golgi of Tangier-macrophages differs in appearance from those of control macrophages. Specifically the trans-cisternae of the Golgi in Tangier-macrophages are markedly dilated. One possible explanation for these changes is that under conditions of a blocked cholesterol transfer an extra demand is placed on the Golgi for production of lysosomal enzymes. A second and more likely possibility is that these morphological changes reflect a reactive overproduction of sphingomyelin and phospholipids. We have shown elsewhere that increased synthesis of these lipids occurs in Tangier-macrophages [12].

Our results indicate that the Golgi apparatus of fibroblasts shows the same characteristic changes in Tangier disease as observed in Tangier-macrophages (Fig. 7B). Tangier-fibroblasts do not, however, show alterations in the lysosomal compartment seen in the macrophages, presumably because of the fundamental differences in the way macrophages and fibroblasts metabolize cholesterol. The fact that Tangier-fibroblasts do express, parallel ultrastructural alterations in the Golgi to those of macrophages, opens the possibility that fibroblast cell cultures could provide a useful model system for investigations in Tangier disease. The advantage of such a system would be the ease of continuous cultivation and the standardization of experimental conditions on a single, defined cell line [24].

2. Mechanisms of cholesterol efflux in macrophages

We have recently shown that there are two major routes, in addition to physicochemical exchange, by which macrophages can release excess cholesterol [20, 21]. The first is a HDL-receptor-dependent secretion of cholesterol, stimulated by ACAT-inhibitors which induce the formation of lamellar bodies originat-

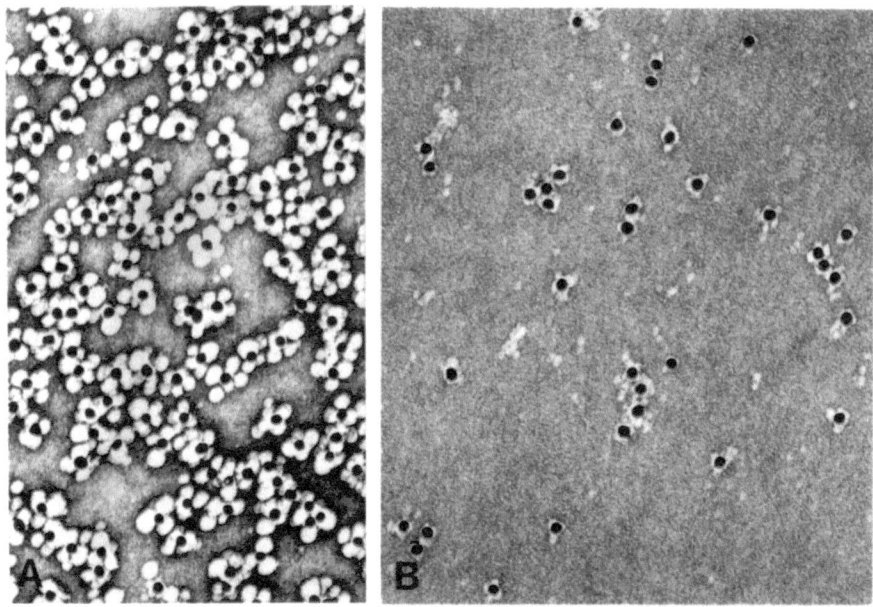

Figure 1: Negative stained LDL-gold conjugates (A) and HDL-gold conjugates (B). X 90.000.

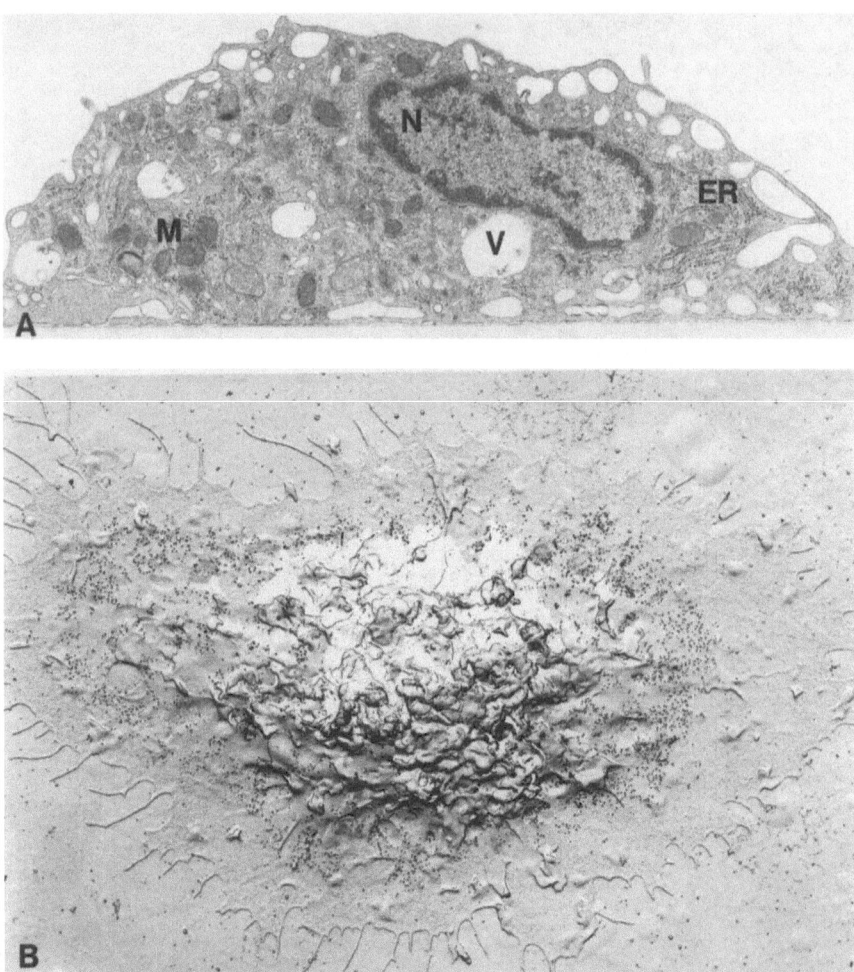

Figure 2: A) Transmission electron micrograph of a mouse peritoneal macrophage cultivated under normal culture conditions for 24 h at 37 °C. The macrophage contains a large nucleus (N), mitochondria (M), rough endoplasmic reticulum (ER) and vacuoles (V). X 14.000
(B) Low magnification surface replica of the plasma membrane of a macrophage showing the distribution of AcLDL-gold complexes after incubation with the respective conjugates for 1 h at 4 °C. X 8.000

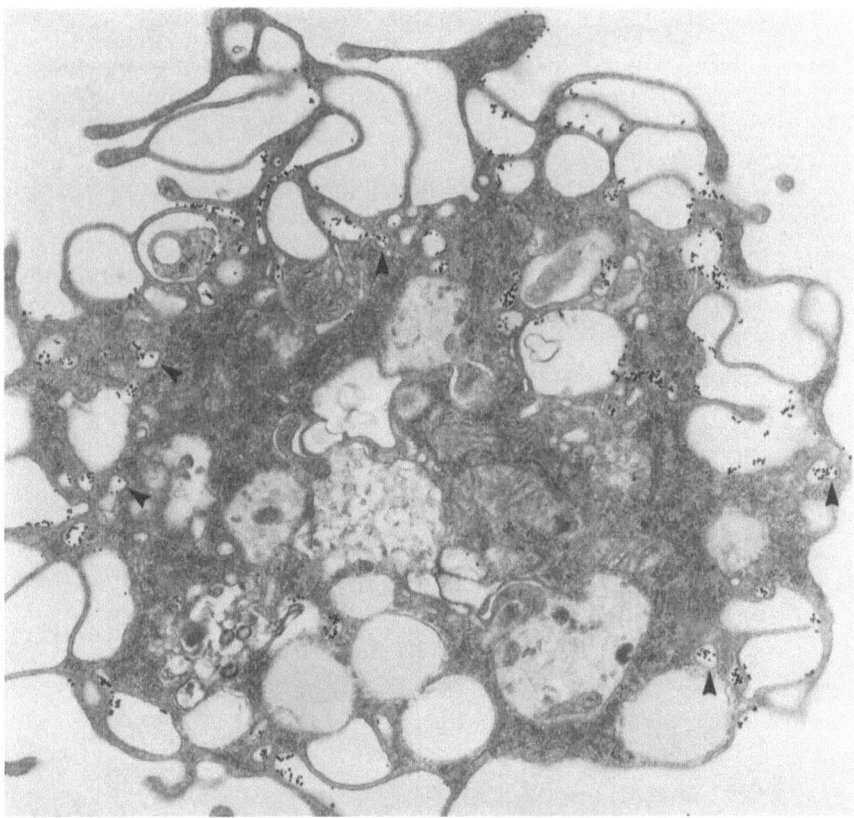

Figure 3: Transmission electron micrograph of a macrophage which was preincubated with 70 μg/ml AcLDL for 12 h at 37 °C, labelled with AcLDL-gold complexes for 1 h at 4 °C and then warmed up to 37 °C for 4 min. The gold label is found in coated pits and coated vesicles (arrow heads) as well as randomly distributed over the plasma membrane. X 22.000

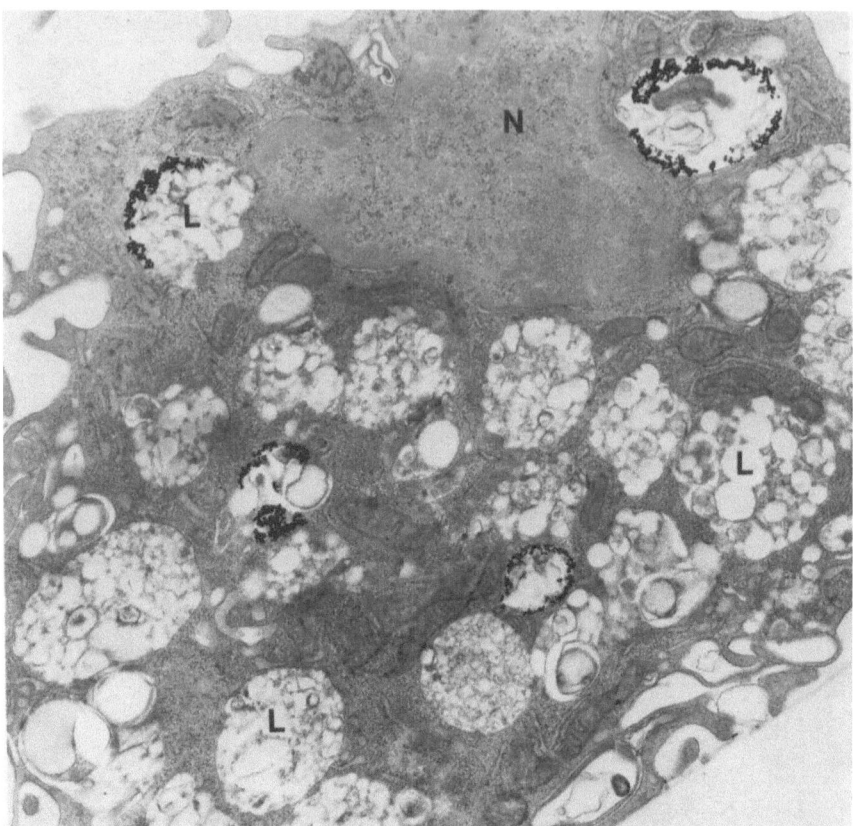

Figure 4: Transmission electron micrograph of a macrophage which was preincubated with 70 μg/ml AcLDL for 12 h at 37 °C, labelled with LDL-gold complexes for 1 h at 4 °C and then warmed up to 37 °C for 15 min. The gold label is found in lysosomes (L). N = nucleus. X 24.000

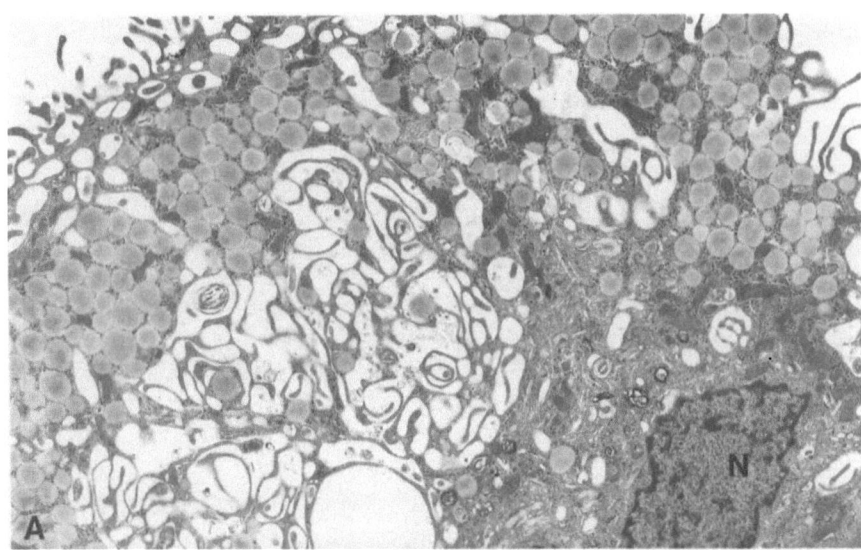

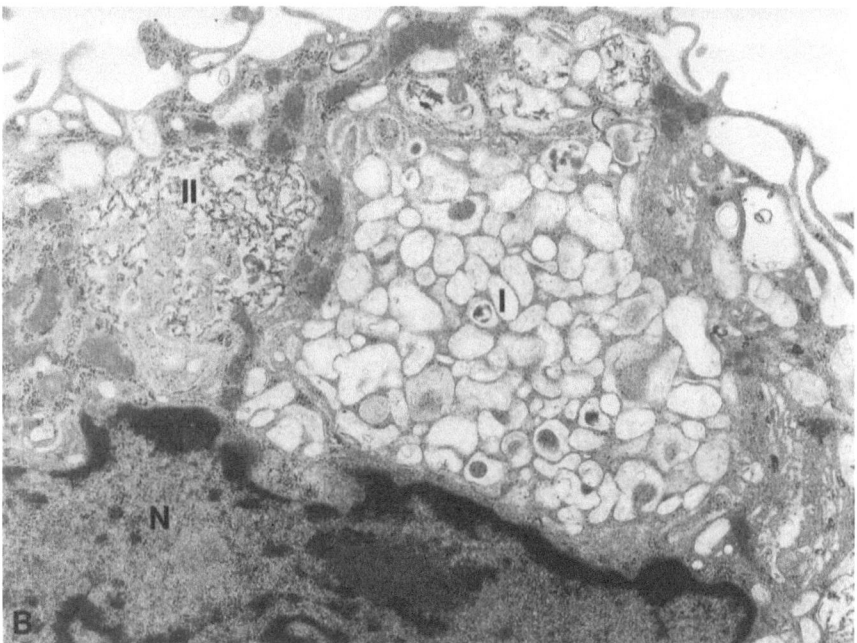

Figure 5: Transmission electron micrograph of a control human monocyte-derived macrophage (A) and Tangier macrophage (B) cultivated in the presence of 70 μg/ml AcLDL for 24 h at 37 °C. The cytoplasm of the normal human macrophage is filled with abundant lipid droplets (A) whereas the Tangier-macrophage contains two types of vacuoles, referred to as type-I-(I)- and type-II-(II) vacuoles. N = nucleus, (A) X 8.000 (B) 17.500

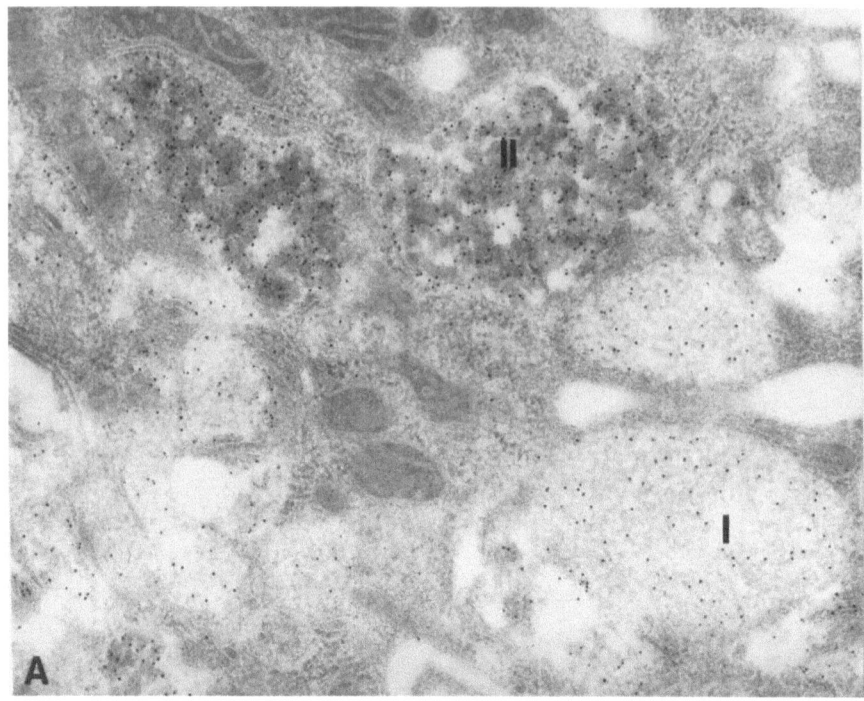

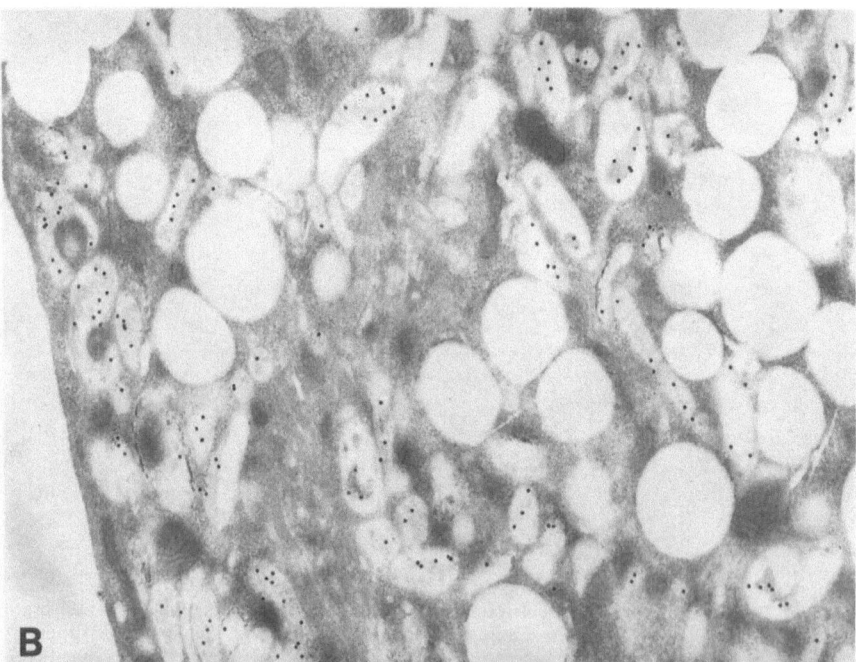

Figure 6: Localization of cathepsin D in a Tangier-macrophage (A) and in a control human monocyte-derived macrophage (B). The cells were cultivated in the presence of 70 µg/ml AcLDL for 24 h at 37 °C. Cathepsin D was revealed by postembedding immunoelectron microscopy with monospecific antibodies against cathepsin D and the protein A-gold technique. Both type-I-(I)- and type-II-(II) vacuoles are found to be intensively and specifically labeled (A). Less gold-label is found in lysosomes of control macrophages (B). (A) X 57.000 (B) 23.000

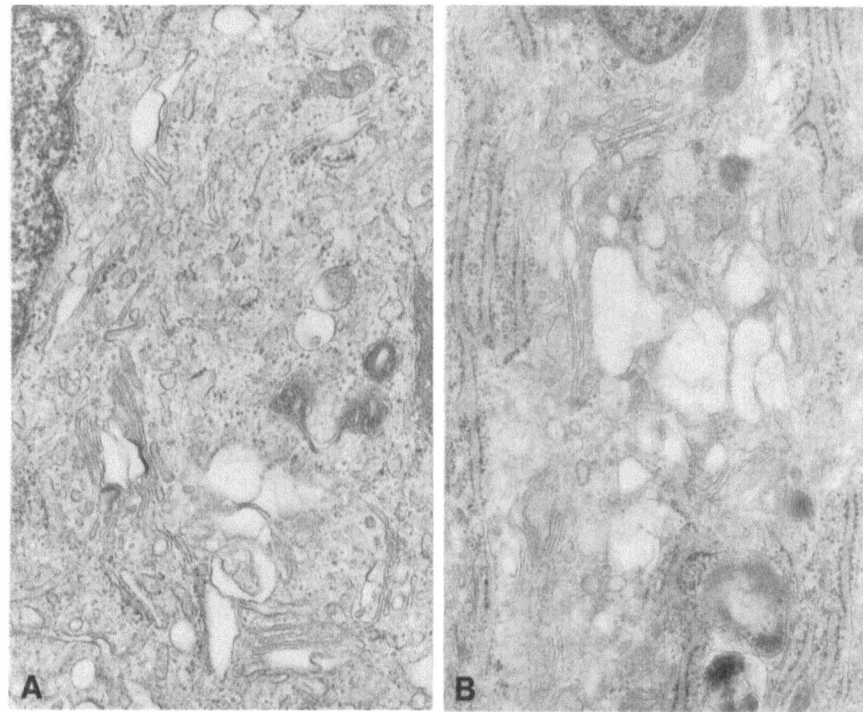

Figure 7: Transmission electron micrographs of a Tangier macrophage (A) and Tangier fibroblast (B) showing a marked hyperplasia of the Golgi-apparatus. (A) X 20.000 (B) X 36.000

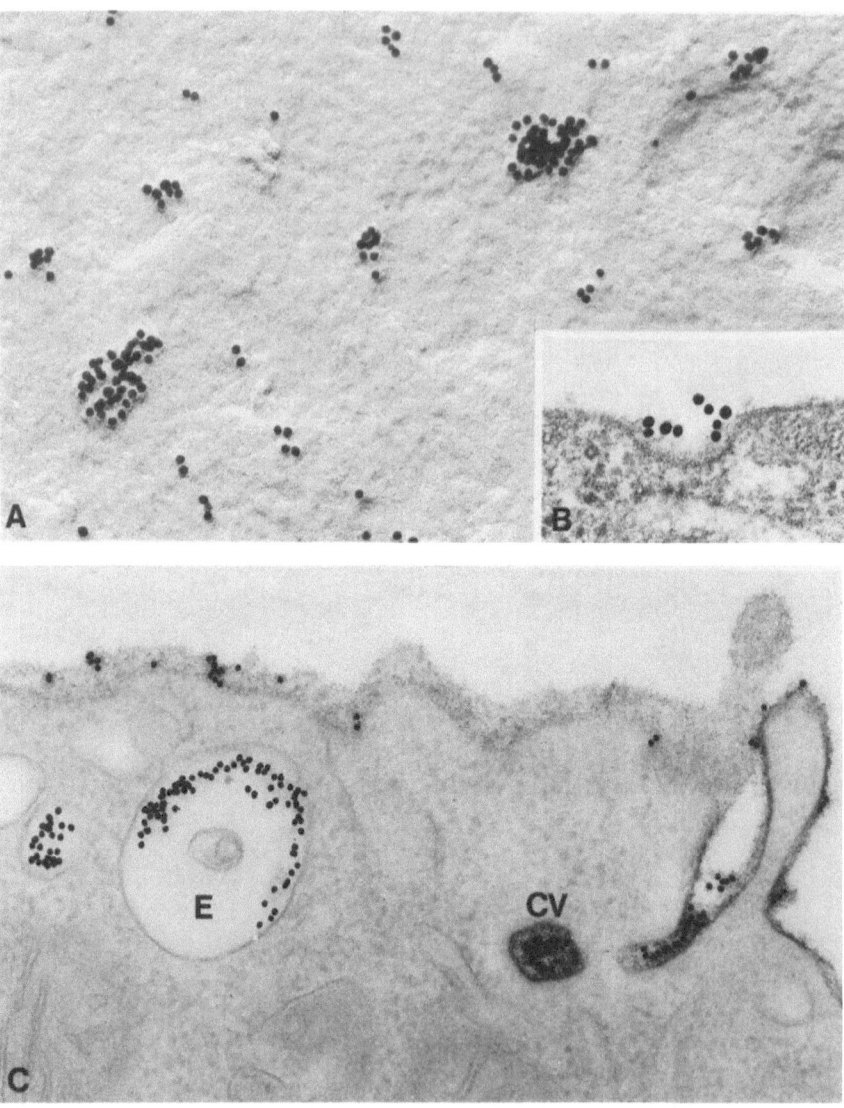

Figure 8: (A) Surface replica of the plasma membrane of a mouse peritoneal macrophage showing the distribution of HDL-gold complexes after incubation with the respective conjugates for 1 h at 4 °C. X 70.000

(B) Transmission electron micrograph showing HDL-gold label in a coated pit. X 90.000

(C) When the incubation temperature was increased to 37 °C, HDL-gold complexes recognized by the HDL-receptor entered the macrophages via coated pits, coated vesicles (CV) and endosomes (E). The cell was stained with ruthenium red. X 43.000

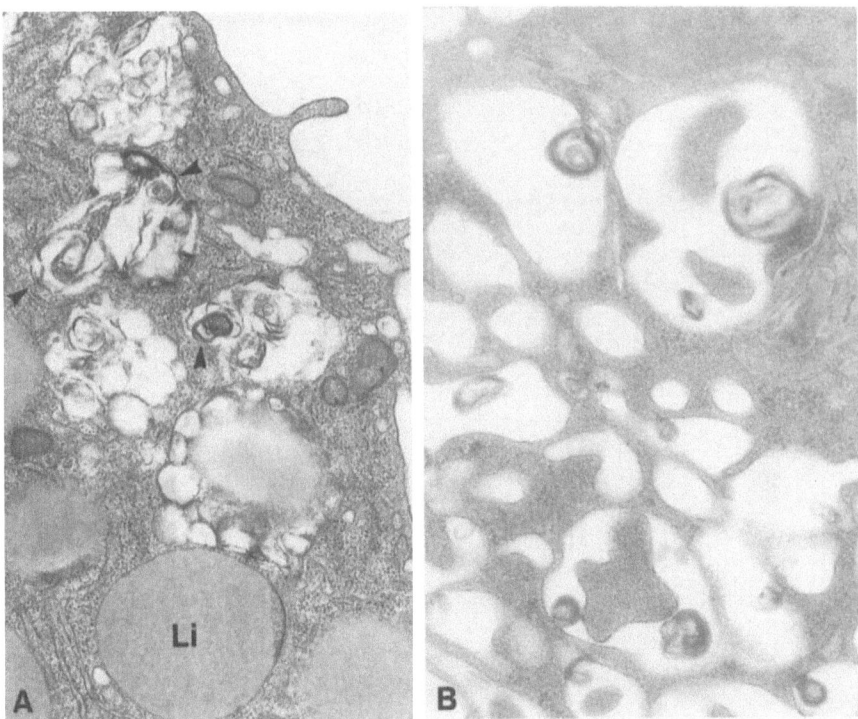

Figure 9: (A) Transmission electron micrograph of a mouse peritoneal macrophage sequentially cultured in the presence of 70 μg/ml AcLDL for 12 h at 37 °C and then in the presence of 2 μmol/l nifedipine for 8 h at 37 °C. The cytoplasm contains many vacuoles with lamellar bodies (arrowheads) and only a few lipid droplets (Li). X 18.000
(B) The lamellar bodies are released by the cells into the extracellular space. X 48.000

ing from lipid droplets or alternatively are released from the trans region of the Golgi apparatus. These lamellar bodies are not directly secreted by the cells. However, when HDL is added to the medium, the lamellar bodies transfer their cholesterol to HDL particles and disappear concomitantly with the HDL-receptor-mediated cholesterol efflux. The second is a HDL-receptor-independent release of cholesterol, stimulated by dihydropyridine Ca^{++}-antagonists which induce the formation of lamellar bodies originating from lysosomes. These lamellar bodies fuse with the cell membrane and can be secreted into the surrounding medium by a HDL-receptor-independent mechanism which appears to be promoted by apo-A-IV and LCAT-rich HDL particles.

HDL-receptor-dependent release of cholesterol

The presence of HDL receptors has been demonstrated in various cells [25–30]. However, a consensus has not been reached as to whether HDL undergoes endocytosis as do ligands known to be endocytosed via the LDL receptor pathway [31–36]. Using morphological methods, we were able to show that apolipoprotein E-depleted HDL particles bind to specific surface receptors on mouse peritoneal and human monocyte-derived macrophages (Figs. 8A–C). Cholesterol loaded macrophages had significantly higher numbers of HDL receptors than did freshly isolated macrophages. Gold-labelled human HDL particles were found pre-clustered and randomly distributed on the cell surface when the experiments were performed at 4 °C. Thus, the native pattern of HDL receptors appeared to be of an intermediate type between exclusive clustering and diffuse distribution. When the incubation temperature was increased to 37 °C, HDL recognized by the receptor entered the macrophages via coated pits and coated vesicles indicating that the uptake of HDL in macrophages occurs by receptor-mediated endocytosis (Figs. 8A, B).

It can be shown with ^{125}I-labelled HDL that the HDL receptor has a high specificity for this lipoprotein, and Scatchard plot analysis reveals high-affinity properties of the ligand-receptor interaction. Apo A-I, the major HDL apolipoprotein, and apo A-IV is probably the ligand of this receptor [37–42]. Normally, only minor amounts of the internalized HDL aggregated in lysosomes. During intracellular processing, the HDL are transported in endosomes, take up unesterified cholesterol from lipid droplets, and are secreted from the cells as cholesterol-rich-HDL particles.

HDL-receptor-independent release of cholesterol

We recently demonstrated that cholesterol efflux from normal macrophages is also facilitated by an HDL-receptor-independent secretion of lamellar bodies which are rich in cholesterol and of lysosomal origin [21]. The Ca^{++}-antagonist nifedipine induced the formation of membrane-surrounded 'lamellar bodies' originating from lysosomes (Fig. 9A). The macrophages secreted these lamellar bodies which were rich in phospholipids and cholesterol, into the culture medium even in the absence of cholesterol acceptors (Fig. 9B). In contrast, the ACAT-inhibitor octimibate induced the formation of lamellar bodies originating from lipid droplets which were also surrounded by membranes. There is strong evidence that these latter membranes were newly synthesized at the margin of the lipid droplets by the endoplasmic reticulum. The lamellar bodies descending from lipid droplets after ACAT-inhibitor treatment were not secreted by the cells. They were stored in the cytoplasmic compartment in the absence of high density lipoproteins. When HDL were added to the medium the lamellar bodies specifically interacted with endosomes containing the internalized HDL particles and disappeared concomitantly with an enhanced HDL-mediated cholesterol efflux.

From our biochemical and morphological data we conclude that macrophages release cholesterol by two major pathways:

1. a HDL-receptor-independent secretion of lamellar bodies containing cholesterol which originate from lysosomes and

2. a HDL-receptor-dependent release of cholesterol via the formation of lamellar bodies descending from lipid droplets which intracellularly fuse with HDL-containing endosomes. The cholesterol-enriched HDL are than secreted as intact lipoproteins.

References

[1] Brown, M.S., Goldstein, J.L.: A receptor-mediated pathway for cholesterol homeostasis. Science 1986; 232: 34–47.

[2] Goldstein, J.L., Brown, M.S., Anderson, R.G.W., Rüssel, D.W., Schneider, W.J.: Receptor-mediated endocytosis: concepts emerging from the LDL receptor system. Ann. Rev. Cell. Biol. 1985; 1: 1–39.

[3] Goldstein, J.L., Anderson, R.G.W., Brown, M.S.: Coated pits, coated vesicles and receptor-mediated endocytosis. Nature 1979; 279: 679–685.

[4] Goldstein, J.L., Brown, M.S.: The low density lipoprotein pathway and its relation to atherosclerosis. Ann. Rev. Biochem. 1977; 46: 897–930.

[5] Brown, M.S., Goldstein, J.L.: How LDL receptors influence cholesterol and atherosclerosis. Sci. Am. 1984; 251: 58–66.

[6] Ross, R.: The pathogenesis of atherosclerosis – an update. New Engl. J. Med. 1986; 314: 488–500.

[7] Ross, R., Masuda, J., Raines, E.W., Gown, A.M., Katsuda, S., Sasahara, M., Malden, L.T., Masuko, H., Sato, H.: Localization of PDGF-B protein in macrophages in all phases of atherogenesis. Science 1990; 248: 1009–1012.

[8] Brown, M.S., and Goldstein, J.L.: Lipoprotein metabolism in the macrophage: implications for cholesterol deposition in atherosclerosis. Ann. Rev. Biochem. 1983; 52: 223–261.

[9] Robenek, H., Schmitz, G.: Receptor domains in the plasma membrane of cultured mouse peritoneal macrophages. Eur. J. Cell. Biol. 1985; 39: 77–85.

[10] Robenek, H.: Topography and internalization of cell surface receptors as analyzed by affinity – and immunolabeling combined with surface replication and ultrathin sectioning techniques. In: Electron Microscopy of Subcellular Dynamics, H. Plattner (ed), CRC Press, Boca Raton USA 1989; 141–163.

[11] Schmitz, G., Beuck, M., Fischer, H., Nowicka, G., Robenek, H.: Regulation of phospholipid biosynthesis during cholesterol influx and high density lipoprotein-mediated cholesterol efflux in macrophages. J. Lipid. Res. 1990; 31: 1741–1752.

[12] Schmitz, G., Fischer, H., Beuck, M., Hoecker, K.P., Robenek, H.: Dysregulation of lipid metabolism in Tangier-monocyte-derived macrophages. Arteriosclerosis 1990; 10: 1010–1019.

[13] Robenek, H., Schmitz, G., Assmann, G.: Topography and dynamics of receptors for acetylated and malondialdehyde-modified low-density lipoprotein in the plasma membrane of mouse peritoneal macrophages as visualized by colloidal gold in conjunction with surface replicas. J. Histochem. Cytochem. 1984; 32: 1017–1027.

[14] Robenek, H., Schmitz, G., Greven H.: Cell surface distribution and intracellular fate of human β-very low density lipoprotein in cultured peritoneal mouse macrophages: a cytochemical and immunocytochemical study. Eur. J. Cell. Biol. 1987; 43: 110–120.

[15] Ho, Y.K., Brown, M.S., Goldstein, J.L.: Hydrolysis and excretion of cytoplasmic cholesteryl esters by macrophages: stimulation by high density lipoproteins and other agents. J. Lipid. Res. 1980; 21: 391–398.

[16] Badimore, J.L., Badimore, L., Galvez, A., Dische, R., Fuster, V.: High density lipoprotein plasma fractions inhibit aortic fatty streaks in cholesterol-fed rabbits. Lab. Invest. 1989; 60: 455–461.

[17] Tabas, J., Tall, A.R.: Mechanism of the association of HDL_3 with endothelial cells, smooth muscle cells and fibroblasts. J. Biol. Chem. 1984; 259: 13897–13905.

[18] Glomset, J.A.: The plasma lecithin: cholesterol acyltransferase reaction. J. Lipid. Res. 1968; 9: 155–167.

[19] Schmitz, G., Robenek, H., Lohmann, U., Assmann, G.: Interaction of high density lipoproteins with cholesterol ester-laden macrophages: biochemical and morphological characterization of cell surface binding, endocytosis and resecretion of high density lipoproteins by macrophages. EMBO J. 1985; 4: 613–622.

[20] Schmitz, G., Robenek, H., Beuck, M., Krause, R., Schurek, A., Niemann, R.: Ca^{++}-antagonists and ACAT-inhibitors promote cholesterol efflux from macrophages by different mechanisms. I. Characterization of intracellular lipid metabolism. Arteriosclerosis 1988; 8: 46–56.

[21] Robenek, H., Schmitz, G.: Ca^{++}-antagonists and ACAT-inhibitors promote cholesterol efflux from macrophages by different mechanisms. II. Characterization of intracellular morphological changes. Arteriosclerosis 1988; 8: 57–67.

[22] Kodama, T., Freeman, M., Rohrer, L., Zabrecky, J., Matsudaira, P., Krieger, M.: Type I macrophage scavenger receptor contains α-helical and collagen-like coiled coils. Nature 1990; 343: 531–535.

[23] Rohrer, L., Freeman, M., Kodama, T., Penman, M., Krieger, M.: Coiled-coil fibrous domains mediate ligand binding by macrophage scavenger receptor type II. Nature 1990; 343: 570–572.

[24] Robenek, H., Schmitz, G.: Abnormal processing of Golgi elements and lysosomes in Tangier disease. Arteriosclerosis 1991; in press.

[25] Oram, J.F., Johnson, C.J., Aulinskas-Brown.: Interaction of high density lipoprotein with its receptor on cultured fibroblasts and macrophages. J. Biol. Chem. 1987; 262: 2405–2410.

[26] Tauber, J.P., Goldminz, D., Gospodarowicz, D.: Up-regulation in endothelial cells of binding sites of high density lipoprotein induced by 25-hydroxy-cholesterol. Eur. J. Biochem. 1981; 119: 327–339.

[27] Fong, B.S., Rodriguez, P.O., Salter, A.M., Yip, B.P., Despres, J.P., Gregg, R., Engel, A.: Characterization of high density lipoprotein binding to human adipocyte plasma membranes. J. Clin. Invest. 1985; 75: 1804–1812.

[28] Gwynne, J.T., Hughes, T., Hess, B.: Characterization of high density lipoprotein binding activity in rat adrenocortical cells. J. Lipid. Res. 1984; 25: 1059–1071.

[29] Hoeg, J.M., Demosky, S.J., Edge, S.B., Gregg, R.E., Osborne, J.C., Brewer, H.B.: Characterization of a human hepatic receptor for high density lipoproteins. Arteriosclerosis 1985; 5: 228–237.

[30] Bachorik, P.S., Virgil, D.G., Kwiterovich, P.O.: Effect of apolipoprotein E-free high density lipoproteins on cholesterol metabolism in cultured pig hepatocytes. J. Biol. Chem. 1987; 262: 13636–13645.

[31] Kambouris, A.M., Roach, P.D., Calvert, G.D., Nestel, P.J.: Retroendocytosis of high density lipoproteins by human hepatoma cell line, HepG2. Arteriosclerosis 1990; 10: 582–590.

[32] Takahashi, K., Fukuda, S., Naito, M., Horiuchi, S., Takata, S., Morino, Y.: Endocytic pathway of high density lipoprotein via trans-Golgi system in rat resident peritoneal macrophages. Lab. Invest. 1989; 61: 270–277.

[33] Takata, K., Horiuchi, S., Torab, A., Rahim, M.A., Morino, Y.: Receptor-mediated internalization of high density lipoprotein by rat sinusoidal liver cells: identification of a non-lysosomal endocytic pathway by fluorescence labeled ligand. J. Lipid. Res. 1988; 29: 1117–1126.

[34] Rinninger, F., Pittman, R.C.: Regulation of the selective uptake of high density lipoprotein-associated cholesteryl esters by human fibroblasts and HepG2 cells. J. Lipid. Res. 1988; 29: 1179–1194.

[35] Bachorik, P.S., Franklin, F.A., Virgil, D.G., Kwiterovich, P.O.: Reversible high affinity uptake of Apo E-free high density lipoproteins in cultured pig hepatocytes. Arteriosclerosis 1985; 5: 142–152.

[36] Alam, R., Yatsu, F.M., Alam, S.: Receptor-mediated uptake and retroendocytosis of high density lipoproteins by cholesterol-loaded human monocyte-derived macrophages: possible role in enhancing reverse cholesterol transport. Biochim. Biophys. Acta. 1989; 1004: 292–299.

[37] Rifici, V.A., Eder, H.A.: A hepatocyte receptor for high density lipoproteins specific for apolipoprotein A-I. J. Biol. Chem. 1984; 25: 13814–13818.

[38] Graham, G.L., Oram, J.F.: Identification and characterization of a high density lipoprotein binding protein in cell membranes by ligand blotting. J. Biol. Chem. 1987; 262: 7439–7442.

[39] Glass, C., Pittman, R.C., Civen, M., Steinberg, D.: Uptake of high density lipoprotein associated apolipoprotein A-I and cholesteryl esters by 16 tissues of the rat in vivo and by adrenal cells and hepatocytes in vitro. J. Biol. Chem. 1985; 260: 744–750.

[40] Fong, B.S., Salter, A.M., Jimenez, Angel, A.: The role of apolipoprotein A-I and apolipoprotein A-II in high density lipoprotein binding to human adipocyte plasma membranes. Biochim. Biophys. Acta 1987; 920: 105–113.

[41] Barbaras, R., Puchois, P., Fruchart, J.C., Ailhaud, G.: Cholesterol efflux from cultured adipose cells is mediated by LpA-I particles but not by LpA-I: A-II particles. Biochim. Biophys. Res. Commun. 1987; 142: 63–69.

[42] Savion, N., Gamliel, A.: Binding of apolipoprotein A-I and apolipoprotein A-IV to cultured bovine aortic endothelial cells. Arteriosclerosis 1988; 8: 178–186.

Participation of Leukocytes in the Development of Experimentally Induced Arteriosclerotic Lesions — Morphological and Functional Aspects

D. Kling[1], H. Heinle[1], J.M. Harlan[2]
[1] Institute of Physiology I, University of Tübingen,
[2] Harborview Medical Center, Seattle, Washington, USA

The occurrence of different types of leukocytes including monocytes, lymphocytes and granulocytes, during the development of atherosclerotic lesions has been numerously reported in both man and animal models [4—6, 13—16, 21, 24, 25, 27]. Various aspects of the possible involvement of these leukocytes in atherogenesis were discussed: e.g., the lipid-scavenging function of monocytes/macrophages [2, 26, 29] and their putative roles in stimulating smooth muscle cell proliferation [7, 8, 22, 23], or the influences of T lymphocytes on growth properties of myocytes [9, 10]. However, it is still impossible to formulate a comprehensive concept on the roles that leukocytes play in the different phases of plaque development.

Our main focus of interest was directed toward an understanding of the dynamics of leukocytes within the lesion as well as of the functional relationship between blood-borne cells and vessel wall components, e.g., smooth muscle cells. Accordingly, two different approaches were taken:

I. The temporal pattern of leukocyte participation was studied from the prelesional state up to the formation of plaques under normo- and hypercholesterolemic conditions.

II. Leukocyte invasion into the intima was inhibited in rabbits by treating them with the monoclonal antibody mAb 60.3 (directed to the adherence-promoting leukocyte glycoprotein CD18), and the effect on migration of medial myocytes was examined.

I. Leukocyte participation in plaque development as influenced by duration of electrostimulation and diet

Methods

The arteriosclerotic lesions were induced by using the method of transmural electrical stimulation (ES) [1, 16]. In brief, the right common carotid artery of male New Zealand rabbits was repeatedly exposed to weak direct current impulses (0.1 mA; 15 ms/imp.; 10 Hz), which were applied via electrodes attached to the adventitia by a teflon cuff. The left carotid artery served as a control; it remained either unmanipulated or it received a so-called "silent" cuff without electrodes. This method was applied to animals fed either a standard diet or a chow, which was supplemented with 1% cholesterol. The feeding of the cholesterol-rich diet started 4d prior to the beginning of the stimulation schedule. In order to establish the time pattern of the changes in the artery wall, the rabbits were exposed to the stimulation schedule for 1, 2, 3, 7, 14 and 28d, resp., with two sessions per day. At the end of the stimulation program the carotid arteries were perfusion-fixed and submitted to procedures either resulting in silver nitrate surface preparations examined at the light microscopic level or in ultrathin sections analyzed by electron microscopy [16, 17]. The morphologic changes described below refer to the anodal site of the stimulated artery segments.

Results

The application of transmural electrical stimulation to rabbit carotid arteries led either to the formation of fibromuscular plaques under standard diet conditions or to so-called lipid-containing plaques under cholesterol-rich chow. The latter advanced to typical atheromatous lesions within 5–6 weeks. The initial events occurring within the first two days in the development of the two types of plaques were characterized by endothelial alterations in conjunction with massive extravasation of leukocytes. Changes of the endothelium were manifest 1) as an increased permeability to macromolecules, detected, e.g., by applying horseradish peroxidase or albumin [12, 17, 18], and 2) as changes in shape, size, argyrophilia and arrangement of the endothelial cells, although they still formed a continuous lining [16, 17]. In association with the functionally and structurally altered endothelium a conspicuous number of leukocytes were observed in the enface-preparations of the stimulated artery segments. Quantitative analysis revealed that in both diet groups the number of leukocytes per standard area of the endothelium ($A = 0.9216$ mm^2) was significantly greater in the stimulated segments than in the controls (standard diet: 362 ± 62 leukocytes/A after 1 d ES vs 27 ± 24 leukocytes/A in controls with "silent" cuffs; cholesterol-rich chow: 414 ± 70 cells/A after 1 d ES vs 42 ± 24 in controls). In the case of cholesterol-rich diet, leukocyte density was indeed larger in comparison to normocholesterolemia, however, the difference was not significant at this time (means were compared with Student's t-test).

As determined by electron microscopy, under both dietary conditions the population of adherent cells consisted of granulocytes, monocytes and lymphocytes. Polymorphonuclear neutrophils and monocytes occurred most frequently. After 1 and 2 d of exposure to the stimulation program, these cells were not only found adhering to the endothelium but also diapedesing through the endothelium or already lying beneath the overtly intact endothelial covering (Plate I). Once they had reached the subendothelium, the leukocytes were arranged in one or two cell layers and formed the major cellular constituents of these early lesions. But at the same time, the first smooth muscle cells (SMC) appeared within the intima. Some of them were just squeezing through pores of the internal elastic lamina, while others were already located in the subendothelium in a longitudinal fashion.

Up to the third day of exposure to ES the sequence of initial events, i.e., endothelial alterations, leukocyte invasion and myocyte migration was very similar in both diet groups. However, within this period particular ultrastructural features could be observed only in association with hypercholesterolemia (Plate II). They are listed in Table 1 together with the time of their first appearance.

The further development of the intimal thickenings, especially the dynamics in the composition of the subendothelial cell population during genesis of the fibromuscular and lipid-containing plaques, are comparatively demonstrated in Fig. 1. Under both diet plans, leukocytes dominated during the first three days in the intimal cell population, consisting of varying proportions of granulocytic and mononuclear cells. (Monocytes and lymphocytes were grouped together as mononuclear cells, since it was sometimes difficult to discriminate between these two cell types.) The first SMC occurred within the subendothelium already after 1 d, and with advancing stimulation time their numbers increased. Accordingly, the relative amount of leukocytes decreased; granulocytes disappeared completely within 14 d. Regarding mononuclear cells, for up to 14 d no significant differences in the respective frequencies were found in the two diet groups. However, comparing the composition of the plaques after 28 d, the percentage of mononuclear cells in the lipid-containing plaque amounted to $18 \pm 5\%$ and was significantly higher than the respective value in the fibromuscular plaque which was $5 \pm 6\%$. (Two-way analysis of variance was performed to test dependence on time and diet; in the case of multiple comparisons, Holm-Bonferroni's correction was used). Various mechanisms may be responsible for this difference. For example, mono-

Table 1: Specific features associated with hypercholesterolemia

Time of ES (days)	Ultrastructural features
1–2	• pronounced accumulation of amorphous, membranous and vesicular material in the subendothelium; often in close contact with mononuclear cells
1–2	• lipid deposition in monocytes/macrophages located in the subendothelium or lying between endothelial cells and emerging into the vessel lumen (macrophage-derived foam cells); platelet association with the exposed lipid-laden macrophages
3	• intimate interdigitations of monocytic foam cells with SMC
3	• occurrence of lipid vacuoles in intimal SMC

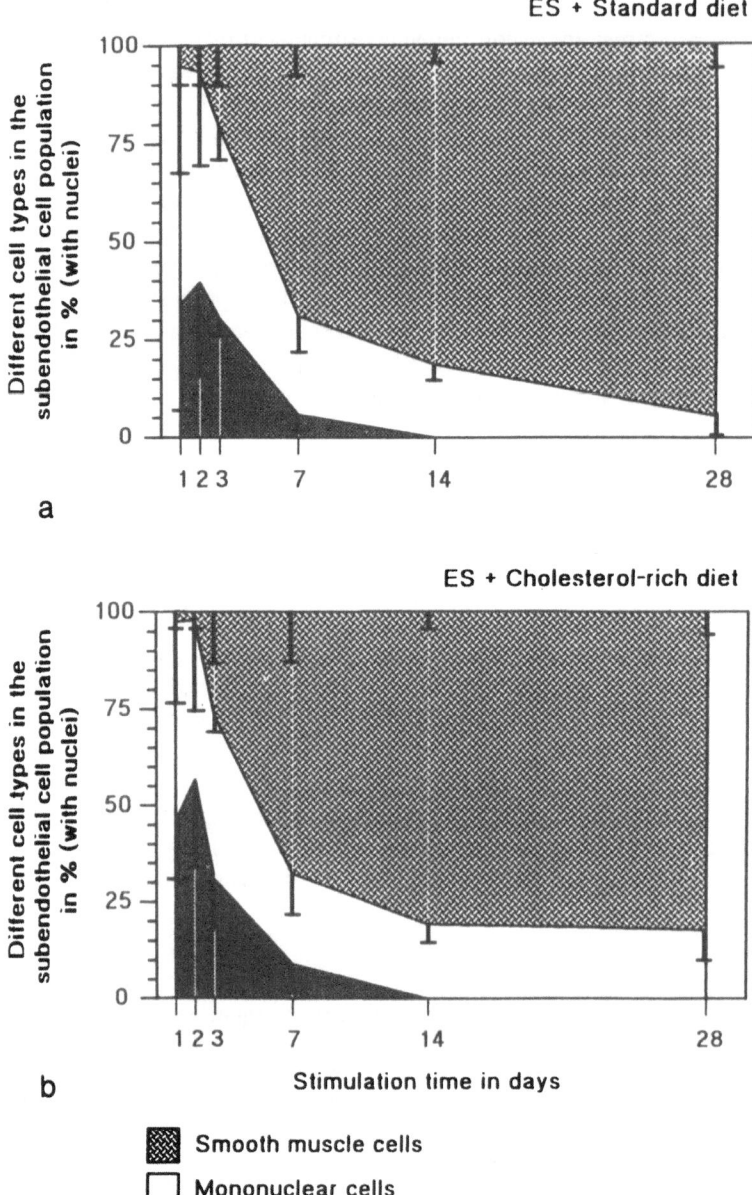

Figure 1: Dynamics in the composition of the subendothelial cell population during genesis of fibromuscular (a) and lipid-containing (b) plaques. The differently marked areas indicate the frequencies of the various cell types determined within the middle region of the forming plaque. Only nucleated cell profiles are included in the count.

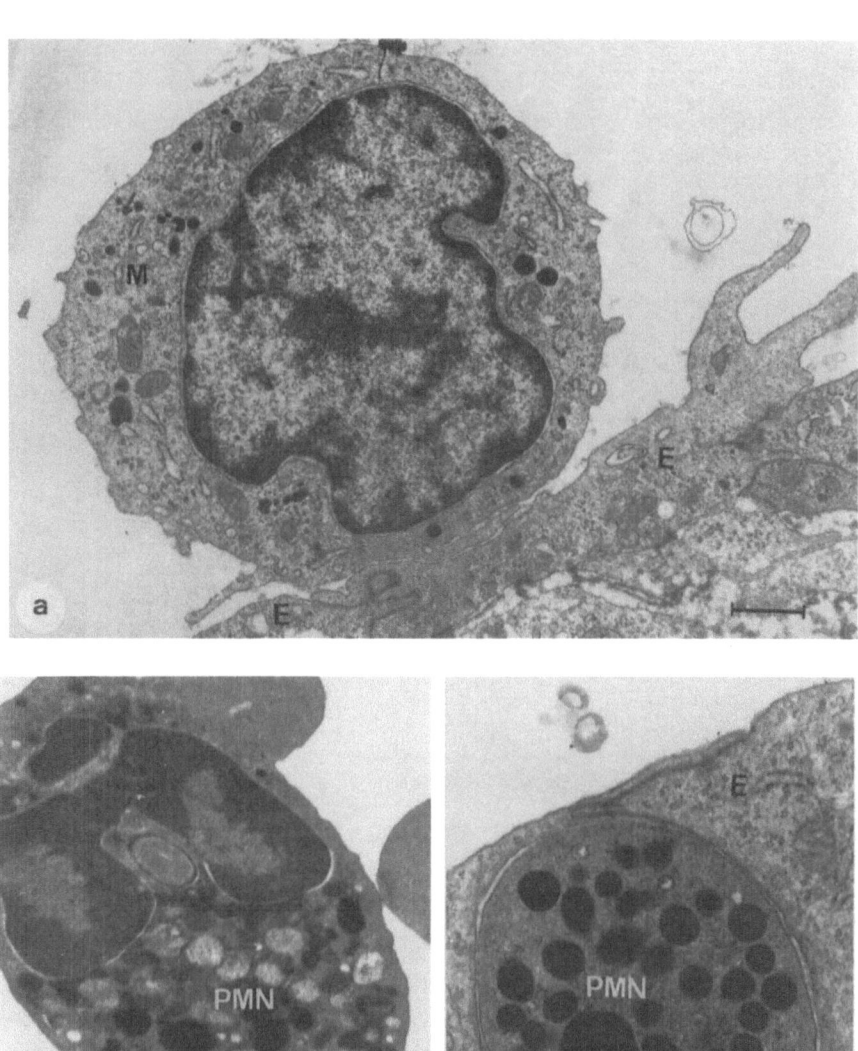

Plate I: Leukocytes associated with the endothelium of electrically stimulated carotid arteries of rabbits exposed to different diets.
a) Monocyte (M) adhering to the endothelium (E); 1 d ES, standard diet. b) Polymorphonuclear granulocyte (PMN) sending a pseudopod into an interendothelial gap. (c) Neutrophil (PMN) located beneath an intact endothelium (E). b) and c) 2 d ES, 6 d cholesterol-rich chow. Bars indicate 1 μm.

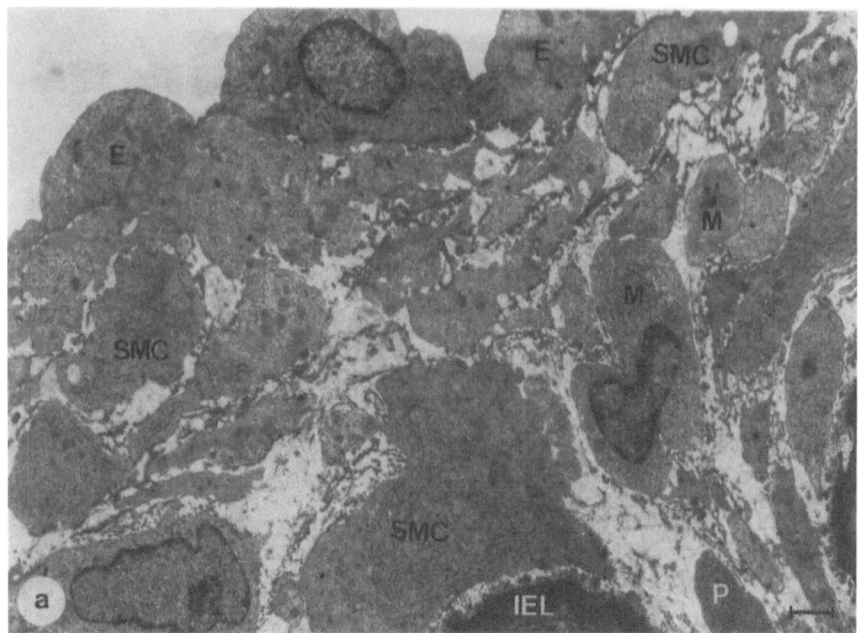

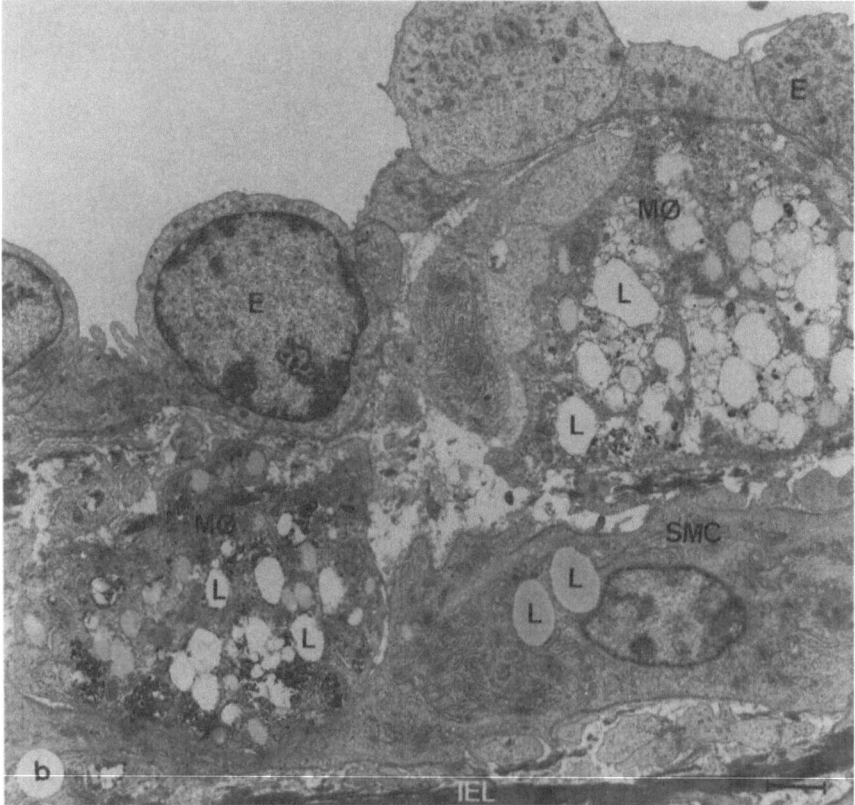

Plate II: Portions of 3-day-old intimal thickenings elicited by electrical stimulation under normocholesterolemic (a) and hypercholesterolemic (b) conditions. Intact endothelial linings cover the lesions consisting of smooth muscle cells (SMC), mononuclear cells (M) and single plasma cells (P). Note lipid vacuoles (L) within macrophages (Mφ; precursors of foam cells) and within smooth muscle cells under hypercholesterolemia. Bars indicate 2 μm.

cytes/macrophages may be trapped within the lipid-containing plaque by oxidatively modified LDL, as proposed by Steinberg and colleagues [26]. Another or even additional possibility is that mononuclear cells continue to invade the artery wall under hypercholesterolemia. The appearance of the endothelial surfaces of the 28-day-old plaques demonstrated that the fibromuscular plaque was covered by a normal-looking endothelium where no or only a few leukocytes were present. In contrast, a large number of mononuclear cells, often containing lipid vacuoles, were associated with the endothelium overlying the lipid-containing plaque. Although it is difficult to decide whether these cells are entering or leaving the artery wall, the findings indicate an increased turnover of leukocytes at the interface blood-vessel wall under prolonged hypercholesterolemia.

Summarizing Remarks I

Initially the sequence of events leading either to fibromuscular plaques (elicited by ES under normocholesterolemia) or to lipid-containing plaques (ES under hypercholesterolemia) was very similar. Under both conditions, enhanced endothelial permeability appeared in conjunction with massive accumulation of granulocytes and mononuclear cells in the arterial intima and was followed by migration and proliferation of SMC, all of which are processes indicating the inflammatory nature of the arteriosclerotic disease.

With prolonged exposure to electrical stimulation and to the different diets the lesions became progressively dissimilar, at least with respect to leukocyte involvement. Thus, under normocholesterolemia after the initial massive invasion of leukocytes, a steady decline in the relative contribution of these cells to the forming fibromuscular plaque was observed. Intimal granulocytes disappeared completely and mononuclear cells finally constituted only a minimal proportion of the intimal cell population. With sustained exposure to electrical stimulation the endothelium regained normal appearance without any adhering mononuclear cells or only a few, a finding which may be interpreted as some kind of adaptation to the applied stimulus. Under hypercholesterolemia, leukocyte involvement was modified in various ways: (1) Intimal mononuclear phagocytes exhibited specific ultrastructural features indicating functions in lipid clearance as well as an accessory role in lipid deposition in SMC. (2) The decline in the contribution of mononuclear cells to the generating plaque was slowed down compared to normocholesterolemia, and they constituted one fifth of the cell population after four weeks. (3) After a protracted period of hypercholesterolemia a large pool of mononuclear cells was associated with the endothelium overlying the atherosclerotic plaque, in contrast to normocholesterolemic conditions.

II. Functional releationship between leukocyte invasion and smooth muscle cell migration

The described temporal sequence of the initial events in the development of electrically induced arteriosclerotic plaques with a massive leukocyte invasion followed by myocyte migration suggests that at least one of the various types of invading leukocytes may promote SMC migration. Especially monocytes/macrophages may be potential promotors since they have been shown to secrete chemotactic and mitogenic substances for SMC [7, 8, 23]. Our aim was to block the extravasation of leukocytes by using the monoclonal antibody mAb 60.3 and to examine the subsequent effect on myocyte migration in the model of transmural electrical stimulation. MAb 60.3 recognizes the membrane glycoprotein CD18 which is involved – in addition to a wide range of other functions – in mediating leukocyte adhesiveness [28, 11]. Numerous in vitro and in vivo studies demonstrated that mouse anti-human mAb 60.3, which cross-reacts with leukocytes from other species, particularly inhibits the binding of neutrophils and monocytes to the endothelium, although to various degrees [reviewed in references 3, 19, 20].

Methods

Normocholesterolemic rabbits (1.6–1.8 kg; n = 3) were exposed to two sessions of electrical stimulation (30 and 15 min per 24 h) and received 3 intravenous mAb injections at a dose of 2 mg/kg at intervals of 12 h. The first dose of mAb was injected during implantation of the electrodes, the second and third approx. two hours before the respective period of electrical stimulation. Immediately before mAb administration blood samples were drawn from an ear vein and analyzed with respect to leukocyte counts and the percentage of different blood cell types. The controls (n = 3) were submitted to the same schedule with corresponding injections of sterile saline. At the end of the experimental period the stimulated carotid arteries of the mAb-treated rabbits and the controls were prepared for transmission electron microscopy, and the composition of the intimal cell population was analyzed. Especially the ratio of the number of intimal cells to the overlying endothelial cells was determined for the different cell types. Note: Rabbit carotid arteries are particularly suitable for migration studies since their subendothelial space is normally void of cells.

Results

The data obtained from the quantitative analysis of the intimal cell populations of the stimulated arteries are summarized in Table 2. In the mAb-treated rabbits, no polymorphonuclear neutrophils were found in the subendothelium after the

Table 2: Analysis of the intimal cell population. Number of intimal cells per overlying endothelial cell determined for different cell types

cell types	number of cells/endothelial cell	
	mAb-treated	controls
neutrophils	0	0.10 ± 0.01
mononuclear cells	0.05 ± 0.02	0.16 ± 0.05
smooth muscle cells	0.15 ± 0.15	0.17 ± 0.01
unident. cells	0.02 ± 0.02	0.02 ± 0.03
Σ subendothelial cells	0.22 ± 0.18	0.45 ± 0.09

applied stimulation program. In the controls, however, intimal neutrophils were present at a ratio of 0.10 ± 0.01, i.e., an average of 10 granulocytes per 100 EC. Regarding mononuclear cells, both monocytes and lymphocytes occurred within the intima of the stimulated rabbits despite administration of mAb. However, their number was clearly reduced compared to the controls. But even an increase in the antibody dose to 3 mg/kg b.wt. was not effective in preventing emigration of monocytes and lymphocytes in this model. The search for SMC within the intima showed that they were present at a very similar ratio in both the mAb-treated animals and the controls.

The findings of complete inhibition of neutrophil emigration and reduced accumulation of mononuclear cells in the intima of the stimulated arteries due to mAb-administration coincide with an increase in the number of peripheral white blood cells to a maximal 4-fold of the baseline during a 36-h period of treatment with mAb 60.3. The white blood picture thereby revealed raised percentages of neutrophils at 12 and 24 hours after the first mAb injection. In addition to neutrophils with nuclei undergoing pyknosis, band or juvenile forms were also observed in the mAb-treated rabbits. In the controls the white blood cell counts increased only up to 1.6 times the baseline and returned to "starting" levels 36 hours after the first saline injection.

Summarizing Remarks II

To test whether leukocyte invasion and SMC migration in the arterial intima are dependent or independent processes in the pathogenesis of arteriosclerosis, we examined the effect of inhibiting leukocyte invasion with mAb 60.3 on the potential of SMC to migrate into the intima in the model of transmural electrical stimulation. The preliminary experiments demonstrated:

(1) Neutrophil migration into the electrically stimulated artery wall is completely abolished by mAb 60.3, suggesting that this process is primarily CD18-dependent.

Additionally, the intimal presence of neutrophils is not necessary to trigger SMC migration, since medial SMC migrated into the intima despite totally blocked neutrophil invasion.

(2) The invasion of mononuclear cells into the stimulated arteries was only partially inhibited by administration of mAb 60.3. This may, for instance, reflect a significant CD18-independent mechanism of emigration of mononuclear cells in this model, indicating that other adhesion molecules which are not recognized by mAb 60.3 are possibly involved. The fact that despite the reduced accumulation of mononuclear cells SMC occurred within the intima leaves the question open as to what role mononuclear cells play in SMC migration. On the one hand, the results allow the interpretation that mononuclear cells are not important for regulating SMC migration. On the other hand, it is also conceivable that even the diminished number of immigrated mononuclear cells provide sufficient amounts of chemoattractants for SMC. To assess the contribution of mononuclear cells to SMC migration and, moreover, to their proliferation, additional experiments are necessary.

Acknowledgement

We thank Marianne Beck for her excellent and skilled technical assistance.

References

[1] Betz, E., Schlote, W.: Responses of vessel walls to chronically applied electrical stimuli. Basic. Res. Cardiol. 1979; 74: 10–20.
[2] Brown, M.S., Goldstein, J.L.: Lipoprotein metabolism in the macrophage: Implications for cholesterol deposition in atherosclerosis. Ann. Review. Biochem. 1983; 52: 223–261.
[3] Carlos, T.M., Harlan, J.M.: Membrane proteins involved in phagocyte adherence to endothelium. Immunol. Rev. 1990; 114: 5–28.
[4] Faggiotto, A., Ross, R., Harker, E.: Studies of hypercholesterolemia in the nonhuman primate. I. Changes that lead to fatty streak formation. Arterioslcerosis 1984; 4: 323–340.
[5] Faggiotto, A., Ross, R.: Studies of hypercholesterolemia in the nonhuman primate. II. Fatty streak conversion to fibrous plaque. Arteriosclerosis 1984; 4: 341–356.
[6] Gerrity, R.G.: The role of the monocyte in atherogenesis. I. Transition of blood-borne monocytes into foam cells in fatty lesions. Am. J. Pathol. 1981; 103: 181–190.
[7] Glenn, K.C., Ross, R.: Human monocyte-derived growth factor(s) for mesenchymal cells: activation of secretion by endotoxin and concanavalin A. Cell 1981; 25: 603–615.
[8] Grotendorst, G.R., Seppa, H.E., Kleinmann, H.K., Martin, G.R.: Attachment of smooth muscle cells to collagen and their migration toward platelet-derived growth factor. Proc. Natl. Acad. Sci. USA 1981; 78: 3669–3672.
[9] Hansson, G.K., Jonasson, L., Holm, J., Clowes, M.M., Clowes, A.W.: Gamma-interferon regulates vascular smooth muscle proliferation and Ia Antigen expression in vivo and in vitro. Circ. Res. 1988; 63: 712–719.
[10] Hansson, G.K., Holm, J., Jonasson, L.: Detection of activated T-lymphocytes in the human atherosclerotic plaque. Am. J. Pathol. 1989; 135: 169–175.

[11] Harlan, J.M., Schwartz, B.R., Wallis, W.J., Pohlmann, T.H.: The role of neutrophil membrane proteins in neutrophil emigration. In: Movat HZ, ed. Leukocyte Emigration and its sequelae. Basel: Karger Press, 1987: 97–104.

[12] Heinle, H., Tarczy, M., Schmid, G., Betz, E.: Morphological and functional alterations in the arterial wall after local electrical stimulation. Biblthca. anat. 1981; 20: 79–82.

[13] Haudenschild, C.C., Prescott, M.F., Chobanian, A.V.: Aortic endothelial and subendothelial cells in experimental hypertension and aging. Hypertension 1981; 3 (suppl. I): 148–153.

[14] Jonasson, L., Holm, J., Skalli, O., Bondjers, G., Hansson, G.K.: Regional accumulations of T cells, macrophages, and smooth muscle cells in the human atherosclerotic plaque. Arteriosclerosis 1986; 6: 131–138.

[15] Joris, J., Zand, T., Nunnari, J.J., Krolikowski, F.J., Majno, G.: Studies on the pathogenesis of atherosclerosis. I. Adhesion and emigration of mononuclear cells in the aorta of hypercholesterolemic rats. Am. J. Pathol. 1983; 113: 341–358.

[16] Kling, D., Holzschuh, T., Betz, E.: Temporal sequence of morphological alterations in artery walls during experimental atherogenesis – occurrence of leukocytes. Res. Exp. Med. 1987; 187: 237–250.

[17] Kling, D., Holzschuh, T., Strohschneider, T., Betz, E.: Enhanced endothelial permeability and invasion of leukocytes into the artery wall as initial events in experimental arteriosclerosis. Inter. Angio. 1987; 6: 21–28.

[18] Kling, D., Holzschuh, T., Betz, E.: Dynamik der Gefäßwandveränderungen bei der Pathogenese der Arteriosklerose. VASA 1988; Suppl. 23: 11–14.

[19] Kuypers, T.W., Roos, D.: Leukocyte membrane adhesion proteins LFA-1, CR3 and p150,95: a review of functional and regulatory aspects. Res. Immunol. 1989; 140: 461–486.

[20] Patarroyo, M., Prieto, J., Rincon, J., Timonen, T., Lundberg, C., Lindbom, L., Asjö, B., Gahmberg, C.G.: Leukocyte cell adhesion: a molecular process fundamental in leukocyte physiology. Immunol. Rev. 1990; 114: 67–109.

[21] Prescott, M.F., Karboski, McBride, C., Court, M.: Development of intimal lesions after leukocyte migration into the vascular wall. Am. J. Pathol. 1989; 135: 835–846.

[22] Rennick, R.E., Campbell, J.H., Campbell, G.R.: Vascular smooth muscle phenotype and growth behavior can be influenced by macrophages in vitro. Atherosclerosis 1988; 71: 35–43.

[23] Ross, R., Masuda, J., Raines, E.W., Gown, A.M., Katsuda, S., Sasahara, M., Malden, L.T., Masuko, H., Sato, H.: Localization of PDGF-B protein in macrophages in all phases of atherogenesis. Science 1990; 248: 1009–1012.

[24] Schwartz, C.J., Sprague, E.A., Kelly, J.L., Valente, A.J., Suenram, C.A.: Aortic intimal monocyte recruitment in the normo and hypercholesterolemic baboon (Papio cynocephalus). An ultrastructural study: Implications in atherogenesis. Virchows Arch. [Pathol. Anat.] 1985; 405: 175–191.

[25] Stary, H.C.: The sequence of cell and matrix changes in atherosclerotic lesions of coronary arteries in the first forty years of life. Eur. Heart. J. 1990; 11 (suppl. E): 3–19.

[26] Steinberg, D., Parthasarathy, S., Carew, T.E., Khoo, J.C., Witztum, J.L.: Beyond cholesterol: Modifications of low density lipoprotein that increase its atherogenicity. New Engl. Med. 1989; 320: 915–924.

[27] Trillo, A.A.: The cell population of aortic fatty streaks in African green monkey with special reference to granulocytic cells. An ultrastructural study. Atherosclerosis 1982; 43: 253–275.

[28] Wallis, W.J., Hickstein, D.D., Schwartz, B.R., June, C.H., Ochs, H.D., Beatty, P.G., Klebanoff, S.J., Harlan, J.M.: Monoclonal antibody-defined functional epitopes on the adhesion-promoting glycoprotein complex (CDw18) of human neutrophils. Blood 1986; 67: 1007–1013.

[29] Watanabe, T., Tokunaga, O., Fan, J., Shimokama, T.: Atherosclerosis and Macrophages. Acta Pathol. Jap. 1989; 39: 473–486.

The Value of Co-Culture Systems in Arteriosclerosis Research

E. Betz

Physiologisches Institut (I), Universität Tübingen

Cultures of EC, SMC and fibroblasts from animal or human arteries have become a tool in atherosclerosis research. Basic problems and therapeutic aspects of growth of cells obtained from normal or atheromatous arteries have been studied in many details. Mass cultures or clone cultures of single cell species are, however, very artificial systems. In these cultures the cells may behave differently than in their normal environment so that efforts have been made to construct cell culture systems that imitate in a better way the conditions which prevail in the walls of arteries and which additionally permit to produce in vitro intimal proliferates or even atheromas. I will present three systems to demonstrate the possiblities which these systems offer.

1. Transfilter culture
2. Transfilter co-culture
3. Sandwich culture.

1. Transfilter culture

For a transfilter culture a Petri dish in which a ring of silicone is cast is provided with a ring shaped frame made of polycarbonate. The ring is used as a frame for a collagen coated polycarbonate filter with pores of a diameter of 5 μm. The filter fits into the silicone ring in such a way that the fluid spaces above the filter and below the filter can be exchanged spearately. For the study of the behaviour of SMC on a filter which serves as an artificial pored lamina interna (however it is not elastic) pieces of media from an artery were placed as explants on the surface of the filter. The explants were obtained by removing the endothelial lining and the adventitia from a longitudinally dissected artery and then cutting the obtained artery media into pieces of 15–20 mm^2. (For technical details see Weber et al. 1986 and Fallier-Becker et al. 1990). It could be seen that the SMC migrate through the pores and formed a multilayer on the other filter side. Plate I a) shows such a typical proliferate after a culturing time of 8 days. If the pores are smaller than 1 μm in diameter the cells can not migrate.

The mitotic rate of SMC can be shown by immunohistolocial staining of the cell nuclei with 5-Bromo-2 -desoxy-Uridine (BrdU). This substance was used as a thymidine analogue. It is incorporated in the DNA of dividing cells in their S-phase. BrdU (30 μM) was added to the culture medium together with 30 mM

PROLIFERATIVE INDEX

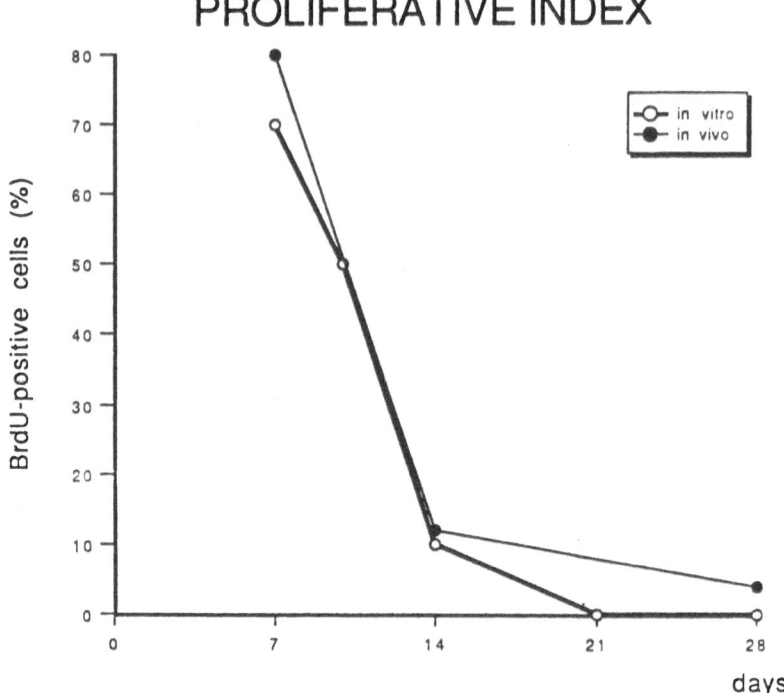

Figure 1: Comparision of mitotic rates in cultures of SMC with mitotic rates in rat carotid arteries after ballooning. -o- transfilterculture "in vitro" incubation time (days); -•- balloon catheter injury "in vivo" (days after injury).

deoxy-Cytidine 18 h prior to fixation of the culture and can be detected by a monoclonal antibody from mouse against BrdU. The second antibody is fluo-rescein conjugated goat anti mouse. Transfilter multilayers contain a great number of dividing cells. The development of the proliferate and the mitotic rate within the proliferate decrease after having reached a maximum after the 5. day in cul-ture. The development of proliferation is nearly identical with that seen in bal-looned arteries of in vivo-experiments. Fig. 1 shows the mitotic rates in transfilter cultures compared with the mitotic rates in rat carotid arteries after ballooning of the artery. This demostrates that the transfilter culture imitates the response of the SMC after balloon angioplasty.

2. Transfilter co-cultures

If on one side of the filter EC were seeded in a sufficient density these cells form a confluent layer within a few days. After turning the filter with its frame

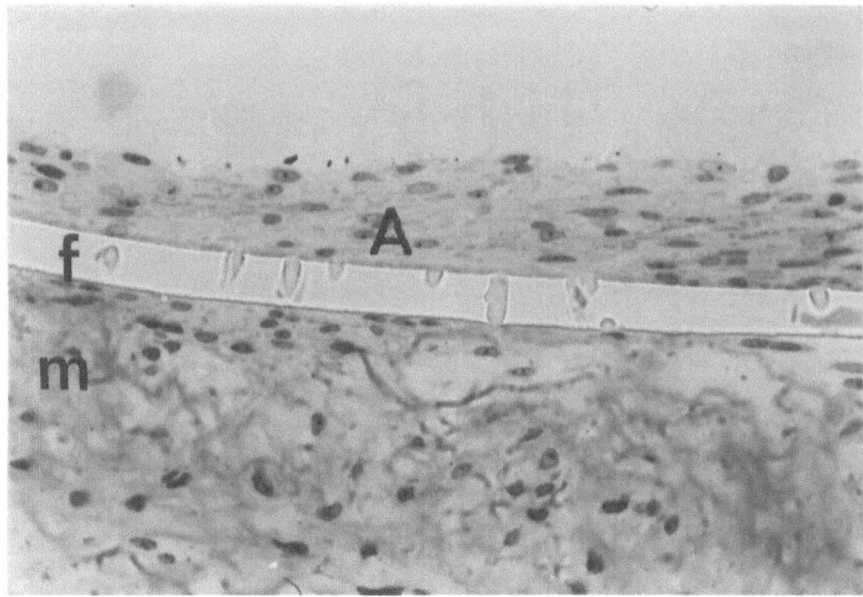

Plate Ia): Semithin section of a transfilter culture after 14 days' incubation time. The proliferate (A) consists of ca. 8–10 SMC layers. f = filter, m = media explant. X 440.

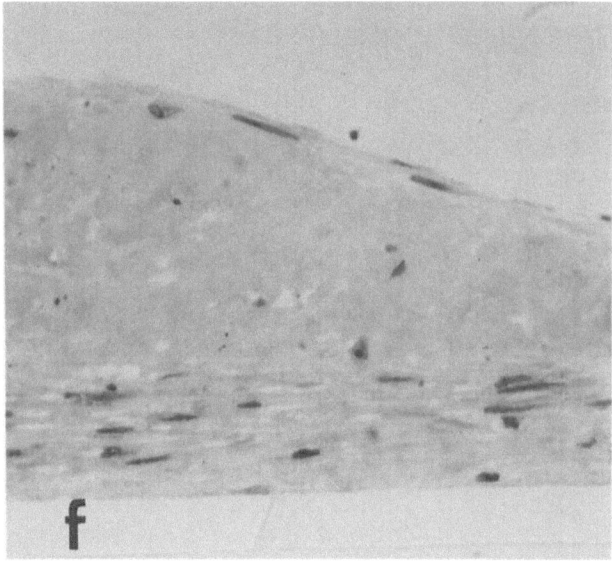

Plate I b): Atheromatous proliferate on a filter (f) 4 weeks after addition of oxidized LDL and monocytes to the culture medium. (From K. Wolburg-Buchholz, P. Fallier-Becker, D.R. Roth, E. Betz: Int. Soc. Appl. Cardiovasc. Biol., II, in press 1991.)

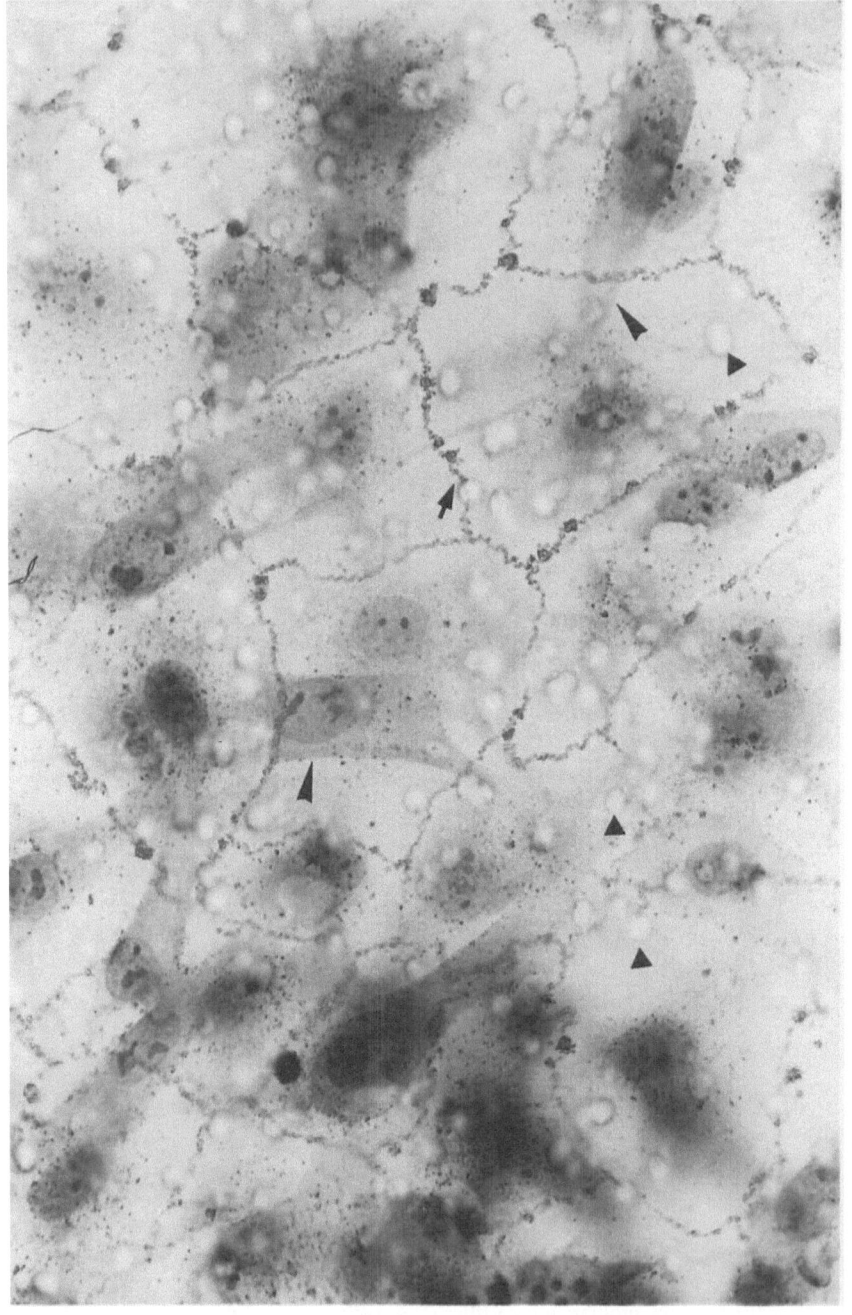

Plate II: Porcine aortic endothelial cells (EC) en face. EC were stained with silver nitrate. The cells are grown on a filter showing the cell borders (arrow). Few SMC (arrow heads) can be seen underneath the EC monolayer. Three filter pores are marked with triangles. X 985.

upside down the endothelial cells remain in the medium below the filter. Media explants are then laid on the upper side of the filter and the system then imitates the two cell species at both sides of the internal elastic lamina in vivo. It could be seen that in contrast to the transfilter cultures without EC the SMC in the co-cultures did not form a multilayer beneath the endothelium on the other side of the filter. Plate II shows the transfilter co-culture 14 days after placing the explant on the filter. There are only few SMC beneath the confluent EC. The contact zones between the confluent EC are stained with silver nitrate. EC form tight junctions, they contain Weibel-Palade-bodies and factor VIII related antigen.

In transfilter co-cultures the confluent endothelial cells do not completely inhibit proliferation of cells below the filter within the media explant. However, the number of dividing cells is somewhat lower and the cells are inhibited to migrate through the filter. This observation has led us to the conclusion that EC inhibit mainly the migratory activity of SMC. In order to prove that the dividing cells are SMC the proliferates were labelled with a monoclonal antibody against SM-α-actin and it was found that in transfilter co-cultures as well as in transfilter cultures without EC within the first days after placing the explant on the filter no or only very few cells of the proliferate contained this cell marker for SMC. However, after 3 weeks of incubation the cells re-expressed SM-α-actin.

3. Sandwich cultures

In vivo the formation of atheromas or fibromuscular proliferates always occurs in the intima. There is no plaque formation near the adventitia of an artery. In order to find out whether the SMC situated in the neighbourhood of the adventitia possess a different proliferative capacity or whether the adventitial tissue influences the mitotic activity of the media we modified the transfilter culture into a so called sandwich culture.

Figure 2 shows the principle. Explants of media tissue are laid between two filters, the endothelial side directed to the upper filter and the adventital side directed to the other filter. The system now forms a sandwich-like arrangement. Fourteen days after the media explants had been laid between the filters the DNA content of the two proliferates which had been formed on the outside of the filters were measured. The DNA content of the proliferate at the endothelial side was 135 ± 10 ng/explant. DNA at the adventitial side of the media explant amounted 139.5 ± 12 ng/explant. There is no significant difference between the DNA contents of both sides. This result demonstrates that the migratory capacity of the adventitial and of the endothelial side of the media is identical in this preparation.

The transfilter cultures and sandwich cultures are simple methods for testing drug effects on migration and on proliferation and on the combination of migration and proliferation of SMC from the media into the intima and to the side

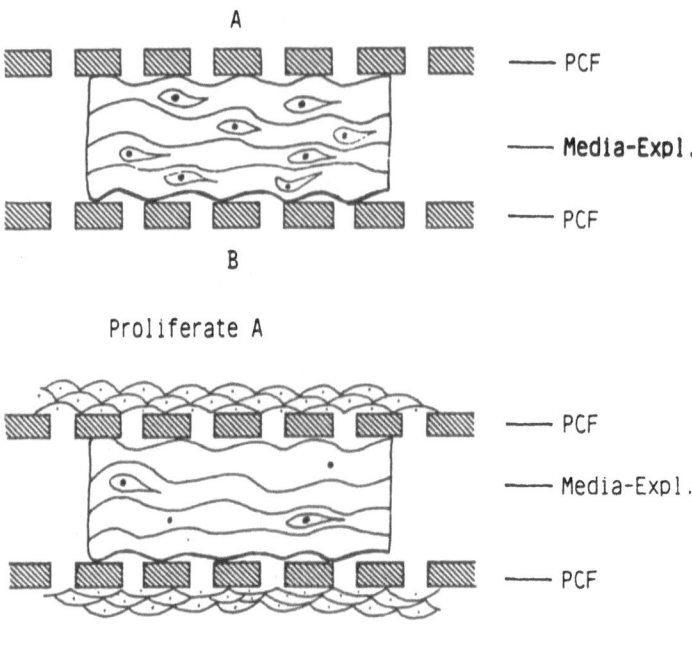

Figure 2: Schematic diagram of a sandwich filter culture. Media explants are placed between two filters having a pore size of 5 μm. Upper figure immediately after explantation, lower figure after 14 days in culture. PCF = polycarbonate filter.

where the adventitia had been. The quantitation of drug actions is possible by a measurement of the DNA content of the proliferate. The method of DNA analysis of cell cultures is based on the technique described by Labarca and Paigen (1980). The amount of DNA is a direct measure of the number of cell nuclei. Figure 3 shows the effect of increasing concentrations of heparin. The drug inhibits in a dose dependent manner the proliferation in the transfilter- and sandwich cultures. Rats in which the carotid artery was ballooned with a F_2-Fogarty catheter received daily a subcutaneous injection of heparin and we found that in comparison to control-animals which received no drugs but in which the carotid artery was ballooned the proliferation is dose dependently suppressed in a similar way as in the transfilter culture.

The sandwich technique enables also to study the effect of adventitial tissue on proliferation and migration of SMC. One of the problems with this technique

ng DNA of the
proliferate/mg tissue

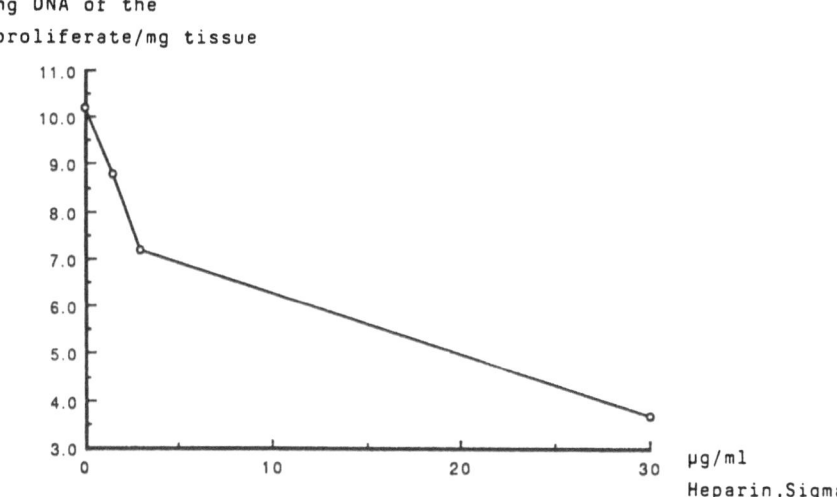

Figure 3: Effect of decreasing concentrations of heparin on migration and proliferation of SMC through the filter pores. Concentration depedent inhibition of SMC proliferation.

concerns the differentiation between fibroblasts of the adventita and SMC of the media. The SMC loose their marker proteins (SM-myosin and α-actin) when they proliferate and regain the ability for the expression of α-actin slowly 14 to 28 days after proliferation through the pores. We therefore used a sandwich filter arrangement in which the filterpores at the endothelial surface of the explant had diameters of 5 μm whereas the pores directed to the adventitial side measured only 0.2 μm. Cells cannot migrate through these narrow pores but fluids can exchange between the compartments on either side of the filter with narrow pores. However, the second filter at the other side allows the passage of the cells if the endothelium is destroyed. The adventitia on the outside of the filter inhibits the migration of SMC through the wide pores of the other filter if it is not covered with EC.

The adventitia has an additional effect on the preservation of α-actin within the media neighboured to the transfilter-adventitial tissue. SM-α-actin is conserved in the cells of the media explant near the adventitia but not at the other side. If endothelium is present as a confluent layer on the other side of the sandwich there occurs no migration through the filter.

With these preparations we have intented to build up a system which allows to study basic mechanisms of atherogenesis not only in vessels of animals but also in imitates of human arteries. The system allows moreover the study of the progression of atheromatous proliferates.

When we added monocytes and oxidized LDL to a transfilter proliferate in culture we observed an immigration of monocytes into the proliferate. 14 days after incubation of the cultures with lipoprotein and monocytes the proliferate contains lipids partially in the fibromuscular proliferates. The similarity of some parts of the proliferate with fresh atheromas was striking (Plate I b). We have not yet been very successful in transforming a fibromuscular transfilter proliferate in such an atheromatous tissue only by addition of lipoproteins without monocytes. However, these studies are ongoing.

References

[1] Fallier-Becker, P., Rupp, J., Fingerle, J., Betz, E.: Smooth Muscle Cells from Rabbit Aorta. In: Cell Culture Techniques in Heart and Vessel Research, ed. by H.M. Piper, Springer-Verlag Berlin, Heidelberg 1990, 247–270.
[2] Labarca, C., Paigen, K.: A Simple, Rapid and Sensitive DNA Assay Procedure. Ann. Biochem. 1980. *102*, 344–352.
[3] Weber, E., Hämmerle, H., Vatti, R., Berti, G., Betz, E.: Co-Cultivation of Endothelial and Smooth Muscle Cells on Opposite Sides of a Porous Membrane. Appl. Pathol. 1986, *4*, 246–252.

11

Local Hormones and the Atherogenic Uptake
of Low Density Lipoprotein in vivo

G.V.R. Born
The William Harvey Research Institute,
St. Bartholomew's Hospital Medical College,
London

Summary

Atherosclerotic disease begins with the accumulation of atherogenic plasma proteins, predominantly low-density lipoprotein (LDL), in the walls of susceptible arteries. One determinant of this accumulation is the LDL concentration in the blood. We are investigating other factors which may influence the uptake of LDL and of fibrinogen, another atherogenic plasma protein, by artery walls from the circulating blood; the mechanism(s) of this uptake; and the rate and magnitude of the accumulation of the atherogenic plasma components in arteries. In order to model human atherogenesis as closely as possible, the experiments are *in vivo* using rabbits in which the initial stages of atherogenesis appear to be similar to those in man.

Up to the present the principal new observations are as follows:

(1) In anaesthetized rabbits, the rate of uptake of LDL related to lumenal surface area is similar in large arteries and large veins, whereas the progressive accumulation of LDL is significantly greater in the arteries than in the veins. This suggests that the accumulation of LDL in arteries but not in veins depends less on haemodynamic than on other differences.

(2) Selective desialation of the endothelial surface of arteries *in vivo* greatly accelerates their LDL uptake. This suggests that the rate of accumulation of LDL may be limited by, *inter alia*, the exceptionally high densities of sialic acids which we had previously demonstrated on the lumenal surface of arteries and veins in several species including man (umbilical vein).

(3) In conscious, restrained rabbits, intravenous infusions of histamine sufficient to produce inter-endothelial gaps throughout the venular systems did not increase the rate constant of the disappearance of LDL from the circulating blood. This makes it improbable that significant quantities of LDL pass out of the blood into vessel walls between endothelial cells and indirectly supports the evidence that LDL leaves the plasma by transcytosis through the endothelial cells.

(4) More recently we discovered that in anaesthetized rabbits the rate of uptake of LDL, methylated to prevent its removal by high-affinity receptors (m-LDL), is significantly increased by noradrenaline and by adrenaline within their physiological concentration ranges in the blood. This appears to be the first direct demonstration of a potentially atherogenic effect of the catecholamines *in vivo* and at physiologically relevant concentrations.

The atherogenic uptake of low-density lipoprotein

Atherosclerosis begins with the accumulation of fatty material, predominantly low-density lipoprotein (LDL), in the walls of arteries susceptible to the disease; the LDL comes from the circulating blood. The mechanism(s) responsible for the accumulation and for its non-uniform distribution are still by no means adequately understood. Specifically, little is known of what determines the rate of atherogenesis, which is very different in different individuals. The only certain determinant is the LDL concentration in the blood plasma because in congenital hyperlipidaemias the disease progresses rapidly and tends to manifest its clinical effects, most commonly angina pectoris and myocardial infarction, at an early age (Goldstein & Brown, 1977; Brown & Goldstein, 1985).

Evidence obtained with several species of experimental animals has shown that LDL enters arterial walls by a mechanism which does not involve the high-affinity LDL receptor, as the uptake of reductively methylated LDL (m-LDL) which does not bind to the LDL receptor (Mahley et al., 1979) is similar to that of native LDL (Wiklund, Carew & Steinberg, 1985). Apparently LDL passes through arterial endothelium by diffusional access limited endo- and transcytosis via plasmalemmal vesicles (Vasile et al., 1983; Simionescu et al., 1986) identical with the pinosomes in which these lipoproteins were observed earlier by autoradiography (Stein and Stein, 1973). Such LDL uptake, which has also been demonstrated with cultured endothelial cells, depends strongly on LDL concentrations (van Hinsbergh, 1984), in agreement with the clinical conclusion (Brown & Goldstein, 1985).

We initiated experiments to find out whether factors other than the blood concentration of LDL affect its uptake and accumulation *in vivo*, as follows:

(1) by comparing uptakes by large arteries and large veins in the same animal;

(2) by modifying the blood/arterial wall interface;

(3) by looking for effects of endogenous and exogenous pharmacological agents.

Each of these approaches has begun to provide new knowledge about the atherogenic process.

Comparisons of large arteries and large veins

The lipid lesions of atherosclerosis occur in arteries but not in veins except when under arterial blood flow conditions. The reasons for this selectivity are not known but could, rather obviously, have to do with differences in haemodynamics; in LDL uptake and degradation; and in vessel structure and properties.

We could find no previous work on this, so we made a beginning by comparing the rates of uptake and degradation of LDL in arteries and veins of rabbits *in vivo* (Shafi, Palinski & Born, 1987). Human and rabbit LDL were isolated by sequential ultracentrifugation (Havel, Eder & Bragdon, 1955). Homologous LDL was labelled with ^{125}I, heterologous LDL was doubly labelled with ^{131}I using iodine monochloride and with [^{125}I] tyramine cellobiose (Pittman, Carew, Glass, Green, Taylor & Attie, 1983) which remains trapped intracellularly. Rabbits were injected with such LDL preparations of high specific activity and after increasing times up to 24 h they were killed with pentobarbital. The systemic circulation was perfused at a pressure of 90 mm Hg via a cannula in the carotid artery and an outlet in the posterior vena cava for 15 min with phosphate-buffered saline to wash out the blood, followed by 2.5% gluteraldehyde for *in situ* fixation. Segments of carotid arteries, jugular veins, aortae, venae cavae and renal arteries and veins were excised and their surface areas, dry weights and radioactivities were measured.

When the uptake of LDL by all arteries was compared with that by all veins on the basis of lumenal surface area, there was no significant difference at any time up to 3.5 h. When the degradation rate of doubly labelled LDL was compared after 24 h on the basis of surface area, there were significant differences between arteries and veins, with all arteries containing about twice as much radioactivities as all veins. When the comparison was based on dry weights of the tissues the differences were not significant. The results suggest that the preferential accumulation of LDL in arteries compared with the veins is due more to the greater thickness and therefore of greater degradation of LDL in arteries than to differences in the rates of uptake.

Modification of the blood/arterial wall interface

From the binding of catonic proteins labelled with colloidal iron or ferritin it has been concluded that the lumenal surface of arterial endothelium has exposed anionic sites (Skutelsky, Rudich & Danon, 1975). Earlier experiments of ours indicated that the endothelial surface of large arteries and veins in several mamma-

lian species, including rabbit and man, actually have exceptionally high negative
charge densities, i.e. from one to two orders of magnitude higher than the surfaces
of other cells such as erythrocytes and lymphocytes; and that these anionic sites,
being removable by neuraminidase, are due to sialic acids (Görög, Schraufstätter
& Born, 1982; Born & Palinski, 1985).

We then showed that the enzymic removal of sialic acids from carotid arteries
in anaesthetized rabbits greatly accelerates the uptake of LDL by the arterial
walls, and somewhat less that of fibrinogen, but not the uptake of plasma albumin
which, unlike LDL and fibrinogen, is not a sialoprotein (Görög & Born, 1982).
Similar results have since been obtained *in vitro* with cultured endothelium (Görög & Pearson, 1984). These observations suggested that the accelerated uptake of
LDL through desialated endothelium is due to diminution of its electrostatic
repulsion towards LDL and fibrinogen which, at physiological pH, are also negatively charged. It appeared, therefore, that one of the factors, possibly a major
one, controlling the rate of accumulation of LDL in artery walls is the net negative charge on their interface with the blood. Somewhat similar conclusions have
been arrived at by the Simionescus who, like ourselves (Görög & Born, 1983),
also demonstrated that arterial sialic acids are distributed non-uniformly, with
lower densities over those areas where lipid accumulations begin (Simionescu and
Simionescu, 1985).

We therefore began to test the hypothesis, *ex vivo* and *in vivo*, that net endothelial surface charge is a determinant of atherogenic LDL uptake by measuring
it under conditions which could also be expected to alter the surface charge. Thus,
there is evidence that vascular endothelium synthesises heparan sulphate which
appears on the surface of the cells (see Rosenberg, Reilly & Fritze, 1985). As
heparan sulphate is highly anionic, it may make a considerable contribution to the
negative charge on arterial endothelium and thereby influence the uptake of the
atherogenic plasma proteins. A possible test of our hypothesis would, therefore,
be to determine the effect on the uptake of m-LDL of the removal of endothelial
heparan sulphate by a specific enzyme *in vivo*. This test would clearly depend in
the first instance on the ability of such an enzyme to reach and act on the heparan
sulphate in living vessels. We have begun to work on this on the strength of elegant
evidence (Marcum, KcKenney, Galli, Jackman and Rosenberg, 1986) that the enzyme heparinase (purified from *flavobacterium*) indeed acts on heparan sulphate
inside living blood vessels. In these experiments, the rapid inactivation of thrombin by antithrombin which occurred when perfused together through the vasculature of the mouse hind-limb was abolished by a preceding perfusion with heparinase, indicating the ability of this enzyme to inactivate heparan sulphate on the
lumenal surfaces.

We have begun our experiments using this enzyme kindly supplied by Prof.
Rosenberg in a newly developed *ex vivo* technique which allows several determinations per animal (instead of our *in vivo* method which allows only one; see
below and Görög and Born, 1982). In this technique, the thoracic aorta from

freshly-killed rabbits is opened longitudinally, washed free of blood, and small, open-ended cylinders, usually eight, are placed on the endothelial surface (away from branch arteries). Some cylinders are filled with heparinase in appropriate medium, others with medium only. After maintaining the preparation at 37° for 30 min, the cylinders are washed out and filled with radiolabelled m-LDL and the preparation is again maintained at 37° for 4 hours. Then the aortic wall beneath each cylinder is cut out, its radioactivity determined and expressed on the basis of exposed endothelial surface area. Initial results with this technique do suggest that exposure to heparinase increases the uptake of m-LDL by the aorta. These results have to be confirmed and extended to different conditions, other enzymes and so on.

Effects of endogenous and exogenous pharmacological agents

There is very little knowledge as to whether and, if so, how endogenous agents such as the catecholamines influence atherogenesis. Such evidence as there is was summarised in an earlier publication of this Academy (see Born 1989).

Increased uptake of methylated low-density lipoprotein induced by
noradrenaline and adrenaline in rabbit carotid arteries

Specifically, it appeared to be unknown whether catecholamines or, indeed, other endogenous mediators influence the removal of LDL from the blood or the accumulation of LDL in arterial walls. In the last three years we have begun to investigate this question, with promising results some of which have been published (Shafi, Cusack and Born, 1989; Born, Shafi and Cusack, 1989).

We have discovered that in anaesthetized rabbits the atherogenic uptake of LDL by arterial walls is accelerated by noradrenaline and by adrenaline at their physiological concentrations in rabbit and human blood. The principle of the experiments was to compare the uptake of intravenously injected, radioactively labelled LDL, methylated to prevent removal by high-affinity receptors, in the two carotid arteries of anaesthetized rabbits after infusing low concentrations of noradrenaline or of adrenaline into one carotid and saline as control into the other, the volume rates of infusion being about 1% of the carotid blood flows. Human LDL, which behaves sufficiently like rabbit LDL for these purposes, was prepared, methylated and radio-iodinated by standard methods. At the end of the infusions, the arteries were excised and their radioactivities determined. Noradrenaline in-fused for 2 h to produce local blood concentrations of nominally 1, 10, 50 and 100 nM significantly increased the LDL radioactivities of the walls of the nor-adrenaline-infused carotids. Concentrations of nominally 100 nM also increased the LDL radioactivities of the walls of the saline-infused carotids; this was associated with significant increases in their blood noradrenaline concentrations (kindly determined by Prof. M. Brown, Department of Clinical Pharmacology in Cambridge).

Infusion of adrenaline gave similar results. They appear to contribute towards an explanation for the accelerated atherosclerosis and the increased incidence of its clinical manifestations in conditions associated with elevated blood noradrenaline concentrations, including the episodic increases associated with stress and cigarette smoking as well as the more persistent increases caused by phaeochromocytoma. Thus, there is the possibility that the slow but continuous passage of LDL into arterial walls depends, at least in part, on the noradrenaline normally present in the circulating blood (Bühler et al., 1978).

The mechanism underlying the accelerating effect of the catecholamines on m-LDL uptake remains to be established. The possibility had to be considered that it is due to their hypertensive effect which could also account for the accelerated atherogenesis associated with pheochromocytoma. The local blood pressure was not significantly increased by noradrenaline infused at nominally 1 and 10 nM and only slightly increased by 100 nM. Thus, the experiments done so far provide no clear evidence on this question, which requires separate investigation.

The catecholamine effect evidently does not involve the high-affinity receptors which, although present on vascular endothelium (Vlodavsky et al., 1978; Carew et al., 1984), do not bind or remove the methylated LDL used here. Another possible route for the movement of LDL from blood into arterial walls is through inter-endothelial junctions. However, this route has been made very unlikely by other recent experiments of ours in which the clearance of LDL from the blood increased not at all when wide inter-endothelial gaps were induced pharmacologically in a large proportion of the rabbit vasculature (Born & Shafi, 1988). This leaves as the predominant if not the only route the passage of LDL by transcytosis through endothelial cells in plasmalemmal vesicles (Stein et al., 1973; Simionescu & Simionescu, 1985). It is therefore reasonable to suggest that it is this process that is somehow accelerated by the catecholamines. As the effect is presumably receptor mediated, the possibility of antagonizing it pharmacologically may provide a new way of slowing the progress of atherosclerosis.

The accelerated LDL uptake here described is brought about by circulating catecholamines in direct and continuous contact with the arterial endothelium where it presumably mediates the effect. Therefore our findings raise the possibility that, as well as the catecholamines, other circulating mediators affect the flux of LDL and of other plasma proteins into arterial walls; these possibilities are being looked into.

Evidence against the atherogenic passage of LDL between endothelial cells

As already said, there is convincing evidence that LDl passes from the blood plasma into arterial walls predominantly *through* the cells of the endothelial layer (Stein *et al.,* 1973; Vasile *et al.,* 1983; Simionescu *et al.,* 1985). This "transcytosis" appears to involve the plasmalemmal vesicles which are characteristic of endothelium; but the actual mechanism is far from being understood. The question remained whether significant amounts of LDL are able also to pass through the junctions *between* endothelial cells. If so, it might be expected that such a passage would become demonstrable *in vivo* as increases in the blood clearances rates of LDL, again methylated to prevent clearance by the high affinity receptors (particularly in the liver), under conditions in which the junctions become widely separated to form inter-endothelial gaps throughout a major part of the circulation, i.e. throughout the venular systems. This can be achieved by various pharmacological agents, e.g. by histamine (Majno, G., Shea, M.S. Leventhal, M., 1969).

We have tested this idea as follows: Unanaesthetized restrained rabbits were injected with human LDL (which for these experiments oculd be considered sufficiently similar to rabbit LDL), methylated and labelled with radio-iodine. By measuring the radioactivity of blood samples taken at frequent intervals over periods of several hours and calculating lines of best fit, rate constants of the *apparent* clearance of m-LDL can be determined with remarkable accuracy, so that even small changes in such rates become evident. Blood samples were taken from a catheter in the central artery of one ear for determinations of radioactivity and haematocrit every 20 min during successive 3 hour periods of infusion (at a rate of 0.05 ml/min) into the marginal vein of the other ear; first of saline, then of histamine (12.5 ug/kg.min) and finally again of saline. The histamine concentrations were chosen to have no significant effect on the heart rate or blood pressure while producing in the venules wide inter-endothelial gaps which were demonstrable morphologically. During histamine infusions the apparent LDL clearance rates, instead of increasing, actually *decreased*. At the same time the histamine infusions also produced the well-established increases in the haematocrit, due to loss of plasma water through the gaps with associated haemoconcentration. This haemoconcentration accounted accurately for the apparent decrease in the rate constant, so that the m-LDL concentration in the plasma increased to exactly the same extent as the red cell concentration. Unless the structure of the intimal tissues underlying the endothelium is very different in veins and arteries, our results make it improbable that significant quantities of LDL pass out of the blood into vessel walls between endothelial cells, and thus give indirect support to the transcytotic pathway in atherogenesis.

References

[1] Battacharya, S.K., Chakravarti, R.N., and Wahi, P.L. (1974): Atherosclerosis, 20, 214.

[2] Born, G.V.R., and Palinski, W. (1985): Br. J. exp. Path., 66, 543.

[3] Born, G.V.R., and Shafi, S. (1988): Abstr. in the Proceedings of the 48th Meeting of the European Atherosclerosis Society, Hamburg.

[4] Born, G.V.R., Shafi, S., and Cusack, N.J. (1989): Transplant Proc., 21, 3660.

[5] Brown, M.A., and Goldstein, J.L. (1985): Annals New York Acad. Sci., 454, 178.

[6] Bühler, H.U., Da Prada, M., Haefely, W., and Picotti, G.B. (1978): J. Physiol. (Lond.), 276, 311.

[7] Carew, T.E., Pittman, R.C., Marchand, E.R., and Steinberg, D. (1984): Arteriosclerosis, 4, 214.

[8] Dimsdale, J.E., and Moss, J. (1980): J.A.M.A., 243, 340.

[9] Goldstein, J.L., and Brown, M.S. (1977): Annu. Rev. Biochem., 46, 897.

[10] Görög, P., Schraufstätter, I., and Born, G.V.R. (1982): Proc. R. Soc. London. B., 214, 471.

[11] Görög, P., and Born, G.V.R. (1982): Br. J. exp. Path., 63, 447.

[12] Görög, P., and Born, G.V.R. (1983): Br. J. exp. Path., 64, 418.

[13] Görög, P., and Pearson, D.J. (1984): Atherosclerosis, 53, 21.

[14] Havel, R.J., Eder, H.A., and Bragdon, J. (1955): J. Clin. Invest., 34, 1345.

[15] Kannel, W.B., Wolf, P.A., Castelli, W.P., D'Agostino, R.B. (1987): J.A.M.A., 258, 1183.

[16] McFarlane, A.S. (1958): Nature Lond., 182, 53.

[17] Mahley, R.W., Weisgraber, K.H., and Innerarity, T.L. (1979): Biochem. Biophys. Acta, 571, 81.

[18] Majno, G., Shea, M.S., and Leventhal, M. (1969): J. Cell. Biol., 42, 647.

[19] Marcum, J.A., McKenney, J.B., Galli, S.J., Jackman, R.W., and Rosenberg, R.D. (1986): Am. J. Physiol., 250, 879.

[20] Meade, T.W., Mellows, S., Brozovic, M., Miller, G.J., Chakrabarti, R., North, W.R.S., Haines, A.P., Stirling, Y., Imeson, J.D., and Thompson, S.G. (1986): Lancet, ii, 533.

[21] Okayama, T., and Satake, K. (1960): J. Biochem., 47, 466.

[22] Osterman, H., and Born, G.V.R. (1986): Proc. Roy. Soc. Lond. B., 227, 17.

[23] Pittman, R.C., Carew, T.E., Glass, C.R., Green, S., Taylor, C.A., and Attie, A.D. (1983): Biochem. J., 212, 791.

[24] Robertson, D., Johnson, G.A., Robertson, R.M., Nies, A.S. Shand, D.G., and Oates, J.A. (1979): Circulation, 54, 637.

[25] Rosenberg, R.D., Reilley, C., and Fritze, L. (1985): Am. New York Acad. Sci., 454, 270.

[26] Shafi, S., Palinski, W., and Born, G.V.R. (1987): Atherosclerosis, 66, 131.

[27] Shafi, S., Cusack, N.J., and Born, G.V.R. (1989): Proc. Roy. Soc. Lond. B., 235, 289.

[28] Simionescu, N., and Simionescu, M. (1985): Microvasc. Res., 30, 314.

[29] Simionescu, N., Vasile, E., Lupu, F., Popescu, G., and Simionescu, M. (1986): Am. J. Pathol., 123, 109.

[30] Skutelsky, E., Rudich, Z., and Danon, D. (1975): Thrombos. Res., 7, 623.

[31] Smith, E.M., and Staples, E.M. (1982): Proc. Roy. Soc. Lond. B., 127, 69.

[32] Stein, Y., and Stein, O. (1973): Ciba Found. Symp., 12, 165.

[33] Stein, O., Stein, Y., and Eisenberg, S. (1973): Z. Zellforsch., mikrosk. Anat., 138, 223.

[34] Vasile, E., Simionescu, M., and Simionescu, N. (1983): J. Cell. Biol., 96, 167.

[35] Vlodavsky, I., Fielding, P.E., Fielding, C.J., and Gospodarowicz, D. (1978): Proc. Natl. Acad. Sci., USA, 75, 356.

[36] Weisgraber, K.H., Innerarity, T.L., and Mahley, R.W. (1978): J. Biol. Chem., 253, 9053.

[37] Wiklund, O., Carew, T.E., and Steinberg, D. (1985): Arteriosclerosis, 5, 135.

Oral Contraceptive Steroids and Arteriosclerosis

Herbert Kuhl

Universitäts-Frauenklinik, Universität Frankfurt/Main

The pattern of plasma lipoprotein levels is to a high degree dependent on endogenous and exogenous sex steroids. As high LDL-cholesterol (CH) and low HDL-CH concentrations are assumed to be involved in the development of arteriosclerosis, attention has to be paid to changes in lipid metabolism on account of alterations in the hormonal status as well as treatment with estrogens, progestogens or androgens.

Lipoprotein pattern during menstrual cycle, pregnancy and menopause

It had been shown that there are considerable fluctuations in lipoprotein levels and composition throughout the menstrual cycle, e.g., a decrease in the LDL-CH level and the hepatic lipase activity during the luteal phase which correlated with the serum concentrations of estradiol [1, 2]. Pregnancy is characterized by a continuous rise in the serum concentrations of estradiol up to 25 ng/ml (luteal phase 0.2 ng/ml) and of progesterone up to 100 ng/ml (luteal phase 20 ng/ml). There is a concomitant increase in the serum levels of total CH (+ 70%), total triglycerides (TG) (+ 200%), total phospholipids (PL) (+ 60%), apolipoproteins A-I (+ 50%), A-II (+ 20%) and B (+ 100%), LDL-CH (+ 80%), HDL-CH (+ 10%) and the LDL/HDL ratio (+ 50%) [3].

The loss of ovarian steroid production after the menopause and oophorectomy is followed by a change in lipoprotein levels, particularly an increase in LDL-CH which is associated with the acceleration of arteriosclerosis [6—8]. On the other hand, estrogen replacement therapy may reverse the abnormal lipoprotein pattern induced by estrogen deficiency [9, 10] and consequently reduce the incidence of atherosclerotic vascular diseases [11]. In order to avoid endometrial hyperplasia induced by long-term unopposed estrogen therapy, the addition of progestogens has been recommended. As progestogens with androgenic activity may counteract the favourable effects of estrogens on lipid metabolism, type and dose of the progestogens has to be chosen in an adequate manner.

Effect of contraceptive steroids on lipid metabolism

Millions of women are taking oral contraceptives for a long period of time. The various formulations contain highly active estrogens and progestogens which may alter lipid metabolism. The changes in the serum concentrations of lipids and the composition of lipoproteins are dependent on the type and dose of the steroids, the route of administration and the duration of treatment [12—18]. The only estrogen used in oral contraceptives, is ethinylestradiol (EE) or mestranol (ME) which becomes hormonally active after demethylation to EE. Contrary to this, a series of different progestogens are contained in the various pill formulations which differ largely in their effect on lipid metabolism. It has to be emphasized that the steroid levels circulating through the liver rather than the dose determine the effect. It is very difficult to find correlations between the serum levels of contraceptive steroids and lipoprotein changes when combinations of estrogens and progestogens are taken which may exert antagonistic effects on lipid metabolism, and the effectiveness of which may reach the end-point due to overdosage in most of the women. A strong inverse correlation has, however, been observed between the serum concentrations of medroxyprogesterone acetate and those of HDL-CH and HDL_2-CH in women treated with depot-medroxyprogesterone acetate [19].

The alterations in lipid parameters during treatment with oral contraceptives mainly reflect the hepatic effects of the oral route of administration. During the first liver passage, the local concentrations in the sinusoids are four- to fivefold those measured in the periphery. Therefore, orally administered steroids exert a much more pronounced change in lipoprotein pattern than those administered parenterally. Contrary to the natural estrogens, e.g. estradiol which is rapidly metabolized after ingestion in the gastrointestinal tract and liver, EE and ME have a strong influence on hepatic metabolism. This is exemplified by the effects of EE on LDL-CH and HDL-CH in postmenopausal women. The dose of 10 μg EE is at least as effective as 1 mg estradiol or 0.625 mg conjugated equine estrogens in reducing LDL-CH levels and in increasing HDL-CH levels. The pronounced effects of the synthetic estrogens is based on the presence of the ethinyl group at position C_{17} which prevents the oxidation of the 17β-hydroxy group and which may inhibit metabolizing enzymes. Treatment of postmenopausal women with the very high dose of 100 μg EE results in an increase of all components of VLDL by more than 100%, of apolipoprotein B (+ 119%) and A-I (+ 27%), total TG (+ 87%), LDL-TG (+ 40%), HDL-TG (+ 173%), HDL-PL (+ 79%), HDL-CH (+ 38%) and HDL_2-CH (+ 150%), while LDL-CH was not altered [20]. Except the strong increase in TG and apolipoprotein B levels, the changes appear to be rather favourable than deleterious with respect to an atherogenic risk. It has, however, to be kept in mind that treatment with high doses of EE is associated with a high incidence of thromboembolic diseases. Therefore, the EE dose in the oral contraceptives has to be reduced as far as possible.

The changes in lipid and lipoprotein pattern observed during treatment with estrogens, reflect the sum of different mechanisms. Estrogens stimulate hepatic synthesis of apolipoprotein A-I and C-II [21] and the production of TG, VLDL and HDL_3 [20, 22—24]. The enhanced lipolysis of higher amounts of VLDL in muscle and fat tissue results in an increased uptake of VLDL fragments by HDL_3 which is transformed to HDL_2. Therefore, the resultant effect may be a rise in HDL_2 but not HDL_3. Estrogens inhibit hepatic TG lipase which degrades mainly the TG and PL of HDL_2, and may also play a role in the rise in HDL_2-CH levels [25–27]. Moreover, estrogens may alter the composition of PL and possibly the membrane fluidity [28, 29].

The most striking effect of the estrogens is the increase in the number or affinity of the LDL (B, E) receptors and the Apo E receptors in the liver which are responsible for the clearance of atherogenic LDL, VLDL remnants and chylomicron remnants [30–35]. Treatment with EE, therefore, increases hepatic uptake of CH-rich VLDL [34, 36], LDL [33] and chylomicron remnants [31, 36]. Although intake of estrogens causes a rise in TG production, the stimulation of hepatic uptake of β-VLDL and chylomicron remnants in women with type III hyperlipoproteinemia results in a decrease in TG and CH levels, a reduction in the CH/TG ratio in VLDL, a decrease in β-VLDL and normalizes lipid composition of abnormal VLDL [36-39]. Similarly, estrogen treatment of women with type II hyperlipoproteinemia also leads to a reduction in LDL-CH and an increase in HDL-CH [40]. Contrary to this, in women with hyperlipoproteinemia type IV or V who are taking estrogens, a massive rise in the CH and TG levels accompanied with pancreatitis may occur which is reversible after discontinuation of hormone treatment [41, 42].

Most of the effects exerted by estrogens are antagonized by progestogens, particularly by nortestosterone derivatives, on account of their anti-estrogenic and/or androgenic properties. Androgens inhibit estrogen-induced synthesis of apolipoproteins A-I and C-II [21], stimulate the acticity of hepatic TG lipase [27], reduce the levels of TG and VLDL [43, 44] and decrease the lecithin content of PL [29]. Treatment with levonorgestrel (LNG) which exerts a relative pronounced androgenic effect, results in a reduction of the serum levels of apolipoprotein A-I, HDL-CH, HDL_2-CH and VLDL-TG but not HDL_3-CH and in an increase in the activity of hepatic TG lipase [45, 46]. Desogestrel (DG) which has less androgenic properties, reduces apolipoprotein A-I and VLDL-TG but not HDL-CH or HDL_2-CH [44]. Contrary to these nortestosterone derivatives, the progesterone derivatives medroxyprogesterone actate and cyproterone acetate do not affect lipid metabolism [45, 47].

The effect of different contraceptive formulations on lipid metabolism

According to the composition of the pill, the resultant effect on lipids and lipoproteins may vary considerably. As oral contraceptives containing high doses of LNG and norethisterone (NET) have been suspected to increase the risk of arteriosclerosis, new progestogens with less androgenic potencies have been developed, e.g. desogestrel, norgestimate and gestodene. The higher the dose of

Table 1: Dependency on the composition of oral contraceptives of changes in lipid metabolism [12, 14, 15]

Formulation	CH	TG	HDL-CH	HDL$_2$-CH	LDL-CH	Apo B	Apo A-I
50 EE/1000 NET	+7%	+45%	–	–	+ 6%		+ 9%
50 EE/1000 EDD	+9%	+57%	–	–	+10%		+11%
35 EE/1000 NET	+9%	+24%	–		+15%	+30%	+12%
35 EE/1000 EDD	+9%	+38%	–		+10%	+29%	+19%
50 EE/250 LNG	+8%	+32%	–13%	–27%	+18%		– 9%
30 EE/250 LNG	–	+17%	–21%				
20 EE/250 LNG	–	+17%	–21%				
30 EE/150 LNG	–	+15%	–10%				

EE: ethinylestradiol; NET: norethisterone; EDD: ethynodiol diacetate;
LNG: levonorgestrel; (doses in μg).

EE, the higher are the levels of total TG, of VLDL-CH and HDL-CH. When the EE dose is reduced, the combination with a progestogen with androgenic side-effects may result in an increase in LDL-CH levels. In fact, treatment with LNG-containing pills caused a rise in LDL-CH which was more pronounced than with formulations containing NET or ethynodiol diacetaté (Table 1) [12—14]. Moreover, the reduction in the HDL-CH levels correlated with the dose of LNG, while preparations containing NET or ethynodiol diacetate have nearly no effect (Table 1) [12, 14, 15].

It is, however, possible to counterbalance this unfavourable effect of LNG on lipid metabolism by a proper composition of the pill, even though the EE dose is reduced. Triphasic formulations containing EE and LNG have been demonstrated not to decrease HDL-CH and not to increase LDL-CH [48]; the effects on various serum parameters of lipid metabolism even indicate a slight overweigh of the action of the estrogen component (Table 2).

The introduction of the new progestogens desogestrel (DG), norgestimate, and gestodene (GSD) with high progestogenic but relatively low androgenic

Table 2: Effect of a triphasic preparation containing 30 μg EE + 50 μg LNG / 40 μg EE + 75 μg LNG / 30 μg EE + 125 μg LNG on various serum parameters of lipid metabolism [48]

Total CH	–	VLDL-CH	–	LDL-CH	–	HDL-CH	–
Total TG	+16%*	VLDL-TG	+17%	LDL-TG	+ 9%	HDL-TG	+52%
Total PL	+ 7%*	VLDL-PL	–	LDL-PL	+19%	HDL-PL	–
Lp(a)	–	Apo B	+ 8%			Apo A-I	+18%*
						Apo A-II	+37%*
						HDL$_3$-CH	+ 6%*

EE: ethinylestradiol; LNG: levonorgestrel. * p < 0.05.

Table 3: Effect of an oral contraceptive containing 30 μg EE + 150 μg DG during 12 treatment cycles on various parameters of lipid metabolism [17]

	Cycle 1	Cycle 3	Cycle 6	Cycle 12
Total CH	–	–	–	–
Total TG	–	–	–	–
Total PL	–	–	–	–
HDL-CH	–	+ 7%	+ 9%	+13%
HDL-TG	+74%	+55%	+69%	+90%
HDL-PL	–	+15%	+15%	+14%
VLDL-CH	–	–	–	+17%
VLDL-TG	–	–	–	–
VLDL-PL	–	–	+37%	+20%
LDL-CH	–14%	–	–	–
LDL-TG	–	–	–	–
LDL-PL	–32%	–25%	–25%	–
HDL$_2$-CH	–	–	–	–
HDL$_2$-PL	–	–	+12%	–
HDL$_3$-CH	–	+12%	+11%	+11%
HDL$_3$-PL	–	+17%	+14%	+10%
Apo A-I	–	–	–	–
Apo A-II	–	+14%	+16%	+20%
Apo B	–	–	+23%	+24%

(Percentage of significant change as compared to the control cycle; mean of the values on day 1, 10 and 21).
EE: ethinylestradiol; DG: desogestrel.

activities rendered it possible to reduce the EE dose of monophasic pills to 30 μg or less without changing the lipoprotein pattern in an adverse manner. This could be demonstrated in our own studies on the effect of low-dose oral contraceptives containing 30 μg EE and 150 μg DG (EE/DG) or 75 μg GSD (EE/GSD) upon 19 serum parameters of lipid metabolism during 12 months of treatment [17] (Table 3 and 4). During a recent study we investigated the changes of lipid and lipoprotein levels during 6 months of treatment with a two-phasic preparation containing 40 μg EE + 25 μg DG (7 days) and 30 μg EE + 125 μg DG (16 days) (Table 5). Material and methods are previously described in detail [17].

The comparison between EE/DG and EE/GSD which was carried out on day 1, 10 and 21 of a preceding control cycle and of the 1st, 3rd, 6th and 12th treatment cycle in 22 volunteers, revealed large intra- and interindividual variations. Therefore, no significant difference between the effects of both oral contraceptives could be found. The changes observed in some parameters during treatment, were to a certain degree dependent on time. In most cases, there was no effect during the first treatment cycle, while during the following cycles significant alterations became discernible. On the other hand, some significant changes occurring during the first treatment cycle, disappeared during the following treat-

Table 4: Effect of an oral contraceptive containing 30 µg EE + 75 µg GSD during 12 treatment cycles on various parameters of lipid metabolism [17]

	Cycle 1	Cycle 3	Cycle 6	Cycle 12
Total CH	—	—	—	—
Total TG	—	+41%	+34%	+32%
Total PL	—	—	—	—
HDL-CH	—	—	+11%	+ 7%
HDL-TG	+65%	+84%	+76%	+114%
HDL-PL	—	+ 7%	+11%	—
VLDL-CH	—	—	+29%	+ 51%
VLDL-TG	—	+35%	—	—
VLDL-PL	—	+30%	+35%	+ 28%
LDL-CH	− 9%	—	—	—
LDL-TG	—	+27%	+24%	—
LDL-PL	−21%	−16%	—	—
HDL$_2$-CH	+16%	—	—	—
HDL$_2$-PL	+21%	—	—	—
HDL$_3$-CH	—	+11%	+13%	+ 7%
HDL$_3$-PL	—	+ 9%	+12%	—
Apo A-I	—	—	—	—
Apo A-II	—	+21%	+26%	+ 24%
Apo B	—	+16%	+20%	+ 22%

(Percentage of significant change as compared to the control cycle; mean of the values on day 1, 10 and 21).
EE: ethinylestradiol; GSD: gestodene.

Table 5: Effect of a two-phasic oral contraceptive containing 40 µg EE + 25 µg DG / 30 µg EE + 125 µg DG during 6 treatment cycles on various parameters of lipid metabolism

	Cycle 1	Cycle 3	Cycle 6
Total CH	—	—	+ 10%
Total TG	+39%	+ 88%	+144%
Total PL	+11%	+ 11%	+ 23%
HDL-CH	+10%	+ 8%	+ 10%
HDL-TG	+ 7%	+ 6%	+ 8%
VLDL-CH	+33%	+ 48%	+ 60%
VLDL-TG	+55%	+ 85%	+111%
LDL-CH	—	—	—
LDL-TG	+83%	+127%	+128%
HDL$_2$-CH	+19%	—	—
HDL$_3$-CH	—	+ 7%	—
Apo A-I	+18%	+ 16%	+ 23%
Apo A-II	+17%	+ 20%	+ 37%
Apo B	—	+ 15%	+ 20%
Apo E	−24%	− 21%	− 24%

ment period. There was no influence of both preparations on total CH and PL, while total TG were considerably elevated with EE/GSD (p $<$ 0.01) (Table 4) and moderately but not significantly with EE/DG (Table 3). The CH content of VLDL was increased after 6 and 12 months, the effect being more pronounced during treatment with EE/GSD. There was also a significant increase in the VLDL-PL and in apolipoprotein B, while that of VLDL-TG was only transitory. LDL-CH and LDL-PL were significantly lower during the first treatment cycle, but there-after the effect extenuated and has disappeared after 12 months of treatment. The increase in LDL-TG during the third and sixth cycle of treatment with EE/GSD was also transitory. There was a significant increase in the CH, TG and PL content of HDL and in the level of apolipoprotein A-II during intake of both formulations which was mainly due to a rise in HDL_3 (Table 3 and 4). Contrary to this, there was no change in HDL_2-CH and HDL_2-PL during the first month of intake of EE/GSD.

During the study with the two-phasic preparation blood samples were taken between day 18 and 22 of a preceding control cycle and of the 1st, 3rd and 6th treatment cycle (Table 5). There was a moderate rise in the levels of total CH and total PL and a doubling of total TG. The CH and TG components of HDL and VLDL increased, whereby the change was more pronounced in VLDL. There was a significant rise in apolipoproteins A-I, A-II and B and a significant reduction in apolipoprotein E. LDL-CH was not altered during treatment, while LDL-TG rose by more than 100%.

Mechanism and significance of changes induced by contraceptive steroids

The increase in total TG, VLDL and apolipoprotein B indicates an overweigh of the effect of EE on lipid metabolism, as estrogens have been shown to stimulate VLDL synthesis and secretion, while progestogens have the opposite effect [49, 50]. The effect was highest using the estrogen-dominant two-phasic pill and lowest with EE/DG. Contrary to this, the increase in apolipoprotein B levels was similar during intake of the three preparations indicating no influence of the progestogen component on apolipoprotein B synthesis. A more or less pronounced elevation of the levels of total TG, VLDL and apolipoprotein B during treatment with modern low-dose oral contraceptives has previously been reported [51−57]. Our results demonstrate that the alterations of some parameters were only transitory, while the effect on some other lipids and lipoproteins was increasing with the duration of treatment. A time-dependent change in lipoprotein pattern has been observed during intake of a combination of EE and LNG [58]

Due to the elevated supply with substrate, the enhanced lipolysis of VLDL leads to an increase in the formation of LDL. As the LDL-CH levels remained unaltered, an increased formation must be counterbalanced by an enhanced clearance of CH-enriched VLDL and LDL in the liver. The CH/TG ratio in VLDL rose during treatment with EE/GSD, was nearly unchanged with EE/DG [18] and decreased with the two-phasic preparation. At the same time, the CH/TG ratio in LDL decreased during treatment with EE/GSD, was not altered with EE/DG and increased strongly with the two-phasic pill. This could be interpreted as reflecting a rise in CH-enriched VLDL or remnants during treatment with EE/GSD and a reduction during intake of the estrogen-dominant two-phasic pill. It is, however, not known whether or not progestogens may modulate or inhibit the estrogen-induced increase in LDL receptors and apo E receptors. In the case of the two-phasic pill, the reduction in the apolipoprotein E concentrations indicate an enhanced removal of VLDL remants.

It could be suggested that the increase in the levels of apolipoprotein A-II, HDL-CH and HDL-PL by 10% and of HDL-TG by 70 to 100% during intake of EE/DG and EE/GSD is based on an increased synthesis of HDL$_3$ which is subsequently converted to HDL$_2$ by assimilation of VLDL fragments, and on an inhibition of hepatic lipase by EE. On the other hand, treatment with the estrogen-dominant two-phasic pill increased HDL-TG only slightly, while the rise in HDL-CH was also in the range of 10%. Therefore, the elevation of HDL-TG and HDL-PL appears not to be the result of an estrogen-induced inhibition of hepatic lipase. In all probability, the hepatic production of apolipoprotein A-II and of HDL$_3$ is not influenced by progestogens [45, 59], and DG has no effect on the activity of hepatic lipase [44]. The increase in the apolipoprotein A-I levels during treatment with the two-phasic pill but not with the monophasic preparations EE/DG and EE/GSD indicate an inhibitory action of DG and GSD on EE-stimulated synthesis of apolipoprotein A-I.

Epidemiologic data suggest an increased risk of coronary heart disease during treatment with high-dosed oral contraceptives [60, 61] which, however, was called in question [62]. Contrary to this, there is no doubt that treatment with EE may trigger thrombotic processes. As the older oral contraceptives containing high doses of NET or LNG caused a reduction in HDL-CH and an increase in LDL-CH (Table 1), it was assumed that this unfavourable change of the lipoprotein pattern led to an accelerated development of arteriosclerosis and consequently to a higher incidence of coronary heart disease. Therefore, new formulations were developed which contain progestogens with relatively weak androgenic properties and do not change lipid metabolism in an adverse manner.

There is, however, no evidence that the reduction in HDL-CH and the increase in LDL-CH levels during long-term treatment with oral contraceptives containing high doses of NET or LNG really accelerated the atherosclerotic process. Angiographic investigations have demonstrated that most women who developed myocardial infarction while receiving oral contraceptives, had no coronary artery atherosclerosis [63]. Recently, the hypothesis of pill-induced arteriosclerosis was investigated in female cynomolgus macaques which were fed a moderately atherogenic diet and were treated with EE and LNG during 24 months [64, 65]. Although HDL-CH serum concentrations were reduced by 27% and total TG were increased by 258%, there was no increase in the prevalence of atherosclerosis and the area of plaques in coronary arteries, but even a marked decrease. Contrary to this, treatment with a vaginal ring releasing estradiol and LNG, caused a similar reduction in HDL-CH but no change in total TG and led to a significant increase in the size of plaques in coronary arteries. The results indicate that oral treatment with EE containing preparations which exerts a strong estrogenic effect on the liver, is not associated with an acceleration of atherosclerosis, even though the HDL-CH levels are reduced. The mechanism of action remains to be elucidated, but it might be speculated that an increase in hepatic LDL receptors and Apo E receptors induced by orally taken EE and which is not antagonized by progestogens, might enhance removal of atherogenic lipoproteins or remnants and thus compensate for the reduction in HDL-CH [31]. In the monkeys, an accelerated coronary artery atherosclerosis could be observed after bilateral oophorectomy. It could also be demonstrated that during pregnancy the extent of diet-induced coronary arteriosclerosis was only half that in non-pregnant animals, although the pregnant monkeys exhibited lower HDL-CH levels [65].

Even though oral contraceptives obviously do not cause arteriosclerosis, formulations should be preferred which do not reduce HDL-CH levels. The favourable effects of HDL are not limited to the reverse cholesterol transport to the liver, but it inhibits proliferation of smooth muscle cells, stimulates endothelial repair, stimulates prostacyclin synthesis in arterial endothelial cells, facilitates fibrinolysis in aggregates and facilitates the catabolism of TG-rich lipoproteins [66].

References

[1] Hemer, H.A., Valles de Bourges, V., Ayala, J.J., Brito, G., Diaz-Sanchez, V., Garza-Flores, J.: Variations in serum lipids and lipoproteins throughout the menstrual cycle. Fertil Steril. 1985; 44: 80–84.

[2] Tikkanen, M.J., Kuusi, T., Nikkilä, E.A., Stenman, U.H.: Variation of postheparin plasma hepatic lipase by menstrual cycle. Metabolism. 1986; 35: 99–104.

[3] Desoye, G., Schweditsch, M.O., Pfeiffer, K.P., Zechner, R., Kostner, G.M.: Correlation of hormones with lipid and lipoprotein levels during normal pregnancy and postpartum. J. Clin. Endocrinol Metab. 1987; 64: 704–712.

[4] Campos, H., McNamara, J.R., Wilson, P.W.F., Ordovas, J.M., Schaefer, E.J.: Differences in low density lipoprotein subfractions and apolipoproteins in premenopausal and postmenopausal women. J. Clin. Endocrinol. Metab. 1988; 67: 30–35.

[5] Witteman, J.C.M., Grobbee, D.E., Kok, F.J., Hofman, A., Valkenburg, H.A.: Increased risk of atherosclerosis in women after the menopause. Br. Med. J. 1989; 298: 642–644.

[6] Parrish, H.M., Carr, C.A., Hall, D.G., King, T.M.: Time interval from castration in premenopausal women to development of excessive coronary atherosclerosis. Am. J. Obstet. Gynecol. 1967; 99: 155–162.

[7] Szajderman, M., Oliver, M.F.: Spontaneous premature menopause, ischaemic heart disease and serum lipids. Lancet. 1963; I: 962–965.

[8] Gordon, T., Kannel, W.B., Hjortland, M.C., McNamara, P.: Menopause and coronary heart disease. The Framingham Study. Ann. Int. Med. 1978; 89: 157–161.

[9] Kuhl, H.: Atherosklerose-Prophylaxe durch Östrogensubstitution? Geburtsh. Frauen-heilk. 1988;48: 747–756.

[10] Fahraeus, L.: The effects of estradiol on blood lipids and lipoproteins in postmenopausal women. Obstet. Gynecol. 1988; 72: 18S–22S.

[11] Knopp, R.H.: The effects of postmenopausal estrogen therapy on the incidence of arteriosclerotic vascular disease. Obstet. Gynecol. 1988; 72: 23S–30S.

[12] Larsson-Cohn, U., Fahraeus, L., Wallentin, L., Zador, G.: Lipoprotein changes may be minimized by proper composition of a combined oral contraceptive. Fertil Steril. 1981; 35: 172–179.

[13] Fotherby, K.: Oral contraceptives, lipids and cardiovascular disease. Contraception. 1985; 31: 367–394.

[14] Lipson, A., Stoy, D.B., LaRosa, J.C. et al.: Progestins and oral contraceptive-induced lipoprotein changes: a prospective study. Contraception. 1986; 34: 121–134.

[15] Burkman, R.T.: Lipid and lipoprotein changes in relation to oral contraception and hormonal replacement therapy. Fertil Steril. 1988; 49: 39S–50S.

[16] Knopp, R.H.: Cardiovascular effects of endogenous and exogenous sex hormones over a woman's lifetime. Am. J. Obstet. Gynecol. 1988; 158: 1630–1643.

[17] März, W., Jung-Hoffmann, C., Heidt, F., Gross, W., Kuhl, H.: Changes in lipid meta-bolism during 12 months of treatment with two oral contraceptives containing 30 μg ethnylestradiol and 75 μg gestodene or 150 μg desogestrel. Contraception. 1990; 41: 245–258.

[18] Kuhl, H., März, W., Jung-Hoffmann, C., Heidt, F., Gross, W.: Time-dependent alterations in lipid metabolism during treatment with low-dose oral contraceptives. Am. J. Obstet. Gynecol. 1990; 163 (Suppl.): 363–369.

[19] Fahraeus, L., Sydsjö, A., Wallentin, L.: Lipoprotein changes during treatment of pelvic endometriosis with medroxyprogesterone acetate. Fertil Steril. 1986; 45: 503–506.

[20] Schaefer, E.J., Foster, D.M., Zech, L.A., Lindgren, F.T., Brewer, H.B., Levy, R.I.: The effects of estrogen administration on plasma lipoprotein metabolism in premenopausal females. J. Clin. Endocrinol. Metab. 1983; 57: 262–267.

[21] Tam, S.P., Archer, T.K., Deeley, R.G.: Effects of estrogen on apolipoprotein secretion by the human hepatocarcinoma cell line, HepG2. J. Biol. Chem. 1985; 260: 1670–1675.

[22] Knopp., R.H., Walden, C.E., Wahl, P.W., Hoover, J.J.: Effects of oral contraceptives on lipoprotein triglyceride and cholesterol: relationships to estrogen and progestin potency. Am. J. Obstet. Gynecol. 1982; 142: 725–731.

[23] Voorhof, L., Rosseneu, M., Caster, H., De Keersgieter, W.: Metabolic effects of a bipha-sic oral contraceptive preparation containing ethinyloestradiol and desogestrel on serum lipoproteins and apolipoproteins. J. Endocrinol. 1986; 111: 191–196.

[24] Glueck, C.J., Fallat, R.W., Scheel, D.: Effects of estrogenic compounds on triglyceride kinetics. Metabolism. 1975; 24: 537–545.

[25] Shirai, K., Barnhart, R.L., Jackson, R.L.: Hydrolysis of human plasma high density lipo-protein$_2$-phospholipids and triglycerides by hepatic lipase. Biochem. Biophys. Res. Commun. 1981; 100: 591–599.

[26] Tikkanen, M.J., Kuusi, T., Nikkilä, E.A., Sane, T.: Very low density lipoprotein tri-glyceride kinetics during hepatic lipase suppression by estrogen. FEBS Letters. 1985; 181: 160–164.

[27] Tikkanen, M.J., Nikkilä, E.A.: Regulation of hepatic lipase and serum lipoproteins by sex steroids. Am. Heart. J. 1987; 113: 562–567.

[28] Silfverstolpe, G., Johnson, P., Samsioe, G., Svanborg, A., Gustafson, A.: Effects induced by two different estrogens on serum individual phospholipids and serum lecithin fatty acid composition. Horm. Metab. Res. 1981; 13: 141–145.

[29] Bagdade, J.D., Subbaiah, P.V.: Influence of low estrogen-containing oral contraceptives on lipoprotein phospholipid composition and mononuclear cell membrane fluidity. J. Clin. Endocrinol. Metab. 1988; 66: 857–861.

[30] Brown, M.S., Goldstein, J.L.: Lipoprotein receptors in the liver. Control signals for plasma cholesterol traffic. J. Clin. Invest. 1983; 72: 743–747.

[31] Berr, F., Eckel, R.H., Kern, F.: Contraceptive steroids increase hepatic uptake of chylomicron remnants in healthy young women. J. Lipid. Res. 1986; 27: 645–651.
[32] Cooper, A.D., Nutik, R., Chen, J.: Characterization of the estrogen induced lipoprotein receptor of rat liver. J. Lipid. Res. 1987; 28: 59–68.
[33] Kovanen, P.T., Brown, M.S., Goldstein, J.L.: Increased binding of low density lipoprotein to liver membranes from rats treated with 17α-ethinyl estradiol. J. Biol. Chem. 1979; 254: 11367–11372.
[34] Floren, C.H., Kushwaha, R.S., Hazzard, W.R., Albers, J.J.: Estrogen-induced increase in uptake of cholesterol-rich very low density lipoproteins in perfused rabbit liver. Metabolism. 1981; 30: 367–375.
[35] Windler, E.E.T., Kovanen, P.T., Chao, Y.S., Brown, M.S., Havel, R.J., Goldstein, J.L.: The estradiol-stimulated lipoprotein receptor of rat liver. J. Biol. Chem. 1980; 255: 10464–10471.
[36] Kushwaha, R.S., Hazzard, W.R., Gagne, C., Chait, A., Albers, J.J.: Type III hyperlipoproteinemia: paradoxical hypolipidemic response to estrogen. Ann. Int. Med. 1977; 87: 517–525.
[37] Stuyt, P.M.J., Demacker, P.N.M., van 't Laar, A.: A study of the hypolipidemic effect of estrogen in type III hyperlipoproteinemia. Horm. metabol. Res. 1986; 18: 607–610.
[38] Knopp, R.H., Heiss, G., Wahl, P.W.: Prevalence and clinical correlates of beta-migrating very-low-density lipoprotein. Am. J. Med. 1986; 81: 493–502.
[39] Chait, A., Brunzell, J.D., Albers, J.J., Hazzard, W.R.: Type-III hyperlipoproteinemia ("remnant removal disease"). Lancet. 1977; I: 1176–1178.
[40] Tikkanen, M.J., Nikkilä, E.A., Vartiainen, E.: Natural oestrogen as an effective treatment for type-II hyperlipoproteinaemia in postmenopausal women. Lancet. 1978; II. 490–491.
[41] Davidoff, F., Tishler, S., Rosoff, C.: Marked hyperlipidemia and pancreatitis associated with oral contraceptive therapy. New. Engl. J. Med. 1973; 289: 552–555.
[42] Glueck, C.J., Scheel, D., Fishback, J., Steiner, P.: Estrogen-induced pancreatitis in patients with previously covert familial type V hyperlipoproteinemia. Metabolism. 1972; 21: 657–666.
[43] Krauss, R.M.: Effects of progestational agents on serum lipids and lipoproteins. J. Reprod. Med. 1982; 8 (Suppl.): 503–510.
[44] Kuusi, T., Nikkilä, E.A., Tikkanen, M.J., Sipinen, S.: Effects of two progestins with different androgenic properties on hepatic endothelial lipase and high density lipoprotein$_2$. Atherosclerosis. 1985; 54: 251–262.
[45] Tikkanen, M.J., Nikkilä, E.A., Kuusi, T., Sipinen, S.: Different effects of two progestins on plasma high density lipoprotein (HDL$_2$) and postheparin plasma hepatic lipase activity. Atherosclerosis. 1981; 40: 365–369.
[46] Crona, N., Silfverstolpe, G., Samsioe, G.: Changes in serum apo-lipoprotein AI and sex-hormone-binding globulin levels after treatment with two different progestins administered alone and in combination with ethinylestradiol. Contraception. 1984; 29: 261–270.
[47] Tikkanen, M.J., Kuusi, T., Nikkilä, E.A., Sipinen, S.: Post-heparin plasma hepatic lipase activity as predictor of high-density lipoprotein response to progestogen therapy: studies with cyproterone acetate. Maturitas. 1987; 9: 81–86.
[48] März, W., Gross, W., Gahn, G., Romberg, G., Taubert, H.D., Kuhl, H.: A randomized crossover comparison of two low-dose contraceptives: effects on serum lipids and lipoproteins. Am. J. Obstet. Gynecol. 1985; 153: 287–293.
[49] Gustafson, A., Svanborg, A.: Gonadal steroid effects on plasma lipoproteins and individual phospholipids. J. Clin. Endocrinol Metab. 1972; 35: 203–207.
[50] Glueck, C.J., Fallat, R.: Gonadal hormones and triglycerides. Proc. Roy. Soc. Med. 1974; 67: 667–669.
[51] Samsioe, G.: Study on the effect of 30 μg ethinylestradiol (EE) + 150 μg desogestrel on lipid and lipoprotein metabolism in healthy volunteers, also in comparison with 30 μg EE + 150 μg levonorgestrel. Acta. Obstet. Gynecol. Scand. Suppl. 1982; 111: 55–60.

[52] Kloosterboer, H.J., van Wayjen, R.G.A., van den Ende, A.: Comparative effects of monophasic desogestrel plus ethinyloestradiol and triphasic levonorgestrel plus ethinyloestradiol on lipid metabolism. Contraception. 1986; 34: 135–144.

[53] Gaspard, U.J., Buret, J., Gillain, D., Romus, M.A., Lambotte, R.: Serum lipid and lipoprotein changes induced by new oral contraceptives containing ethinylestradiol plus levonorgestrel or desogestrel. Contraception. 1985; 31: 395–408.

[54] Harvengt, C., Desager, J.P., Gaspard, U., Lepot, M.: Changes in lipoprotein composition in women receiving two low-dose oral contraceptives containing ethinylestradiol and gonane progestins. Contraception. 1988; 37: 565–575.

[55] Bergink, E.W., Kloosterboer, H.J., Lund, L., Nummi, S.: Effects of levonorgestrel and desogestrel in low-dose oral contraceptive combinations on serum lipids, apolipoproteins A-I and B and glycosylated proteins. Contraception. 1984; 30: 61–72.

[56] Bertolini, S., Elicio, N., Cordera, R., Gapitanio, G.L., Montagna, G., Crose, S., Saturnino, M., Balestreri, R., De Cecco, L.: Effects of three low-dose oral contraceptive formulations on lipid metabolism. Acta. Obstet. Gynecol. Scand. 1987; 66: 327–332.

[57] Van der Vange, N., Kloosterboer, H.J., Haspels, A.A.: Effects of seven low dose combined oral contraceptives on high density lipoprotein subfractions. Brit. J. Obstet. Gynaecol. 1987; 94: 559–567.

[58] Ahren, T., Lithell, H., Victor, A., Vessby, B., Johansson, E.D.B.: Comparison of the metabolic effects of two hormonal contraceptive methods: an oral formulation and a vaginal ring. II. Serum lipoproteins and apolipoproteins. Contraception. 1981; 24: 451–468.

[59] La Rosa, J.C.: The varying effects of progestins on lipid levels and cardiovascular disease. Am. J. Obstet. Gynecol. 1988; 158: 1621–1629.

[60] Mann, J.I., Inman, W.H.W., Thorogood, M.: Oral contraceptive use in older women and fatal myocardial infarction. Brit. Med. J. 1976; II: 445–447.

[61] Shapiro, S., Rosenberg, L., Slone, D., Kaufman, D.W., Stolley, P.D., Miettinen, O.S.: Oral-contraceptive use in relation to myocardial infarction. Lancet. 1979; I: 743–746.

[62] Realini, J.P., Goldzieher, J.W.: Oral contraceptives and cardiovascular disease: a critique of the epidemiologic studies. Am. J. Obstet. Gynecol. 1985; 152: 729–798.

[63] Engel, H.J., Engel, E., Behnke, K., Lichtlen, P.: Angiographische Befunde nach Herzinfarkt junger Frauen: Die Rolle oraler Kontrazeptiva. Herz. 1987; 12: 290–295.

[64] Adams, M.R., Clarkson, T.B., Koritnik, D.R., Nash, H.A.: Contraceptive steroids and coronary artery atherosclerosis in cynomolgus macaques. Fertil Steril. 1987; 47: 1010–1018.

[65] Clarkson, T.B., Adams, M.R., Kaplan, J.R., Shively, C.A., Koritnik, D.R.: From menarche to menopause: Coronary artery atherosclerosis and protection in cynomolgus monkeys. Am. J. Obstet. Gynecol. 1989; 160: 1280–1285.

[66] Glueck, C.J.: Nonpharmacologic and pharmacologic alteration of high-density cholesterol: Therapeutic approaches to prevention of atherosclerosis. Am. Heart. J. 1985; 110: 1107–1115.

Parathormone, Calcium Imbalance and Atherogenesis

H. Raidt[1], *F. Baumgarten*[1], *H.-J. Bauch*[2], *K. Langer*[1],
U. Graefe[1], *W.H. Hauss*[2] :
[1] Nephrologisches Institut an der Universität Münster
[2] Institut für Arterioskleroseforschung an der Universität Münster

Introduction

Arteriosclerosis is very strongly connected with the aging process. The lots of theories over the last 170 years elucidate two crucial problems of arteriosclerosis research:

1. Arteriosclerosis (AS) is generated by *multiple* endogenous and exogenous factors influencing differently the progression of the disease.

2. Arteriosclerosis develops *very slowly over decades*. That means the causing biochemical agents may show only minimal deviations from normal range at any given time of the pathogenesis.

Only few of these many risk factors, as for example diabetes mellitus or hypertension, are thougt to produce AS on their own. Even these factors are in need of cofactors and mediators. In this multifactorial network of pathogenetic agents it may be more efficient, not just to summarize risk factors but to search for synergisms between them (Hauss 1970, Ross 1986).

In this context *calcium* experiences a renaissance whenever the pathogenesis of AS is under discussion.

Plate I demonstrates why the German common language is using "Arterienverkalkung" (arterial calcification) as a synonym for "arteriosclerosis". This may be inaccurate, but it is characterizing the visible storage of calcium salts into the vessel walls whereas the bones are softening in aging process. The deposition of calcium into the arterial media is known as "Mönckeberg's Mediasclerosis" and is usually not narrowing the vascular lumen. This phenomenon is also common in scar formation and aging.

Calcium as Intracellular Messenger

Newer findings suggest that calcium is not simply deposited in the extracellular spaces of the vascular media as inactive mineral salt, leading to nonstenosing mediasclerosis according to the left branch of Fig. 1.

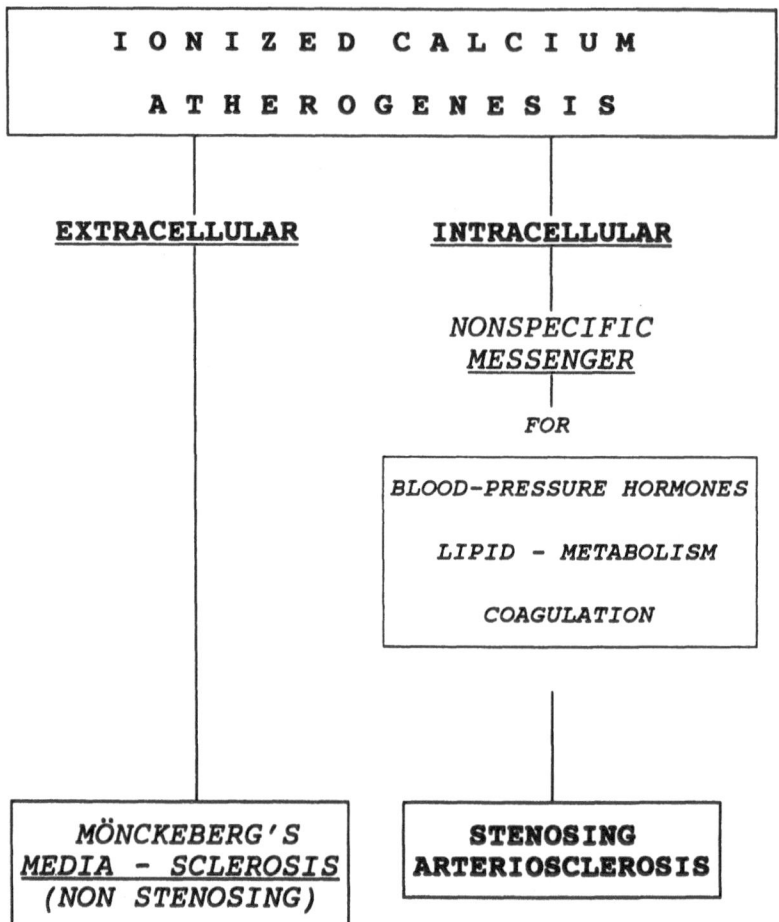

Figure 1: Extracellular and intracellular participation of Ca²⁺ on the pathogenesis of arteriosclerosis. The extracellular calcium is deposited as mineral salt in the arterial media (plate I),
whereas intracellular calcium is acting as amplifiing mediator of several primary atherogenic
risk factors.

Calcium is rather acting as an *universal unspecific second messenger inside the
cell,* as demonstrated in the right branch of Fig. 1. Intracellular ionized Ca^{2+} influences for example the synthesis and receptor activity of blood pressure hormones, the activity of lipid turnover and the coagulation system (Rasmussen
1986). By the way of this signal transfer Ca^{2+} may well contribute to progressive
stenosing AS (Henry 1985, Cheung 1986).

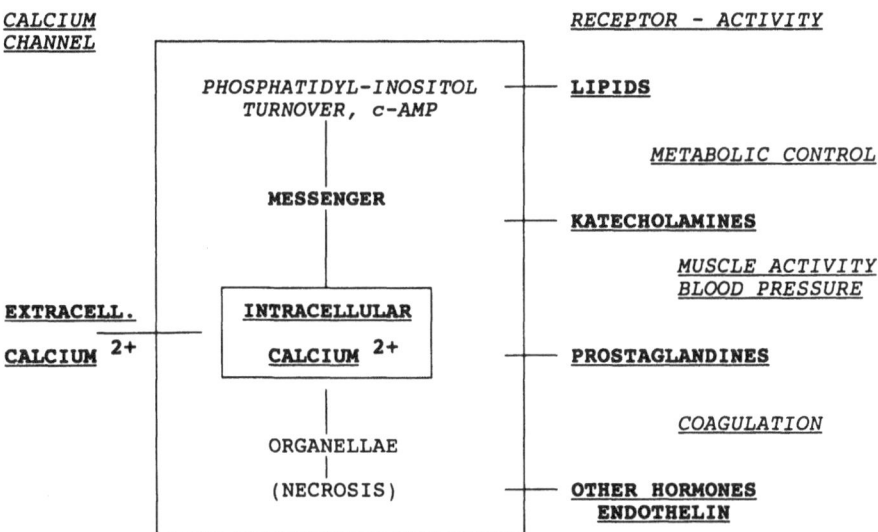

Figure 2: The right side of this Figure demonstrates the receptor activities for several atherogenic factors and their effects dependant on the level of intracellular ionized calcium. The symbolized cell shows the pathways of intracellular Ca^{2+} action. This study focuses on mechanisms and substances influencing the intra-extracellular Ca^{2+} exchange via cell membrane-calcium channels.

Figure 2 exhibits an overview over several cellular activities which are controlled by intracellular Ca^{2+} as second messenger for other primary signals resp. in connection with cAMP-activation and the phosphatidyl-inositol-turnover. This Ca^{2+} dependant intracellular regulation-mechanism is found in all cells of higher animals (Rasmussen 1986). The effects (shown on the right side of Fig. 2) are dependant on the cell species. As far as the cells of atherogenesis, smooth muscle and endothelial cells, macrophages, thrombocytes, fibroblasts, endocrine and neurocrine cells are concerned, Ca^{2+} is involved in the regulation of the most discussed mechanisms of pathogenesis. The receptor activity and thus the turnover of lipids, the synthesis and activity of katecholamines and other pressor hormones and thus blood pressure and smooth muscle activity, the prostaglandin system and thus coagulation and other local vascular repair mechanisms at least other local hormones like endothelin are dependant on the level of intracellular free Ca^{2+}.

In general,, the higher the intracellular Ca^{2+} level, the more active are the systems mentioned (Rasmussen 1986, Henry 1985, Rüegg 1986, Yanagisawa 1988, Kai 1989, Sugiura 1989).

It cannot be the intention of a clinician to unravel this complex network at a cellular or molecular basis. The figure is just presented to elucidate a *potential central role of intracellular Ca^{2+}* in atherogenesis.

```
------------------------------------
              INTRACELLULAR

           CALCIUM  ²⁺  LEVEL
------------------------------------
       INCREASED by          DECREASED by
       -----------           -----------


   Ca²⁺ ENRICHED FOOD        Ca²⁺ CHANNEL

                               BLOCKERS

       VITAMINE D₃          (NIFEDIPINE)


      PARATHORMONE


      ENDOTHELINE


      CHOLESTEROL(?)
```

Figure 3: Overview on substances increasing or decreasing the intracellular Ca^{2+} level.

The question we will focus on is given on the left side of Figure 2: Are there any factors in humans which open calcium channels thus elevating the intracellular free Ca^{2+} concentration and possibly contributing to AS?

The concentration of Ca^{2+} is altered by several substances, some of which are listed in Figure 3. Most of them act via a receptor dependant opening of the plasma membrane calcium channels. Some of them are also believed to release stored intracellular calcium from the organellae.

An *increase* of intracellular calcium is observed under the influence of vitamine D_3, parathormone, probably cholesterol and the recently discovered tissue hormone endothelin (Cavallero 1973, Kramsch 1980, Morrison 1972, Henry 1985, Mundy 1989, Raisz 1980, Karpf 1990, Müller 1988, Brickman 1987, Yanagisawa 1988, Sugiura 1989, Hirata 1988, Kai 1989).

A *decrease* of intracellular free Ca^{2+} is found under the influence of chemically different drugs called *"calcium channel blockers"* as for example nifedipine or verapamil, only to name the worldwide most used drugs of this group in clinical medicine (Fleckenstein 1969, 1984, 1986, Morrison 1972, Henry 1981, 1985, Kramsch 1980, Snyder 1985).

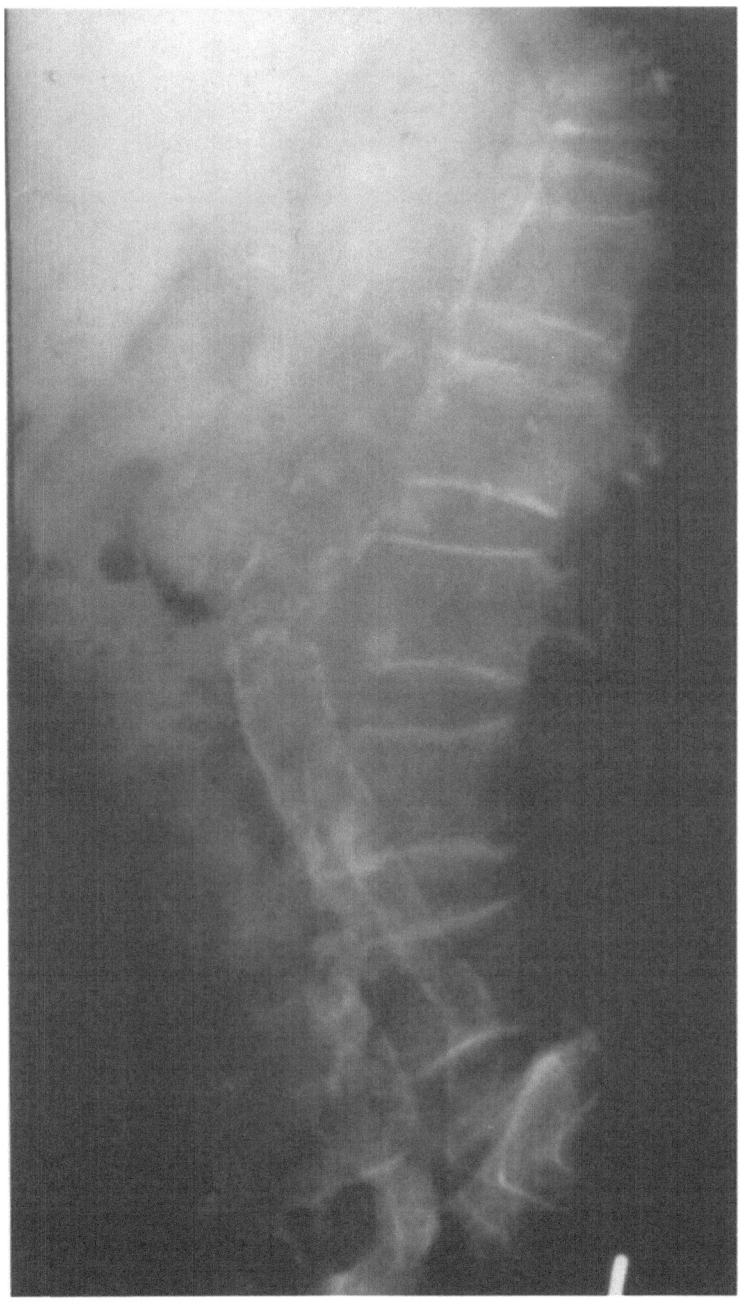

Plate I: Example of a typical media-sclerosis of the abdominal aorta and the iliacal arteries of a woman aged 67 years.

STRUCTURE: PROTEOHORMONE OF THE
                          PARATHYREOID GLANDS (84 AA)

STIMULATION: BY LOW SERUM Ca^{2+} LEVELS

FUNCTION: UPREGULATION OF SERUM Ca^{2+}
                          (TOG.WITH VITAMINE D_3 AND CALCITONIN)

TARGET ORGANS: BONE, KIDNEYS, INTESTINE

Figure 4: Characterization of parathormone.

Parathormone

Vitamine D_3 or parathormone together with cholesterol – rich food are used to develop experimental atherosclerosis (Morrison 1972, Borle 1968, Kramsch 1980, Henry 1985). Vitamine D_3 excess is usually due to drug overdosage and therefore a seldom phenomenon in humans. Parathormone (PTH) excess occurs more frequently as autonomous or reactive hyperfunction of the parathyreoid glands (Raisz 1983, Reichel 1989, Schmidt-Gayk 1990).

The release of this proteohormone is stimulated through a lowered level of ionized calcium in serum. Its purpose is the upregulation of serum calcium by releasing calcium from the bone and stimulating calcium backresorption in the kidneys (Fig. 4) (Raisz 1983).

Parathormone is binding to a membrane receptor and in this way opening the membrane Ca^{2+} channels (Fig. 5). The effect is an increase in intracellular free

Figure 5: Properties and target cells of parathormone.

PROPERTIES: RECEPTOR DEPENDANT **OPENING**
                 OF MEMBRANE Ca^{2+} - **CHANNELS**

                 = **INCREASE IN INTRACELL.** Ca^{2+}

TARGET CELLS: - BONE CELLS
(RECEPTOR POSITIVE)
                     - KIDNEY CELLS

                     - SMOOTH MUSCLE CELLS

                     - FIBROBLASTS

                     - ERYTHROCYTES

calcium. The classical target cells, in which this Ca^{2+} influx takes place, are bone and kidney cells. But also other cells are targets of this effect: It should be emphasized that at least two cell types with PTH-receptors described above, *smooth muscle cells* and *fibroblasts,* are major actors in the arteriosclerotic process as well. Erythrocytes bearing also PTH receptors may be used as simply available test cells. Vitamine D_3, by the way, has a similar distribution of receptor positive cells and is working synergistically with PTH (Borle 1968, Hehrmann 1980, Raisz 1983, Schmidt-Gayk 1990, Karpf 1990).

Parathormone excess and Cholesterol in Humans

As described above a cholesterol rich food together with parathormone or vitamine D_3 produces arteriosclerosis in experimental animals. It has to be asked wether conditions like that may likewise naturally occur in humans and whether those groups present a high prevalence of arteriosclerosis (Fig. 6).

These atherogenetic factors in experimental animals are indeed coming together in patients with terminal renal insufficiency surviving only by means of chronic dialysis treatment (Fig. 6). It is well established that *uraemic patients* exhibit a moderate *hypercholesterolaemia* with an unfavourable ratio between total cholesterol and HDL-cholesterol.

Most of these patients develop *hypocalcaemia* due to a vitamine D_3 deficiency and hyperphosphataemia what again — as mentioned above — is the *stimulus for parathormone excess.* In other words, they demonstrate a high prevalence of reactive *hyperparathyreoidism.*

Figure 6: Synopsis of factors enhancing the calcium influx through calcium channels into cells and possibly thus contributing to atherogenesis (HPT = hyperparathyreoidism = parathormone excess). This constellation of risk factors is frequently found in chronic dialysis patients.

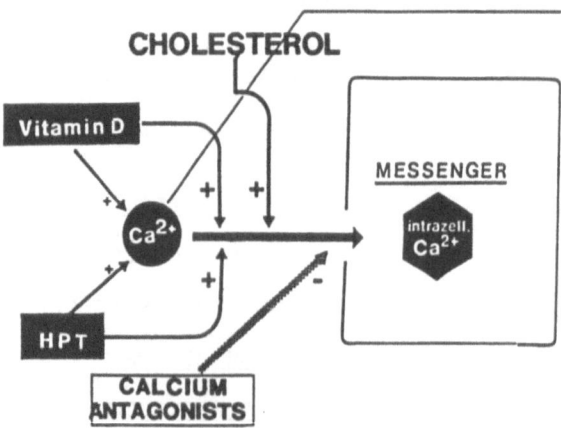

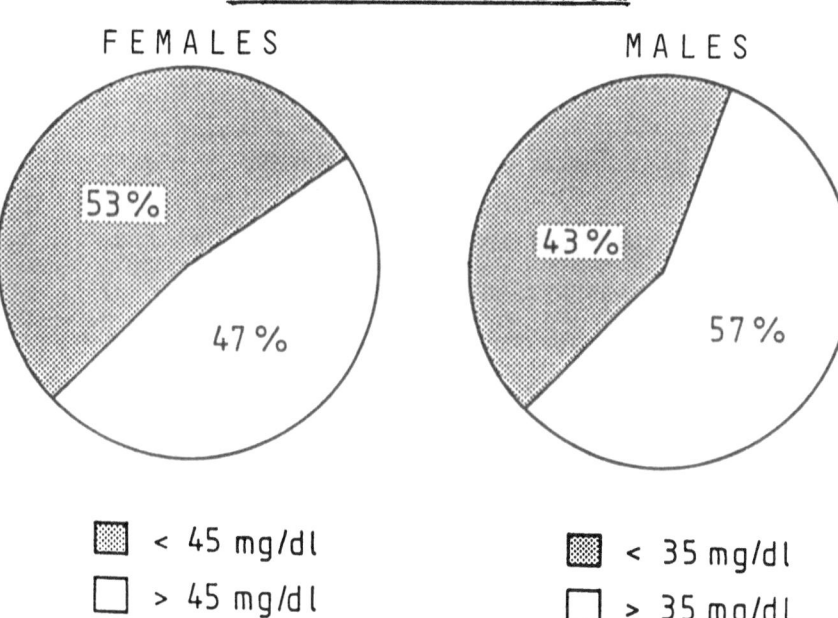

Figure 7: High frequency of lowered HDL-cholesterol levels in 105 male and female dialysis patients.

Finally dialysis patients show a high prevalence of *artiosclerosis* with early onset and rapid progression.

Figure 7 demonstrates an unfavourable level of HDL-cholesterol measured in about 50% of 105 unselected uraemic patients. In more than 50% of this group a total cholesterol level above 220 mg/dl was found. In addition it is remarkable that this hyperlipidaemia is seen likewise in males and females. An impaired lipid metabolism of this kind in uremic patients is confirmed by the results of many other authors (Green 1984, Goldberg 1983, Bagdade 1983, Grützmacher 1984, Hahn 1983, Lindner 1981, Mordasini 1982, Raidt 1987, Ritz 1985, Rapoport 1978, Rostand 1984, Nestel 1982).

It is well established that uremic patients undergoing dialysis have a very high prevalence of severe AS (Lindner 1981, Nestel 1982, Goldberg 1983, Brunner 1979, 1985, Bagdade 1983, Hahn 1983, Green 1983, Grützmacher 1984, Rostand 1984, Ritz 1985, Raidt 1987).

Therefore it was not surprising to find in a retrospective analysis of 215 uremic patients with a mean age of 45 years (range 17–73 years) and a mean dialysis treatment of 65 months *47 patients (22%) with moderate AS and 67 patients (31%) with severe AS*. 44 patients of the latter group had already suffered from myocardial infarction, in the remainder severe AS was ascertained by stroke

HYPERPARATHYREOIDISM (HPT) AND ACCELERATED

ARTERIOSCLEROSIS (AS) IN UREMIC PATIENTS

----

215 DIALYSIS PATIENTS (MEAN AGE 45 YEARS,
MEAN TIME ON RENAL REPLACEMENT THERAPY 65 MONTHS)

GROUP I   (WITHOUT ARTERIOSCLEROSIS)   N = 101

GROUP II   (MODERATE ARTERIOSCLEROSIS)   N = 47

GROUP III (SEVERE ARTERIOSCLEROSIS)   N = 67
     (SUBGROUP: MYOCARDIAL INFARCTION   N = 44)

HYPERPARATHYREOIDISM   N = 87/215

Figure 8: Long term observation of 215 dialysis patients demonstrating moderate or severe arteriosclerosis in 53%. All 67 patients with severe AS (group III) had already suffered from diseases secondary to AS, for example 44 patients from myocardial infarction.
87 of the 215 patients (40.4%) had developed secondary hyperparathyreoidism.

events, peripheral arterial occlusive disease, angiography or during surgery (Fig. 8) (Raidt 1987).

Parallel to that we revealed a prevalence of hyperparathyreoidism (PTH-excess) in 87 patients (40.5%) (Fig. 8). Such a high rate of secondary HPT is found in all dialysis populations, since nearly all uremic patients develop calcium-phosphate imbalance which again is the stimulus for PTH-excess (Slatopolsky 1980, Hehrmann 1980, Rambausek 1982, Green 1983, Raidt 1987).

Only to demonstrate the enormous prevalence of AS in dialysis patients Figure 9 presents a rough comparison of the myocardial infarction rate in the Münster-PROCAM-study and in our dialysis-study in the same region. The PROCAM study on 1674 males aged 40–65 years recorded 45 infarction events over a period of 4 years, whereas in only 215 male and female dialysis patients nearly the same amount of 41 infarction events was observed over 7.4 years (Assmann 1980, 1983, Raidt 1987).

This is even true for the total European dialysis and transplant population of about 80.000 patients annually registered in the EDTA registry also with their secondary diseases. In 1978 and again in 1985 their annual rate of letal myocardial infarctions was compared with that of the general population of the FRG (Fig. 10).

This data revealed a 173 times higher relative risk for young kidney patients to expire with letal infarction as compared to the general population. For patients between 35 and 54 years the risk is 20 times and for patients over 54 years still 10 times higher (Brunner 1979, 1985).

MYOCARDIAL INFARCTION RATE

PROCAM STUDY   VS   DIALYSIS PATIENTS

MYOCARDIAL INFARCTION

	YES	NO	TOTAL
PROCAM (*MALES, 40-65 years*)	45 (2.7%)	1629 (97.3%)	1674
DIALYSIS PTS (*MALES,FEMALES, mean age 45 y*)	41 ** (19%)	174 (81%)	215

Figure 9: Comparison of the myocardial infartion rate in the Münster-PROCAM-study (only males, 4 years follow up) and the dialysis-study Münster (males *and* females, 7.4 years follow up) showing an infarction rate in dialysis pts. high above the expected level (**). (Assmann 1980, 1983, Raidt 1987).

Figure 10: Comparison of the letal myocardial infarction (MI) rate in the Western German general population and the European dialysis and transplant population of about 80.000 patients and the elevated relative MI-risk for the latter in different age groups. (mod. Brunner 1979, 1985).

ANNUAL LETAL MYOCARDIAL INFARCTIONS PER 1000 INHABITANTS

mod.EDTA 1978

	AGE		
	15 - 34	**35 - 54**	**> 54**
TOTAL POPULATION F R G	0.015	0.5	2.7
DIALYSIS/TRANSPLANT EUROPE	2.6	10.0	25.1
RELATIVE RISK	173x	20x	9.3x

Arteriosclerosis and Parathormone Excess (HPT)

If dialysis patients have a high prevalence of AS on one hand and HPT on the other, the question will arise whether or not these conditions are connected with each other (Horsch 1981, Grützmacher 1986).

As Figure 11 points out they indeed are statistically coincident: The group with HPT demonstrates a significant higher rate of AS than the group without PTH-excess. Also myocardial infarctions were more frequent in the HPT-group (28% vs. 16%) (not significant in our population: p = 0.051).

Multifactorial discriminant analyses are used to find out stepwise which risk factor is the most relevant, the next relevant and so on, to classify people with or without a given attribute correctly to their subgroups. The result of this meanwhile common biostatistical tool is a list of the relative *statistical weight* of several risk factors.

Figure 11: Statistical coincidence of hyperparathyreoidism (HPT) with a high prevalence of arteriosclerotic disease (AS) in 215 dialysis patients (Raidt 1987).

ARTERIOSCLEROSIS (AS)

HYPERPARATHYREOIDISM (HPT)

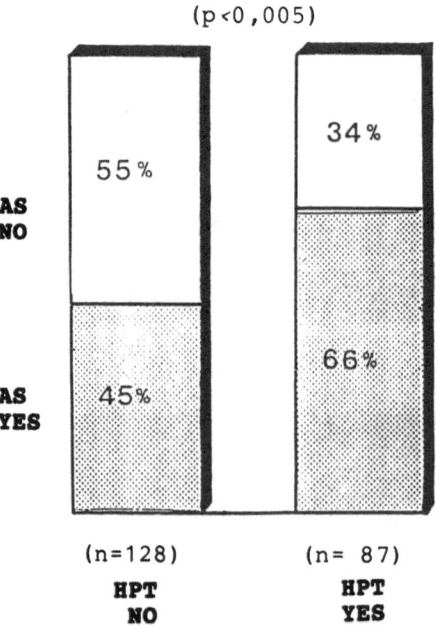

(p<0,005)

To discriminate in our patients between those without AS and those with severe AS hyperparathyreoidism (HPT) was the third strongest factor for the whole group after age and diabetes as shown in the left column of Figure 12 and the strongest differentiating factor for patients of medium age and those without hypertension as demonstrated in the middle and right column of Figure 12 (Raidt 1987).

Conclusions

All these observations suggest that dialysis patients may be a suitable "model" to study the influence of calcium on atherogenesis. But nevertheless, is this model, bearing several metabolic abnormities due to uremia, really comparable to conditions found in the general population?

First of all it is a *human model* similar to those of familiar homocystinuria or genetic receptor defects in lipid metabolism. Therefore this may be another chance to find more marked risk factors of AS (Assmann 1982).

The special features ·of uremic patients, severe calcium imbalance, PTH excess, moderate hypercholesterolemia and premature AS are described uniformly in all dialysis populations (Green 1983).

Since geriatric medicine is developing as own subspeciality more attention is paid to particular conditions in the elderly. Several authors describe an apparently very frequent rise of PTH serum levels in older and otherwise healthy people. This is probably due to a relative vitamine D_3 deficiency in part caused by low sex hormone levels. In addition some authors found elevated PTH levels patients with

Figure 12: Stepwise discriminant analyses to evaluate the relative statistical risk of probably atherogenic factors in 215 dialysis patients. Only patients with ascertained severe AS (n = 67, group III) were compared with 101 pts. without AS (group I). HPT (hyperparathyreoidism = PTH-excess) seems to be one of the most valid factors for the whole group (left column), for the medium aged (middle column) and for those with normal blood pressure (BP) (right column) (Raidt 1987).

DISCRIMINANT ANALYSIS OF ATHEROGENIC RISK FACTORS

A R T E R I O S C L E R O S I S

NO/SEVERE	NO/SEVERE (AGED 35-54Y)	NO/SEVERE (NORMAL BP)
1 AGE	1 HPT	1 HPT
2 DIABETES	2 DIABETES	2 DIABETES
3 HPT	3 TIME ON RRT	3 HEMATOCRITE
4 CALCIUM	4 HYPERTENSION	4 TIME ON RRT
5 DURATION OF RENAL DISEASE	5 HEMATOCRITE	5 HYPERTENSION BEFORE RRT

essential hypertension (Parrot-Garcia 1984, Krall 1989, Petersen 1983, Sokoll 1988, Oster 1990).

Finally several older and recent studies support the hypothesis that Ca^{2+} channel blockers may prevent the progression of AS also in humans *at normal doses*. This emphasizes the role of elevated intracellular Ca^{2+} as important co-factor or mediator to primary atherogenetic agents (Kramsch 1980, Henry 1985, Lichtlen 1990). Moreover it seems promising to investigate other factors opening the Ca^{2+} channels besides PTH in arteriosclerotic subjects.

Calcium imbalance is probably of some influence on atherogenesis and therefore more extensive studies on the beneficial effect of calcium channel blockers as antiatherogenetic agents may be useful (Lichtlen 1990).

Another clinical implication of the data presented here is the demand of careful monitoring calcium and vitamine D therapy of postmenopausal bone loss. Up to now it is not safely excluded that this may promote atherogenesis.

At least we believe that further research on the premature and rapidly progredient AS of uremic patients is worthwile, since the observation time in intervention studies may be shortened due to more rapid atherogenesis and since they present their network of atherogenetic risk factors much more pronounced than the general population.

References

[1] Assmann, G., Oberwittler, W., Schulte, H., Schriewer, H., Funke, H., Epping, P.H., Hauss, W.H.: Prädiktion und Früherkennung der koronaren Herzkrankheit − Prospektive epidemiologische Studie bei Betriebsangehörigen im Raum Westfalen. Internist. 1980; 21: 446−459.

[2] Assmann, G.: Lipid metabolism and atherosclerosis. Schattauer Stuttgart, New York 1982.

[3] Assmann, G., Schulte, H.: Prediction and early detection of coronary heart disease. Rhein.-Westfäl. Akad. der Wissenschaften. Abhandlung Bd. 70, Westdeutscher Verlag 1983.

[4] Bagdade, J.D.: Hyperlipidemia and atherosclerosis in chronic dialysis patients. In: Drukker, W. et al. (Ed.): Replacement of renal function by dialysis. Martinus Nijhoff Publ. Bosten, Den Haag 1983; II. Edition: 588−594.

[5] Borle, A.B.: Calcium metabolism in hela cells and the effects of parathyreoid hormone. Journal Cell. Biol. 1968; 36: 567−582.

[6] Brunner, F.P., Brynger, H., Chantler, C., Donckerwolcke, R.A., Hathway, R.A., Jacobs, C., Selwood, N.H., Wing, A.J.: Combined report on regular dialysis and transplantation in Europe IX, 1978: Proc. EDTA 1979; 16: 2−70.

[7] Cavallero, C., Di Tondo, U., Mingazzini, P., Pesando, P., Spagnoli, L.: Cell proliferation in the atherosclerotic lesions of cholesterol-fed rabbits. Atherosclerosis 1973; 17: 49−62.

[8] Cheung, J.Y., Bonventre, J.V., Malis, C.D., Leaf, A.: Calcium and ischemic injury. N. Engl. J. Med. 1986; 314: 1670−1676.

[9] Fleckenstein, A., Tritthard, H., Fleckenstein, B., Herbst, A., Grün, G.: A new group of competitive Ca-antagonists (Iproveratril, D600, Prenylamine) with highly potent inhibitory effects on excitation-contractation coupling in mammalian myocardium. Pflügers Arch. Ges. Physiol. 1969; 307: R 25.

[10] Fleckenstein, A.: Calcium antagonism: history and prospects for a multifacted pharmacodynamic principle. In: Calcium antagonists and cardiovascular Disease; Opie LH (Ed.), Raven Press. New York 1984; 9–28.

[11] Fleckenstein, A., Frey, M., Zorn, J., Fleckenstein-Grün, G.: Antihypertensive anticalcitonische und antiarteriosklerotische Effekte von Calcium-Antagonisten. Modell-Experimente an spontan-hypertensiven Ratten (SHR). In: Distler A. (Ed.): Calcium-Antagonisten in der Hochdrucktherapie. Schattauer-Verlag Stuttgart, New York 1986; 3–24.

[12] Goldberg, A.P., Harter, H.R., Patsch, W., Schechtman, K.B., Province, M., Weerts, C., Kuisk, I., McCrate, M.: Racial differences in plasma high density lipoproteins in patients receiving hemodialysis. N. Engl. J. Med. 1983; 308: 1245–1252.

[13] Green, D., Stone, N.J., Krumlovsky, F.A.: Putative atherogenic factors in patients with chronic renal failure. Prog. Cardiovasc. Dis. 1983; 26: 133–144.

[14] Grützmacher, P., Radtke, H.W., Schieferdecker, E., Peschke, B., Riepenhausen, J., Fassbinder, W., Schoeppe, W.: Early changes of plasma lipid status and glucose tolerance during the course of chronical renal failure. Contr. Nephrol. 1984; 41: 332–336.

[15] Grützmacher, P.: Is hyperparathyroidism a risk factor for atherosclerosic disease in RDT patients. Nephrol. Dial. Transplant. 1986; 1: 122–123.

[16] Hahn, R., Oette, K., Mondorf, H., Finke, K., Sieberth, H.G.: Analysis of cardiovascular risk factors in chronic hemodialysis patients with special attention to the hyperlipoproteinamias. Atherosclerosis 1983; 48: 279–288.

[17] Hauss, W.H.: Über Entstehung und Verhütung der Arteriosklerose. Arbeitsgemeinschaft für Forschung des Landes NRW, Heft N 197: 7–33. Westdeutscher Verlag Köln-Opladen 1970.

[18] Hehrmann, R.: Plasma-Parathormon: Methodik, Pathphysiologie und Klinik. Urban & Schwarzenberg Verlag München–Wien 1980.

[19] Henry, P.D.: Atherosclerosis, calcium and calcium antagonists. Circulation 1985; 72: 456–569.

[20] Henry, P.D., Bentley, K.I.: Suppression of atherogenesis in cholesterol-fed rabbit treated with nifedipine. J. Clin. Invest. 1981; 68: 1366–1369.

[21] Hirata, Y., Yoshimi, H., Takata, S., Watanabe, T.X., Kumegai, S., Nakajima, K., Sakakibara, S.: Cellular mechanism of action by a novel vasoconstrictor endothelin in cultured rat vascular smooth muscle cells. Biochem. Biophys. Res. Commun. 1988; 154: 868–875.

[22] Horsch, A., Ritz, E., Heuck, C.C., Hofmann, W., Kühne, E., Bisson, M.: Atherogenesis in experimental uremia. Atherosis 1981; 40: 279–289.

[23] Kai, H., Kanaide, H., Nakamura, M.: Endothelin-sensitive intracellular Ca store overlaps with caffeine-sensitive one in rat aortic smooth muscle cells in primary culture. Biochem. Biophys. Res. Commun. 1989; 158: 235–243.

[24] Karpf, D.B., Bambino, T., Arnaud, D.C., Nissenson, R.A.: Molecular determinants of parathyroid hormone receptor function. In: Cohn, D.V., Charieur, F.H., Martin, T.J. (Ed.): Calcium regulation and bone metabolism, Elsevier Science Publishers 1990.

[25] Krall, E.A., Sahyoun, N., Tannenbaum, S., Dallai, G.E., Dawson-Hughes, B.: Effect of vitamin D intake on seasonal variations in parathyreiod hormone secretion in postmenopausal women. N. Engl. J. Med. 1989; 321: 1777–1783.

[26] Kramsch, D.M., Aspen, A.J., Apstein, C.S.: Suppression of experimental atherosclerosis by the Ca-Antagonist Lanthanum. J. Clin. Invest. 1980; 65: 976–981.

[27] Lichtlen, P.R., Hugenholtz, P.G., Raffenbeul, W., Hecker, H., Jost, S., Deckers, J.W.: Retardation of angiographic progression of coronary artery disease by nifedipine. Lancet 1990; 335: 1109–1113.

[28] Lindner, A., Haas, L., Sherrard, D.J.: Atherosclerosis in uremia. "The seattle experience re-visited". Panel conference Trans. ASAIO 1981; XXVII: 669–670.

[29] Mordasini, R.: Sekundäre Hyperlipoproteinämien bei chronischen Nierenkrankheiten. Verlag Hans Huber Bern–Stuttgart–Wien 1982.

[30] Morrisson, L.M., Bajwa, G.S., Alfin-Slater, R.B., Ershoff, B.H.: Prevention of vascular lesions by chondroitin sulfate a in the coronary artery and aorta of rats induced by a hypervitaminosis D, cholesterol-containing diet. Atherosclerosis 1972; 16: 105–118.

[31] Müller, O.A., van Werder, K.: Rezeptorstörungen in der Endokrinologie. Internist. 1988; 29: 445–454.

[32] Mundy, G.R.: Calcium homeostasis: hypercalcemia and hypocalcemia. Martin Dunitz, London 1989; 149.

[33] Nestel, P.J., Fidge, N.H., Tan M.H.: Increased lipoprotein-remnant formation in chronic renal failure. N. Engl. J. Med. 1982; 307: 329–333.

[34] Oster, P., Müller, T., Schmidt-Gayk, H., Schlierf, G.: Parathyreoid hormone, 25-hyroxyvitamin D and 1,25-dihydroxy-vitamin D concentration in elderly patients. Klin. Wochenschr. 1990; 68: 421–426.

[35] Parrot-Garcia, M., McCarron, D.A.: Calcium and hypertension. Nutrition Rev. 1984; 42: 205–213.

[36] Petersen, M.M., Briggs, R.S., Ashby, M.A., Reid, R.I., Hall, M.R., Wood, P.J., Clayton, B.E.: Parathyreoid hormone and 25-hydrxyvitamin D concentrations in sick and normal elderly people. Brit. Med. J. 1983; 287: 521–523.

[37] Raidt, H.: Untersuchungen zur Atherogenese bei dialysepflichtiger Niereninsuffizienz. Habilitationsschrift; Universität Münster 1987.

[38] Raidt, H., Langer, K., Baumgarten, F. et al.: Hyperparathyreoidism and accelerated arteriosclerosis in uraemic patients. Nephrol. Dial. Transplant. 1987; 2: 418.

[39] Raisz, L.G., Kream, B.E.: Regulation of bone formation. N. Engl. J. Med. 1983; 1: 29–35.

[40] Rambausek, M., Ritz, E., Rascher, W., Kreusser, W., Mann, J.F.E., Kreye, V.A.W., Mehls, O.: Vascular effects of paratyreiod hormone. Adv. Exp. Med. Biol. 1982; 151: 619–632.

[41] Rapoport, J., Aviram, M., Chaimovitz, C., Brook, J.G.: Defective high-density lipoprotein composition in patients on chronic hemodialysis. N. Engl. J. Med. 1978; 299: 1326–1329.

[42] Rasmussen, H.: The calcium messenger system. First part. N. Engl. J. Med. 1986; 314: 1094–1101.

[43] Rasmussen, H.: The calcium messenger system Second Part. N. Engl. J. Med. 1986; 314: 1164–1170.

[44] Reichel, H., Koeffler, H.P., Norman, A.W.: The role of the vitamin D endocrine system in health and disease. N. Engl. J. Med. 1989; 320: 980–991.

[45] Ritz, E., Augustin, J., Bommer, J., Gnasso, A., Haberbosch, W.: Should hyperlipidemia of renal failure be treated? Kidney Int. 1985; 28, Suppl.: 84–87.

[46] Ross, R.: The pathogenesis of atherosclerosis an update. N. Engl. J. Med. 1986; 314: 488–500.

[47] Rostand, S.G., Kirk, K.A., Rutsky, E.A.: Dialysis-associated ischemic heart disease: Insights from coronary angiography. Kidney Int. 1984; 25: 653–659.

[48] Rüegg, J.C.: Calcium in muscle activation. Springer-Verlag Berlin, Heidelberg, New York 1986.

[49] Slatopolsky, E., Martin, K., Hruska, K.: Parathyreoid hormone metabolism and its potential role as a uremic toxin. Am. J. Physiol. 1980; 239: 1–11.

[50] Snyder, S.H., Reynolds, I.J.: Calcium-antagonist drugs: Receptor-interactions that clarify therapeutic effects. N. Engl. J. Med. 1985; 313: 995–1002.

[51] Sokoll, L.J., Morrow, F.D., Quirbach, D.M., Dawson-Hughes, B.: Intact parathyrin in postmenopausal women. Clin. Chem. 1988; 34: 407–410.

[52] Sugiura, M., Inagami, T., Hare, G.M.T., Johns, J.A.: Endothelin action: Inhibition by a proteinkinase C inhibitor and involvement of phosphoinositols. Biochem. Biophys. Res. Commun. 1989; 58: 170–176.

[53] Yanagisawa, M., Inoue, A., Ischikawa, T., Kasuya, Y, Kimura, S., Kumagaye, S.I., Nakjima, K., Watanabe, T.X., Sakakibara, S., Goto, K., Masaki, T.: Promary structure, synthesis and biological activity of rat endothelin, an endothelium-derived vasoconstrictor peptide. Proc. Natl. Acad. Sci. USA 1988; 85: 6964–6967.

14

Nicht-medikamentöse Therapie von ventrikulären Tachyarrhythmien

Günter Breithardt, Martin Borggrefe, Christine Hief,
Michael Block und H.H. Scheld*
Medizinische Klinik und Poliklinik,
Innere Medizin C (Kardiologie/Angiologie)
und *Klinik für Herz-, Thorax- und Gefäßchirurgie,
Westfälische Wilhelms-Universität Münster

Während der letzten zehn Jahre sind die Probleme und Limitierungen der medikamentösen antiarrhythmischen Therapie bewußt geworden [1, 2]. Bei Patienten mit dokumentierten anhaltenen Kammertachykardien oder Kammerflimmern, die nicht während der Akutphase eines frischen Infarktes aufgetreten sind, wird die medikamentöse antiarrhythmische Therapie üblicherweise durch serielle elektrophysiologische Testungen auf ihre Wirksamkeit überprüft [3, 4]. Unglücklicherweise sprechen jedoch nur etwa 30% der Patienten während serieller elektrophysiologischer Testungen auf Antiarrhythmika an [1, 3, 4]. Insbesondere bei Patienten mit einer eingeschränkten linksventrikulären Funktion läßt sich wesentlich seltener ein Antiarrhythmikum finden, welches die Auslösbarkeit der Tachykardien unterdrückt oder zumindest erschwert, als bei Patienten mit guter linksventrikulärer Funktion [5]. Aufgrund von Verlaufsbeobachtungen bieten sich serielle elektrophysiologische Untersuchungen dafür an, einerseits diejenigen Patienten zu identifizieren, bei denen unter antiarrhythmischer Therapie eine gute Prognose zu erwarten ist, andererseits solche Patienten, die trotz antiarrhythmischer Therapie eine hohe Sterblichkeit, insbesondere als Folge von rhythmusbedingten Komplikationen aufweisen. Das Bestreben geht dahin, bei letzteren Patienten neue Interventionstechniken wie Katheterablation, gezielte antitachykarde Operation und implantierbare Kardioverter/Defibrillatoren einzusetzen [6, 7, 8].

Indikation für nicht-medikamentöse antiarrhythmische Therapie

Die Hauptindikation für nicht-medikamentöse antiarrhythmische Maßnahmen sind:

1. vorangegangener Herzstillstand
2. hämodynamisch beeinträchtigende anhaltende Kammertachykardie.

Beide Rhythmusstörungen sollten außerhalb der Akutphase eines Infarktes (aus rhythmologischer Sicht nach mehr als 48 Stunden) aufgetreten sein, da dann mit einer hohen Rezidivquote zu rechnen ist. Zusätzlich sollten sich diese Rhythmusstörungen als medikamentös therapieresistent erwiesen haben, und die Lebenserwartung des Patienten sollte mindestens sechs Monate betragen. Es ist bisher nicht entschieden, ob auch asymptomatische Kammertachykardien, die somit nicht zu hämodynamischen Beeinträchtigungen oder sogar zu Synkopen oder Herzstillstand geführt haben, in der gleichen Weise behandelt werden sollen.

Die nicht-medikamentöse Therapie kann in kurative Verfahren (z.B. Katheterablation oder gezielte antitachykarde Operation) und palliative Verfahren (z.B. implantierbare Kardioverter/Defibrillatoren oder antitachykarde Schrittmacher mit sog. "back-up" Kardioversion/Defibrillation) eingeteilt werden. Im letzteren Fall treten die Tachykardien auf und werden durch antitachykardie Stimulation oder Defibrillation beendet.

Der Nucleus der Arbeitsgruppe "Arrhythmien" der Deutschen Gesellschaft für Herz- und Kreislaufforschung hat kürzlich Empfehlungen zur Implantation von Defibrillatoren verabschiedet,, die bald veröffentlicht werden [9]. Diese Indikationen unterscheiden zwischen gesicherten, möglichen und "keinen" Indikationen. Diese drei verschiedenen Kategorien der Implantationsstellung, die durch die Autoren etwas modifiziert worden sind, sind in den Tabellen 1 bis 3 wiedergegeben.

Tabelle 1: "Gesicherte Indikationen" für die Implantation eines Kardioverter/Defibrillators (ICD) auf der Basis der Empfehlungen des Nucleus der Arbeitsgruppe "Arrhythmiediagnostik" der Deutschen Gesellschaft für Herz- und Kreislaufforschung".

Indikationen für ICD

A. gesicherte Indikationen:

anhaltende Kammertachykardie mit hämodynamischer Beeinträchtigung oder primäres Kammerflimmern oder Flimmern

- eine oder mehrere Episoden, induzierbar
- mindestens zwei Episoden, nicht-induzierbar
- eine Episode, nicht-induzierbar, eingeschränkte linksventrikuläre Funktion oder positive Familienanamnese im Hinblick auf akuten Herztod

wenn

- nicht während der Akutphase eines Infarktes auftretend
- keine behebbare Ursache vorliegt (Medikamente, Elektrolytstörungen, Ischämie, Herzinsuffizienz)
- refraktär gegenüber Antiarrhythmika oder hierunter nicht tolerable Nebenwirkungen
- kein Kandidat für Katheterablation oder antitachykarde Operation

---

Tabelle 2: "Mögliche Indikationen" für die Implantation eines Kardioverter/Defibrillators (ICD) auf der Basis der Empfehlungen des Nucleus der Arbeitsgruppe "Arrhythmiediagnostik" der Deutschen Gesellschaft für Herz- und Kreislaufforschung".

Indikationen für ICD

B. Mögliche Indikationen

- ansonsten nicht erklärbare Synkopen bei induzierbaren monomorphen Kammertachykardien (Kammerflimmern?), therapieresistent gegenüber Antiarrhythmika und nicht geeignet für Katheterablation oder antitachykarde Chirurgie
- nach erfolgloser gezielter antitachykarder Operation mit weiterhin auslösbaren (klinischen) Kammertachykardien
- als "Back-up"-Behandlung unter Antiarrhythmika oder nach antitachykarder Operation, wenn der Erfolg dieser Maßnahmen nicht eindeutig zu sichern ist

Tabelle 3: Situationen, bei denen "keine Indikation" für die Implantation eines Kardioverter/Defibrillators (ICD) gesehen wird, basierend auf den Empfehlungen vorläufiger Vorschläge des Nucleus der Arbeitsgruppe "Arrhythmiediagnostik" der Deutschen Gesellschaft für Herz- und Kreislaufforschung".

Indikationen für ICD

C. Keine Indikationen
- Kammertachykardien mit keinen oder nur geringen Symptomen
- nicht-anhaltende Kammertachykardien
- medikamenten-induzierte Kammertachykardie oder Kammerflimmern (arrhythmogene Wirkung)
- Synkopen ohne induzierbare Kammertachykardien oder -flimmern
- hartnäckige ("incessant") Kammertachykardien oder sehr häufig auftretende Anfälle
- behebbare Ursache der Kammertachykardien oder des -flimmerns
- Kammertachykardie/-flimmern, welches einer Katheterablation oder einer antitachykardien Chirurgie zugänglich ist
- schwere Begleiterkrankungen
- Herzinsuffizienz im Stadium IV (NYHA)

Es ist vorgeschlagen worden, den implantierbaren Kardioverter/Defibrillator als eine Überbrückungsmaßnahme bis zu einer späteren Herztransplantation bei Patienten mit erheblich eingeschränkter linksventrikulärer Funktion und ventrikulären Arrhythmien, die im Augenblick zu "gut" für eine sofortige Transplantation sind, einzusetzen. Diese Patienten haben eine verhältnismäßig hohe Häufigkeit des akuten Herztodes, wenn sie (nur) mit Antiarrhythmika behandelt werden. Diese spezielle Patientengruppe verlangt in Zukunft sicherlich größerer Beachtung.
    Es erscheint wichtig zu betonen, daß keine Indikation für die Implantation eines Kardioverter/Defibrillators existiert, wenn Kammertachykardien oder Kammerflimmern einer Katheterablation oder einer gezielten antitachykarden Operation zugänglich sind [9, 10]. Somit sollte zunächst ein kuratives (operatives oder

abladierendes) Vorgehen in Betracht gezogen werden, bevor die Entscheidung zur
Implantation eines Defibrillators gefällt wird.

Verschiedene Parameter beeinflussen den Entscheidungsprozeß. Diese beziehen
sich auf die Frage, ob die zugrunde liegende Herzerkrankung durch chirurgische
Maßnahmen (z.B. Aneurysmektomie und/oder Bypass-Implantation) verbessert
oder korrigiert werden kann. In diesem Fall ist wichtig zu wissen, ob ein umschrie-
benes arrhythmogenes Substrat, das durch endokardiales Kathetermapping oder
intraoperatives Mapping lokalisiert werden kann, vorliegt. Gelingt es, den "Ursprungsort" der Kammertachykardie auf diese Weise zu lokalisieren, stellt dies
eine wichtige Voraussetzung für eine gezielte antitachykarde Operation unter Einsatz des intraoperativen Mappings dar. Grundsätzlich muß das Risiko der einzelnen zur Verfügung stehenden Interventionen gegeneinander abgewogen werden,
wobei bei operativen Maßnahmen vor allem das Ausmaß der linksventrikulären
Funktionsstörung entscheidend ist [11].

Bei der Entscheidung zur Implantation eines Kardioverter/Defibrillators müssen
auch die psychologischen Folgen berücksichtigt werden, die bei u.U. häufig notwendigen Schockabgaben auftreten können. In manchen Fällen gelingt es, die
Häufigkeit dieser Attacken durch eine begleitende antiarrhythmische Therapie zu
reduzieren. Die Bedeutung psychologischer Beeinträchtigungen sind durch Cooper
und Mitarbeiter aufgezeichnet worden [12]. Ein großer Teil ihrer Patienten berich-
tete über anhaltende Angst vor der Schockabgabe, über tägliches Bewußtsein des
implantierten Gerätes und über Angst vor vorzeitiger Batterieerschöpfung. Viele
Patienten zeigten eine verminderte Aktivität und Abnahme oder Abstinenz bei
sexueller Aktivität. Dieses Spektrum an psychischen Störungen dürfte sich in der
Zukunft bei immer vielseitigeren Geräten verringern lassen, derzeit stellt es jedoch
noch ein ernstes Problem dar. Schließlich sollten die Kosten einer Implantation
und eines Geräteaustausches berücksichtigt werden [13, 14].

Durch die jetzt zur Verfügung stehenden Geräte, die antitachykarde Stimulation mit Kardioversion/Defibrillation verbinden [15, 16], dürften auch häufige
Anfälle von Kammertachykardien kein großes Problem mehr darstellen, wenn
diese zuverlässig durch antitachykarde Stimulation beendet werden können. Im
Falle einer Akzeleration der Tachykardie steht dann die "Back-up" Kardioversion/
Defibrillation zur Verfügung. Situationen, in denen die Implantation eines Kardio-
verter/Defibrillators vorzuziehen ist, liegen bei Fehlen eines lokalisierbaren arrhythmogenen Substrates, bei wegen ihrer hohen Frequenz durch Kathetermapping und intraoperatives Mapping nicht lokalisierbaren Kammertachykardien, bei
nicht-auslösbaren Kammertachykardien, bei diffuser linksventrikulärer Funktionsstörung und bei einer vorangegangenen, erfolglosen antitachykarden Operation
vor. Argumente zugunsten einer Katheterablation sind schwerwiegende Begleiterkrankungen, das Alter des Patienten, eine sehr schlechte linksventrikuläre Funktion und eine verhältnismäßig langsame Frequenz der Kammertachykardie. Auch
wenn Patienten mit nur einer Morphologie der Kammertachykardie die idealen
Kandidaten für eine Lokalisationsdiagnostik (Mapping) sind, können auch Patien-

ten mit mehreren Morphologien und damit der Möglichkeit verschiedener Ursprungsorte erfolgreich durch Katheterablation behandelt werden [17].

Algorithmus für nicht-medikamentöse antiarrhythmische Maßnahmen

Der Algorithmus, den wir während der letzten Jahre bei Patienten mit entweder anhaltenden und/oder induzierbaren Kammertachykardien oder Kammerflimmern trotz antiarrhythmischer Therapie oder bei Patienten mit sog. hartnäckigen ("incessant") Kammertachykardien zugrunde gelegt haben, ist in Abbildung 1 und 2 dargestellt. Die Hauptkriterien in diesem Algorithmus sind das Ausmaß der linksventrikulären Funktionsstörung und die Möglichkeit des Kathetermappings, um den sog. Ursprungsort der Kammertachykardie zu lokalisieren. Bei denjenigen Patienten, bei denen eine primäre Indikation für eine Herzoperation wegen z.B. eines großen Vorderwandaneurysmas und einer begleitenden Zwei- oder Dreigefäßerkrankung besteht, wird die Entscheidung für die begleitende anti-

Abb. 1: Algorithmus für die nicht-medikamentöse Therapie anhaltender Kammertachykardien oder von Kammerflimmern (außerhalb der Akutphase des Infarktes auftretend) bei Patienten mit induzierbaren Kammertachykardien, die nicht auf eine medikamentöse antiarrhythmische Therapie ansprechen. Zum Vorgehen bei Patienten mit dokumentierter Kammertachykardie, die im Rahmen elektrophysiologischer Untersuchungen nicht auslösbar ist, siehe Tabelle 1. Abkürzungen: KT = Kammertachykardie; KF = Kammerflimmern; LV = linker Ventrikel; ICD = implantierbarer Kardioverter/Defibrillator; HTP oder HTX = Herztransplantation.

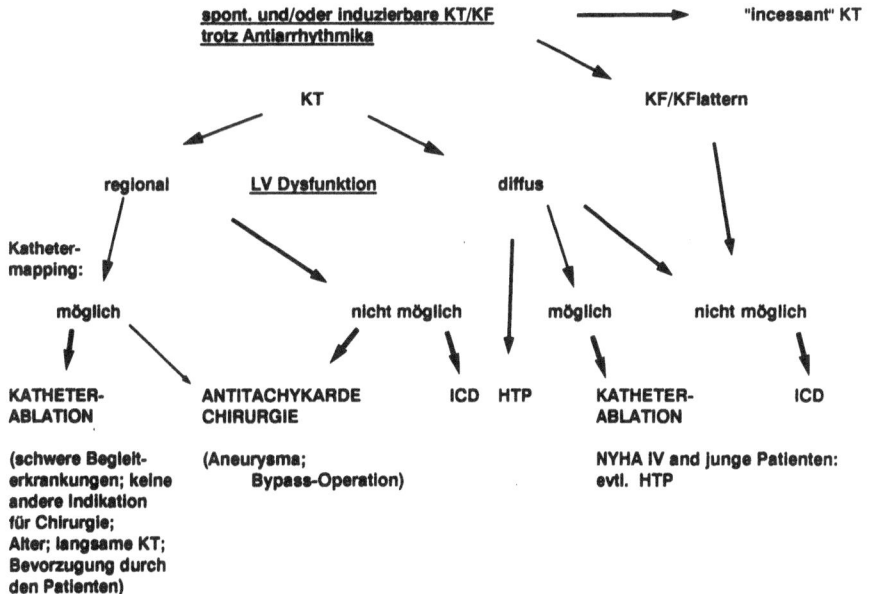

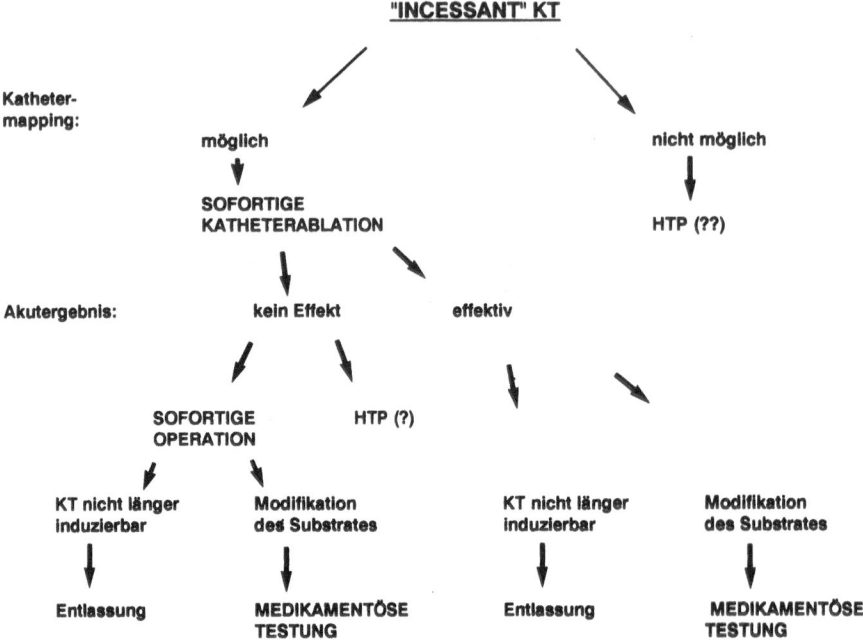

Abb. 2: Algorithmus für die nicht-medikamentöse Therapie von anhaltenden Kammertachykardien oder von Kammerflimmern (außerhalb der Akutphase des Infarktes auftretend) bei
Patienten, die medikamentös therapieresistent sind und die sog. hartnäckige ("incessant")
Kammertachykardien haben. "Incessant" Kammertachykardie wird definiert als eine Tachykardie, die entweder durch Stimulation oder Kardioversion nicht beendet werden kann, oder
die zwar kurzfristig beendet werden kann, aber nach im allgemeinen wenigen Sinusaktionen
wieder anfängt, und die während mehr als 50% der Zeit vorhanden ist. Abkürzungen: siehe
Abb. 1.

tachykarde Chirurgie nach sorgfältiger präoperativer elektrophysiologischer und
angiographischer Diagnostik gestellt. Bei allen anderen Patienten wird erst ver-
sucht, eine wirksame medikamentöse antiarrhythmische Therapie durch serielle
elektrophysiologische Testung herauszufinden [3, 4]. Dieser Algorithmus sieht auf
den ersten Blick sehr einleuchtend aus; es sollte aber nicht vergessen werden, daß
die Entscheidung im Einzelfall auf der Basis zahlreicher zusätzlicher klinischer
Kriterien und unter Berücksichtigung auch der Einstellung der Patienten gefällt
wird.

Literatur

[1] Breithardt, G., Borggrefe, M., Zipes, D.P.: Current aspects of pharmacological and non-pharmacological therapy of tachyarrhythmias. In: Breithardt, G., Borggrefe, M., Zipes, D.P. (eds.). Nonpharmacological Therapy of Tachyarrhythmias. 1987, Mount Kisco, NY: Futura Publishing, 1987, pp. 1.

[2] CAST-Investigators. Preliminary Report: Effect of encainide and flecainide on mortality in a randomized trial of arrhythmia suppression after myocardial infarction. N. Engl. J. Med. 1989; 321: 406.

[3] Breithardt, G., Borggrefe, M., Seipel, L.: Selection of optimal drug treatment of ventricular tachycardia by programmed electrical stimulation of the heart. In: Clinical Aspects of Life-threatening Arrhythmias. Ann. NY Acad. Sci. 1984; 427: 49.

[4] Borggrefe, M., Trampisch, H.J., Breithardt, G.: Reappraisal of criteria for assessing drug efficacy in patients with ventricular tachyarrhythmias: complete versus partial suppression of inducible arrhythmias. J. Am. Coll. Cardiol. 1988; 12: 140.

[5] Podczeck, A., Borggrefe, M., Bartels, K., Breithardt, G.: Efficacy of flecainide in pacing-induced sustained ventricular tachyarrhythmias: correlation to clinical parameters and tachycardia-characteristics. Eur. Heart. J. 1989; 10: 928.

[6] Saksena, S., Goldschlager, N. (eds.): Electrical therapy for cardiac arrhythmias. Pacing, antitachycardia devices, catheter ablation. W.B. Saunders Company, Philadelphia, 1990.

[7] Breithardt, G., Borggrefe, M., Zipes, D.P. (eds.): Nonpharmacological Therapy of Tachyarrhythmias. 1987, Mount Kisco, NY: Futura Publishing, 1987.

[8] Borggrefe, M., Hindricks, G., Haverkamp, W., Budde, Th., Breithardt, G.: Radiofrequency ablation. In: Cardiac Electrophysiology. From Cell to Bedside. D.P. Zipes, J. Jalife, eds., 1990: 997.

[9] Steinbeck, G., Meinertz, T., Andresen, D., Borggrefe, M., Brachmann, J., Gonska, B.-D., Klein, H., Kuck, K.-H., Manz, M.: Empfehlungen zur Implantation von Defibrillatoren, herausgegeben von der Arbeitsgruppe "Herzrhythmusstörungen" der deutschen Gesellschaft für Herz- und Kreislaufforschung. In preparation.

[10] Cox, J.L.: Patient selection criteria and results of surgery for refractory ischemic ventricular tachycardia. Circulation 1989; 79 (suppl. I): 163.

[11] Borggrefe, M., Podczeck, A., Ostermeyer, J., Breithardt, G., and the Surgical Ablation Registry. In: Breithardt, G., Borggrefe, M., Zipes, D.P. (eds.): Nonpharmacological Therapy of Tachyarrhythmias. 1987, Mount Kisco, NY: Futura Publishing, 1987, 109.

[12] Cooper, D., Luceri, R.M., Thurer, R.J., Myerburg, R.J.: The impact of the automatic implantable cardioverter defibrillator on quality of life. Clin. Progr. Electrophysiol. Pacing 1986; 4: 306.

[13] Kuppermann, M., Luce, B.R., McGovern, B., Podrid, P.J., Bigger, J.Th. Jr., Ruskin, J.N.: An analysis of the cost effectiveness of the implantable defibrillator. Circulation 1990; 81: 91.

[14] Campbell, R.W.F.: Life at a price: the implantable defibrillator. Br. Heart. J. 1990; 64: 171.

[15] Block, M., Borggrefe, M., Hammel, D., Hief, C., Scheld, H.H., Breithardt, G.: First experience with an implantable antitachycardia system featuring antitachycardia stimulation, cardioversion and defibrillation. Eur. Heart. J. 1990; 11: abstract suppl., 405.

[16] Block, M., Borggrefe, M., Budde, T., Hachenberg, T., Hammel, D., Hief, C., Scheld, H.H.: Transvenous-subcutaneous implantation of pacer-cardioverter-defibrillator in patients with prior cardiac surgery (submitted for publication).

[17] Borggrefe, M., Breithardt, G., Podczeck, A., Rohner, D., Budde, T., Martinez-Rubio, A.: Catheter ablation of ventricular tachycardia using defibrillator pulses: electrophysiological findings and long-term results. Eur. Heart. J. 1989; 10: 591.

Folgezustände nach Herzinfarkt

G. Junge-Hülsing
Medizinische Klinik
Städt. Kliniken Osnabrück

Kurzreferat

In den nachfolgenden Referaten im Rahmen der Themen über Therapie und Prävention von Folgezuständen nach Herzinfarkt wird auf die Behandlung von Herz- und Coronarinsuffizienz, von Rhythmusstörungen, auf die Frage der chirurgischen Intervention und die Therapie mentaler Risikofaktoren detailliert eingegangen. Diese Themen werden folglich bei der Besprechung der Folgezustände nach Herzinfarkt ausgespart.

Hingegen werden die Prophylaxe und Therapie der Risikofaktoren und Fragen der medikamentösen Prophylaxe ausführlicher, die Therapie reaktiv-depressiver Folgezustände nach Herzinfarkt nur kurz gestreift.

Die Bedeutung der *Risikofaktoren* für die Entstehung von Arteriosklerose bzw. Coronarsklerose und Herzinfarkt wird anhand von Beispielen aufgezeigt und der Mechanismus der Entstehung der Coronarsklerose diskutiert.

Für die Prophylaxe und Behandlung der Folgezustände nach Herzinfarkt wie insbesondere auch nach erfolgreicher Bypass-Operation und PTCA ergeben sich aus den Beobachtungen über den Entstehungsmechanismus der Coronarsklerose wesentliche Konsequenzen: der Bluthochdruck muß extrem gut eingestellt sein; die Cholesterinwerte sollten nach entsprechender diätetischer und ggf. medikamentöser Therapie deutlich unterhalb der Normwerte liegen; der Diabetes, auch der sog. präklinische Diabetes mellitus muß oft unter Einsatz von Insulin so reguliert sein, daß auch bei Tagesprofilkontrollen keine nennenswerten erhöhten Blutzuckerwerte vorhanden sind; Zigarettenkonsum und Übergewicht sollten vollständig beseitigt und die Lebensführung mit Durchführung eines körperlichen Trainings und Einhaltung von Arbeitspausen so reguliert sein, daß insgesamt die beeinflußbaren Risikokrankheiten und die Faktoren der Lebensführung keine Gefährdung des Patienten mehr beinhalten.

Regelmäßige Gespräche mit den Patienten und engmaschige Kontrollen über den Erfolg oder den Mißerfolg der Behandlung der Risikofaktoren sind unbedingte Pflicht des behandelnden Arztes.

Die *medikamentöse Prophylaxe* nach Herzinfarkt wird recht unterschiedlich bewertet, dies bezieht sich sowohl auf die Therapie der Frühphase wie auch auf die der Folgezustände nach Herzinfarkt.

Unter Zusammenfassung aller Beobachtungen erscheint es heute sinnvoll, unter Beachtung gewisser Kontraindikationen, eine vorsichtige und möglichst niedrig-dosierte Therapie sowohl mit Beta-Blockern wie auch mit Diltiazem zu empfehlen.

Unterschiedliche Ergebnisse liegen über die Langzeitwirkung anderer Medika-mente wie Calciumantagonisten vom Typ des Verapamil oder Nifedipin vor, eben-so sind die Urteile im Hinblick auf die protektive Wirkung der Nitropräparate nicht einheitlich.

In welcher Form neuere sog. Calciumantagonisten vom Typ des Nisoldipin oder die Gruppe der sog. ACE-Hemmer über die Entlastung des Herzens mit Senkung der Vorlast und selektive Verbesserung der Coronardurchblutung zu einer günsti-geren Prognose der Folgezustände nach Herzinfarkt führen werden, ist sicherlich noch den Ergebnissen weiterer Langzeitstudien vorbehalten.

Auf die Verhütung und Behandlung *mentaler Risikofaktoren* nach Herzinfarkt wird ebenfalls in einem nachfolgenden Referat näher eingegangen. Für die tägliche Praxis erscheint es notwendig, die jeweils für die Patienten spezifischen psycho-so-zialen Streßformen herauszuarbeiten und eine Lösung der oft komplizierten Kon-fliktsituationen herbeizuführen. Ebenso notwendig ist es, mehr als bisher, insbe-sondere bei den Patienten nach operativen Eingriffen am Herzen, die oft nur la-viert vorhandenen depressiven Verstimmungen herauszufinden. Nach neueren Untersuchungen erscheint ein sehr hoher Prozentsatz von Patienten nach Herz-infarkt, insbesondere aber nach operativen Eingriffen, in dem Sinne einer depres-siven Verstimmung gefährdet zu sein.

Gespräche mit den Patienten und den Partnerinnen oder Partnern über Beruf, Partnerbeziehung, Belastbarkeit und Schonung, über neue Lebensqualität sind er-forderlich. Vielfach ist auch der vorsichtige Einsatz antidepressiver Medikamente sinnvoll und notwendig.

Grenzprobleme zwischen chirurgischer und internistischer Therapie bei Koronarkranken

H. H. Scheld, D. Hammel
Klinik und Poliklinik für
Thorax-, Herz- und Gefäßchirurgie der
Westfälischen Wilhelms Universität Münster

Einleitung

Die koronare Herzerkrankung manifestiert sich heutzutage im 5. und 6. Lebensjahrzehnt meist in Form der Angina pectoris oder des Myokardinfarktes. Herzinsuffizienz oder Herzrhythmusstörungen sind seltenere Erstsymptome dieser Erkrankung.

Diagnostisch ist ein abgestuftes Instrumentarium verfügbar, hier sind für den Chirurgen Lävokardiographie und Coronarangiographie entscheidend. Ein breites Spektrum von Behandlungsmethoden konnte etabliert werden, jedoch kommt der Prävention, als Gesundheitserziehung im Sinne der *Primärprävention* oder der Einstellung der koronaren Risikofaktoren als *Sekundärprävention*, in Anbetracht der weiten Verbreitung der Erkrankung der größte Stellenwert zu.

Neben der „klassischen" medikamentösen Therapie sind die Verfahren der interventionellen Kardiologie seit Ende der 70er Jahre ständig verbessert worden. Die von Grüntzig [21] für die 1-Gefäßerkrankung eingeführte Technik der percutanen transaortalen Coronarangioplastie wird mittlerweile auch mit großem Erfolg bei der 2- und 3-Gefäß-KHK eingesetzt. Technische Weiterentwicklungen stellen die Rotationsangioplastie und die intraluminale Laser-Applikation dar.

Nach ersten chirurgischen Behandlungsansätzen mit Denervierung des Herzens oder Einpflanzung der Arteria mammaria interna ins Myokard ist mit der Einführung der aortocoronaren Bypasschirurgie durch Favaloro [13] eine rasante Entwicklung eingeleitet worden, die die operative Myokardrevaskularisierung als Standardtherapie in der Behandlung der medikamentös nicht mehr behandelbaren koronaren Herzerkrankung etabliert hat. Aortocoronare Bypassanlagen mittels autologer Saphena magna-Transplantate oder Verwendung der inneren Brustarterie werden heute durch die koronare Endarteriektomieverfahren [39] (Abb. 1), intra-operative Coronardilatation und Lasertechnik ergänzt. Additive Verfahren, wie Klappenrekonstruktion oder Klappenersatz bei ischämischer Mitralinsuffizienz, Aneurysmaresektionen und antitachycarde Prozeduren vervollständigen das chirurgische Therapiespektrum.

Die Indikationsstellung zum Einsatz des für den jeweiligen Patienten optimalsten Therapieverfahrens ist nicht immer einfach. Idealerweise sollte die Behandlungsform gewählt werden, die mit der geringsten Invasivität den größtmöglichen therapeutischen Nutzen in Form von Beschwerdebesserung und/oder Lebensverlängerung erreicht.

Eine Graduierung bezüglich der Invasivität der Methodik bietet sicherlich keine Schwierigkeiten. Ist die medikamentöse Therapie, trotz einiger Nebenwirkungen am Ende der Invasivitäts-Skala einzuordnen, so ist die chirurgische Intervention schon alleine durch den notwendigen Zugang zum Herzen die invasivste Prozedur.

Bezüglich der Lebensverlängerung ist die Beurteilung der Methoden nicht immer einfach: Die medikamentöse Therapie kennt praktisch keine Akutletalität, hingegen kann die perioperative Letalität für die einzelnen Operationsverfahren genau bestimmt werden. Sie wird von allen Beteiligten sehr sensibel registriert. Für interventionelle Verfahren ist die Situation nicht so eindeutig, hier sei beispielhaft ein perioperativer Todesfall nach Akutrevaskularisation im Anschluß an eine Angioplastie angeführt. Ist ein solcher Patient an den Folgen der operativen Intervention oder der vorausgegangenen Angioplastie verstorben?

Zur chirurgischen Mortalität seien an dieser Stelle einige theoretische Bemerkungen erlaubt. Determinanten der Sterblichkeit stellen:
— Erfahrung der Chirurgen und der „Mannschaft",
— Nebenerkrankungen und Alter des Patienten,
— Schwere der kardialen Grunderkrankung und
— „Unwägbarkeiten" dar.

Die Unwägbarkeiten (seltene Nebenwirkungen, z.B. allergische Reaktionen, etc.) machen den geringsten Anteil aus und sind nicht zu beeinflussen. Bei optimierter Erfahrung wird die Letalität also im wesentlichen durch die Nebenerkrankungen und die Schwere der Herzerkrankung bestimmt [24]. An dieser Stelle wird die operative Sterblichkeit durch eine entsprechende Patientenauswahl beeinflußt.

Koronarkranke mit nicht sehr fortgeschrittener Erkrankung kann man mit niedrigerem Risiko operieren als solche mit sehr diffusem Gefäßbefall oder deutlich eingeschränkter linksventrikulärer Funktion. Andererseits ist bekannt, daß Patienten mit fortgeschrittener Erkrankung nach erfolgreicher Operation mehr von dem Eingriff, im Sinne einer Lebensverlängerung, profitieren als solche mit nur umschriebenen Veränderungen. Eine restriktive Einstellung zur Operationsindikation bei fortgeschrittener Erkrankung wird somit die operative Sterblichkeit reduzieren auf Kosten einer erhöhten Letalität im Gesamtkollektiv.

Bei Grenzproblemen zwischen chirurgischer und internistischer Therapie handelt es sich häufig um Notfallsituationen bzw. um fortgeschrittene Erkrankungsformen. Hier ist speziell der Chirurg, dessen Ergebnisse unabhängig vom Einzelfall an der Operations-Letalität gemessen werden, gefordert, trotz des erhöhten Risikos die im Sinne des Patienten richtige Entscheidung zu treffen.

Behandlung von Koronarstenosen

Durchgängigkeit von Venenbypasses

Ende der sechziger Jahre wurde die Verwendung von Saphena magna Transplantaten und die Verwendung der A. mammaria interna zur Umgehung von Koronarstenosen von Favaloro [13] bzw. Green et al. [18] beschrieben. Aufgrund von Untersuchungen in den frühen siebziger Jahren, die die Vene bedingt durch einen höheren Blutfluß und die damit verbundene bessere Patency-rate gegenüber der IMA favorisierten, wurden IMA-Grafts nur selten verwandt. Trotz neuerer Untersuchungen, die eindeutige Vorteile (längeres ereignisfreies Intervall nach OP, höhere Patency, Fehlen von arteriosklerotischen Veränderungen) für IMA-Transplantate nachweisen [19], werden auch heute noch mehr Koronarstenosen mit Venengrafts als mit IMA-Transplantaten überbrückt. Bei der zur Zeit geübten Technik wird die linke Mammaria zur Revaskularisierung des größten Koronargefäßes, meist der LAD benutzt, die übrigen Stenoses werden dann durch V. saphena magna Transplantate versorgt. Die angeführten Studien, die die Überlegenheit von IMA-Transplantaten belegen, werden relativiert, wenn man Mammaria- und Venen-LAD-Bypass vergleicht. Die Arbeitsgruppe aus Cleveland (1989) sah bei 1-Gefäß-KHK (LAD) keinen Unterschied bezüglich IMA- und Venen-Graft [26].

Man schätzt, daß in der frühen postoperativen Phase 8–12% und in den ersten 12 Monaten weitere 5–8% der Venengrafts verschließen. Am Ende des ersten Jahres sind somit 12–20% der Venen-Bypasses occludiert. In den folgenden Jahren

Tabelle 1: Durchgängigkeit von Venen-Transplantaten

	Time after Surgery		
	1 Month	**1 Year**	**10 Years**
No. of patients studied	207	162	58
No. of grafts studied	366	276	96
Percent occluded	10,6 %	14,5%	31,2 %
Percent with atherosclerosis	--	—	43,6 %

Grondin et al. Circulation 1984; 70 (Suppl I): I-208 - I-212

muß mit einer jährlichen Verschlußrate von 2% gerechnet werden, so daß nach 5 Jahren ca. 22--30% verschlossen sind [20]. Grondin und Mitarbeiter haben 1984 eine Studie vorgelegt, die neben der Durchgängigkeit auch das Auftreten arteriosklerotischer Veränderungen untersuchte. Er findet für sein Kollektiv 11% bzw. 15% Verschlüsse nach 1 Monat bzw. Jahr. Nahezu 70% der Grafts waren nach 10 Jahren noch durchgängig, wobei allerdings 44% arteriosklerotische Veränderungen in den Transplantaten aufwiesen [19] (Tab. 1).

Gründe für das Versagen der Venentransplantate sind neben technischen Problemen und Bedingungen der Konorarmorphologie in strukturellen und physiologischen Veränderungen nach Einbindung der Venen ins arterielle System zu suchen [4, 6, 16, 29, 38] (Abb. 3 + 4).

Operation versus medikamentöse Therapie

Die operative Behandlung von Koronarstenosen stellt für den Patienten eine erhebliche Belastung in psychischer und physischer Hinsicht dar. Die Legitimation eines solchen Behandlungsverfahrens sind Lebensverlängerung und Besserung der Lebensqualität.

In den siebziger Jahren wurden weltweit verschiedene Studien begonnen, um chirurgische und medikamentöse Behandlung in ihrer Wertigkeit zu vergleichen. Die Veterans Administration Cooperative Study (VA study) [32, 33], die European Coronary Surgery Study (ECSS) [12] und die Coronary Artery Surgery Study (CASS) [7, 8] sind die fundiertesten Untersuchungen. Es konnte gezeigt werden, daß operierte Patienten durch eine Beschwerdebesserung von der Operatin profitieren [5, 8, 17, 35]. Für Patienten mit eingeschränkter linksventrikulärer Funktion (CASS) [31, 34] und für Patienten mit Mehrgefäßerkrankungen war eine Lebensverlängerung nachweisbar. Am eindrucksvollsten ist dies bei der Hauptstammstenose der linken Kranzarterie (Abb. 5). Unabhängig vom Bestehen subjektiver Beschwerden leben nach 5 Jahren noch 80% der chirurgischen behandelten Patienten, aber nur noch weniger als 60% der medikamentös therapierten [41, 43].

Angioplastie versus operative Myocardrevaskularisation

Seit Einführung der percutanen transluminalen Coronarangioplastie durch Grüntzig [21] ist über ein Jahrzehnt vergangen. Der Wert der Methode ist heute unumstritten, wobei allerdings eine endgültige Beurteilung für bestimmte Patientenuntergruppen noch aussteht.

Prospektive randomisierte multizentrische Studien sind begonnen worden, um Angioplastie und Operation in ihrer Wertigkeit zu vergleichen (Emory Angioplasty Surgery Trial [EAST], Bypass Angioplasty Revascularization Investigation [BARI], Randomized Intervention in the Treatment of Angina [RITA], Coronary

Artery Bypass Revasculariziation Investigation [CABRI], German Angioplasty Bypass Investigation [GABI], Angioplasty Compared to Medicine [ACME]).

Die Arbeitsgruppe um Floyd D. Loop und Delos M. Cosgrove [26] aus Cleveland hat 1989 erste Ergebnisse einer retrospektiven Studie von 781 konsekutiven Patienten veröffentlicht, die bei isolierter LAD-Stenose zwischen 1980 und 1984 mit PTCA bzw. ACVB behandelt wurden. 5 Jahre nach PTCA bzw. Bypass waren 76% der mit PTCA behandelten und 78% der operierten Patienten beschwerdefrei. Bei vergleichbarem Ergebnis in diesen Patientengruppen war die PTCA die weniger invasive, mit kürzerem stationären Aufenthalt belastete und kostengünstigere Methode für den Patienten. Wurde bei den PTCA-Patienten eine Notfall-Bypassoperatin notwendig, war diese mit höherer Mortalität und einem erhöhten Infarktrisiko belastet. Das ereignisfreie Fünfjahresüberleben (Tod, Infarkt oder ACVB-Operaton nach Entlassung aus stationärer Behandlung) war mit 94,6% in der operierten Gruppe signifikant besser als in der PTCA-Gruppe mit 87,1%.

Zusammenfassend stellten die Untersucher fest, daß die operative Behandlung der isolierten LAD-Stenose im Vergleich zur Angioplastie die besseren Langzeitergebnisse ausweist und die Vorteile der PTCA (geringere Invasivität, kürzere Verweildauer, niedrigere Kosten) hierdurch relativiert werden.

Notfall Revaskularisation nach PTCA

Mit der immer häufigeren Anwendung von percutanen Angioplastietechniken, auch bei Mehrgefäßerkrankungen, wird immer öfter der Chirurg gefordert, akut eine operative Revaskularisation durchzuführen. Tally und Mitarbeiter [42] konnten zeigen, daß es bei diesen Notfallpatienten signifikant häufiger zum Auftreten von perioperativen Infarkten kommt, Katecholamine und die intraaortale Ballongegenpulsation werden häufiger gebraucht. In Tab. 2 sind Häufigkeit von periope-

Tabelle 2: OP-Ergebnisse bei Notfall-Bypass nach PTCA

		Total Group (no.)	Emergency CABG (no.)	Q-Vave MI (no.)	Mortality (no.)
Cowley	(1984)	3079	202 (6,6%)	52 (25,7%)	13 (6,4%)
Golding	(1986)	1831	81 (4,4%)	37 (46 %)	2 (2,5%)
Kiken	(1985)	3000	115 (3,8%)	50 (43,5%)	13 (11,3%)
Reul	(1984)	518	70 (13,5%)	8 (11,4%)	4 (5,7%)
Total		8428	468 (5,6%)	147 (31,4%)	32 (6,8%)

rativen Infarkten und Mortalität aus der Literatur zusammengestellt. Von 8428 Operationen mußten 5,6% notfallmäßig nach PTCA durchgeführt werden. Bei 31,4% der Patienten waren perioperativ Myokardinfarkte nachweisbar, die Mortalität lag bei 6,3%.

Verbesserungen in diesem Bereich sind durch die Verwendung von Perfusions-PTCA-Kathetern, den frühzeitigen, schon präoperativen Einsatz der IABP und eine sehr rasche chirurgische Versorgung zu erwarten.

Notfall Revaskularisation bei instabiler Angina pectoris

Die instabile Angina pectoris dürfte die Hauptindikation für ein notfallmäßiges operatives Handeln in der Herzchirurgie darstellen. Die Diagnose einer instabilen Situation ist sehr vom jeweiligen Untersucher abhängig. Folgende allgemeingültige Kriterien weisen einen Patienten mit instabiler Anginasymptomatik aus: Aufnahme in einer Intensiveinheit zum Ausschluß eines Myocardinfarktes, über 15minütiger Ruhe-Anginaschmerz trotz entsprechender Therapie, Endstreckenveränderungen in Standard-EKG, Einsatz einer intravenösen Therapie mit Heparin und Nitrokörpern.

Kaiser und Mitarbeiter [25] haben 1989 die Daten von 6136 wegen instabiler Angina operierter Patienten aus der Literatur zusammengestellt. Die mittlere Operationsletalität betrug 3,7% (1,2–8,5%), perioperative Infarkte traten mit 9,9% relativ häufig auf und auch ein Low-cardiac-output-Syndrom wurde mit 16% der Fälle relativ häufig gesehen. Im weiteren Verlauf konnten dann keine signifikanten Unterschiede zum Vergleichskollektiv (ACVB wegen stabiler Angina) gesehen werden. Im Rahmen der Veterans Administration Cooperative Study Group wurde in einer kontrollierten und randomisierten Studie von Parisi und Mitarbeitern (1989) [33] die Wertigkeit von chirurgischer und medikamentöser Therapie der instabilen Angina pectoris verglichen. Für Patienten mit 3-Gefäß-Erkrankung ergaben sich im 60monatigen Follow up deutliche Unterschiede. Das Überleben der chirurgisch behandelten Patienten war mit 89% signifikant besser als in der medikamentös behandelten Gruppe mit 75%. Weiterhin war in dieser Gruppe seltener eine Hospitalisierung nach initialer chirurgischer Therapie notwendig als in der medikamentös behandelten.

Operative Revaskularisation bei diffuser koronarer Herzerkrankung

Die Möglichkeit einer konventionellen Bypassanlage wird durch die diffuse Verkalkung eines Kranzgefäßes limitiert. Einerseits können lokale Wandverkalkungen eine Anastomosierung technisch unmöglich machen, andererseits begünstigt der schlechte Abfluß in solchen Gefäßen einen frühzeitigen Bypassverschluß.

Für diese Patientengruppe eröffnet die koronare Endarteriektomie eine Behandlungsperspektive [27, 30, 36]. Nach Eröffnung des Gefäßes wird der verkalkte Intimazylinder vorsichtig extrahiert, wobei auf das Miterfassen von Seitenästen Wert gelegt werden muß. Abgeschlossen wird die Prozedur mit der Bypassversorgung des jetzt entkalkten Gefäßes. Kardiogreenflußprobe und angioskopische Kontrolle bestätigen die Durchgängigkeit des Gefäßes (Abb. 2).

Noch in Gießen haben wir ein Kollektiv von 2415 Patienten, die zur operativen Revaskularisierung anstanden, untersucht [39]. Bei 16,4% (397) mußte wegen diffusem Gefäßbefall eine Endarteriektomie vorgenommen werden. Das RCA-System war in 57,9%, das linke Koronarsystem in 30,8% und beide in 8,3% betroffen. Die 30 Tage Mortalität war in diesem speziellen Krankengut mit 3,8% leicht erhöht, auch traten mehr perioperative Infarkte (9,3%) als im Vergleichskollektiv auf. Im Langzeitverlauf waren 92% zur Zeit der Nachuntersuchung (6–60 Monate post OP) beschwerdefrei und besser belastbar.

Behandlung von Folgen der koronaren Herzerkrankung

Störungen der Koronarzirkulation führen zu strukturellen Schäden am Myokard. Stellt der akute Myokardinfarkt eine Indikation zum konservativen Vorgehen dar, gewinnt die chirurgische Therapie von Infarktfolgen immer größeren Stellenwert. Das Behandlungsspektrum reicht von der Aneurysmaresektion bishin zur Herztransplantation bei terminaler myocardialer Insuffizienz.

Tabelle 3: OP-Ergebnisse bei VSD-Verschluß im kardiogenen Schock

Autor		Patients (no.)	Survivors (no.)
Windsor	(1982)	12	7
Feneley	(1983)	13	3
Scanlon	(1985)	20	12
Weintraub	(1986)	10	5
Moore	(1986)	8	1
Personal experience		2	1
Total		65	29 (44,6 %)

Behandlung von infarktbedingten Herzscheidewanddefekten

Man rechnet mit dem Auftreten eines Ventrikelseptumdefektes beim akuten Myokardinfarkt in 2% der Fälle. Meist tritt der Defekt am 2. oder 3. Tag nach dem Infarktereignis auf, Ventrikelseptumdefekte können aber noch bis zur 2. Woche nach dem Ereignis entstehen. Bei konservativer Behandlung ist die Mortalität extrem hoch. 25% sterben in den ersten 24 Stunden, 50% innerhalb einer Woche und nahezu 85% in den ersten beiden Monaten [23]. Ist der Patient mit konservativen Maßnahmen zu stabilisieren, wird man die Intervalloperation anstreben. Im kardiogenen Schock ist dies naturgemäß nicht möglich, hier hat sich der präoperativ begonnene Einsatz der diastolischen Augmentation als hilfreich erwiesen. In der Literatur wird nur über jeweils sehr kleine Patientenserien berichtet (Tab. 3). Von 65 Patienten, die im cardiogenen Schock wegen eines Infarkt-VSD operiert wurden, konnten 29 (44,6%) nach Hause entlassen werden [2].

Noch düsterer als bei Infarkt-VSD ist die Prognose bei einer infarktbedingten Ruptur der Ventrikelwand. Die meisten Patienten versterben hier sofort beim Auftreten des Wanddefektes unter dem Bilde einer akuten Pericardtamponade. Kommen diese Patienten zur operativen Versorgung, bessert sich die Prognose. Von 20 in der Literatur berichteten Fällen wurden 12 (60%) erfolgreich versorgt [2].

Behandlung von infarktbedingter Mitralinsuffizienz

Die ischämische Mitralinsuffizienz ist definiert als im Rahmen eines Infarktgeschehens auftretende Schlußunfähigkeit der Mitralklappe bei vorher intakter Klappe. Man findet diesen Befund bei 5% der Infarktpatienten in der ersten Woche nach dem akuten Ereignis. Häufig sieht man als Ursache der Insuffizienz einen abgerissenen hinteren Papillarmuskel, es kommen aber auch narbige Schrumpfungen des Halteapparates oder Anulusdilatationen vor. Eingriffe bei ischämischer Mitralinsuffizienz sind mit einem hohen Risiko belastet, das um 20% abzuschätzen ist, im Gegensatz zu einem 12% Risiko für KHK-Patienten mit zusätzlichem rheumatischen oder degenerativen Klappenfehler [37].

Bei der akuten Insuffizienz tritt meist ein Lungenödem auf, die Ausbildung eines cardiogenen Schocks ist nicht selten. Nachlastsenkung, medikamentös und/oder mittels IABP sind Therapie der Wahl. Nach Sicherung der Diagnose sind die Patienten sofort der operativen Versorgung zuzuführen, wobei den Klappen erhaltenden OP-Verfahren vor dem Klappenaustausch der Vorzug gegeben wird. Aufgrund des kleinen linken Vorhofes bei der akuten Mitralinsuffizienz bietet der Eingriff technische Probleme. Bei der Operation sollte gleichzeitig die Revaskularisation angestrebt werden. Insgesamt ist die Prognose in Fällen, die im cardiogenen Schock operiert werden, schlecht. Tab. 4 gibt eine Übersicht von in der Literatur berichteten Fällen. Die Erfolgsaussicht scheint mit ca. 50% eher gering, wobei die Prognose nicht so sehr durch die kardiale Problematik, als vielmehr durch die Einbeziehung anderer Organsysteme in den Schockzustand belastet wird [2].

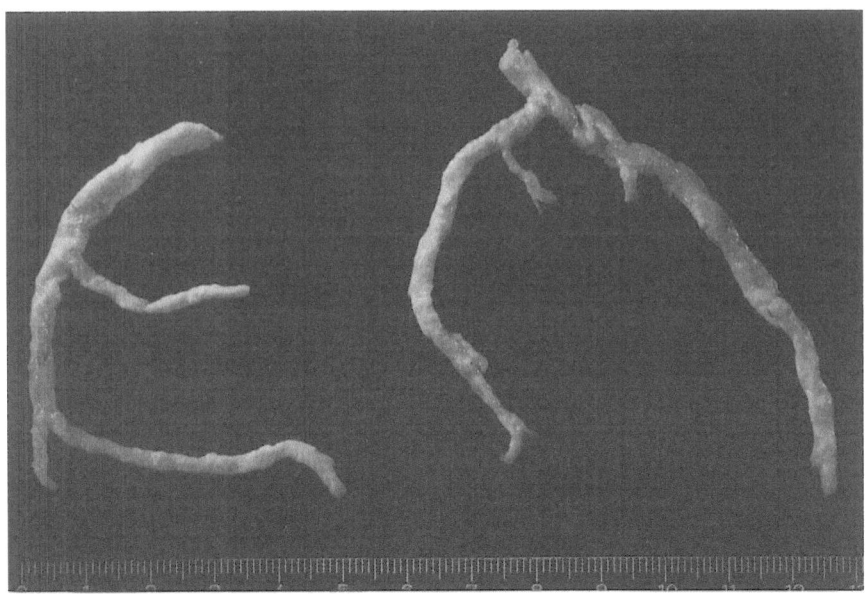

Abb. 1: Endarteriektomie Präparate, links: rechte Kranzarterie, rechts: linke Kranzarterie.

Abb. 2: Operationssitus nach Endarteriektomie der rechten Kranzarterie, Bildausschnitt unten rechts: angioskopische Kontrolle.

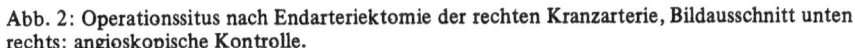

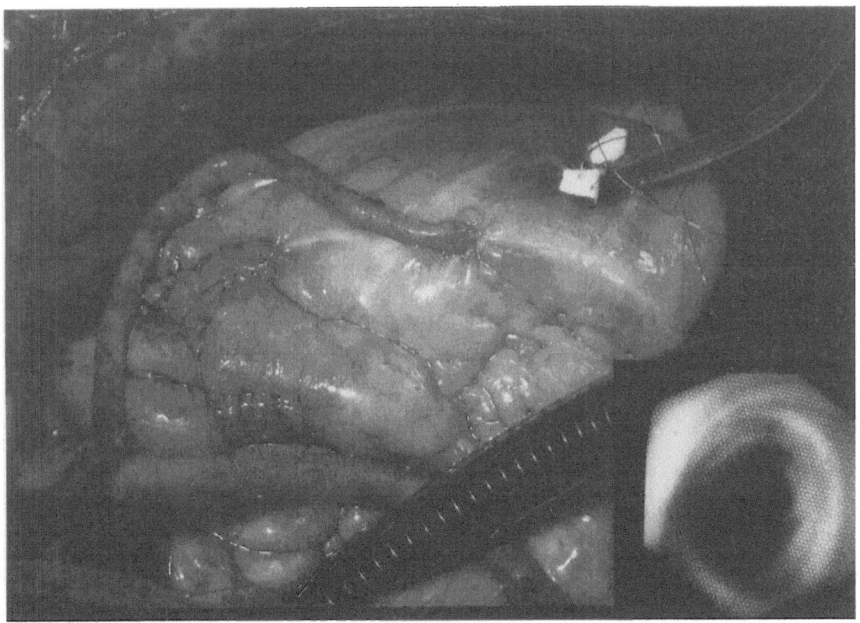

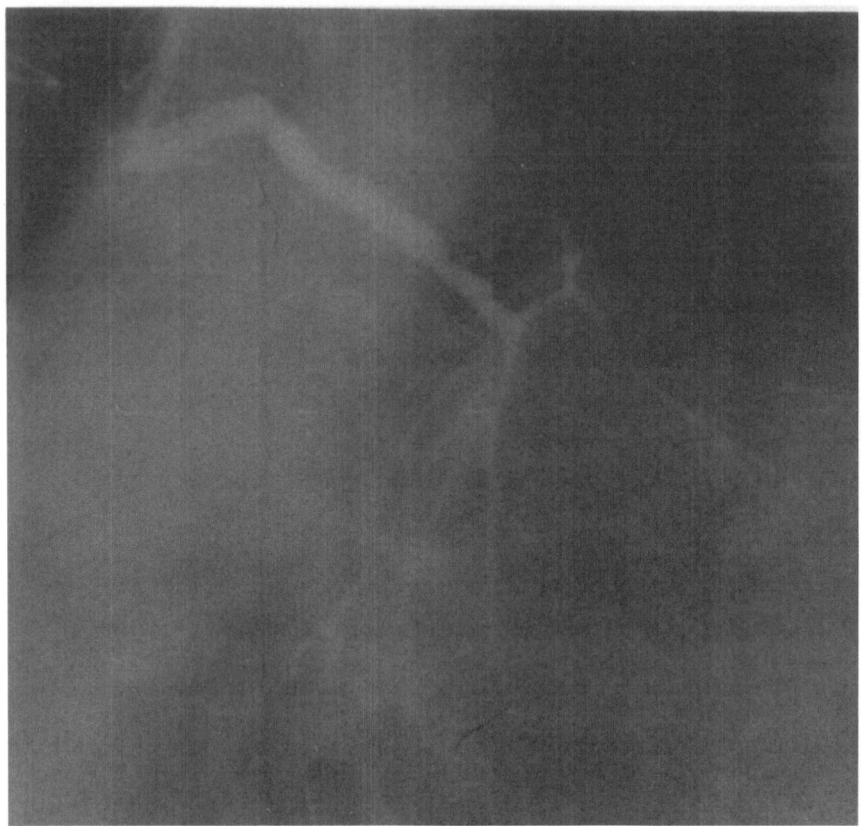

Abb. 3: Arterisklerotische Veränderungen im RIVA-Bypass 4 Jahre nach Operation.

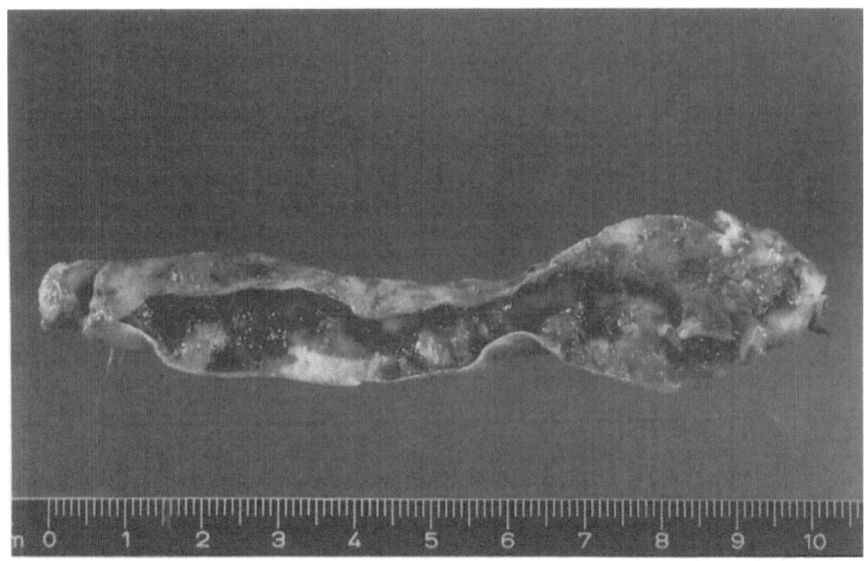

Abb. 4: Arteriosklerose in einem verschlossenen Saphena magna Transplantat (OP-Präparat).

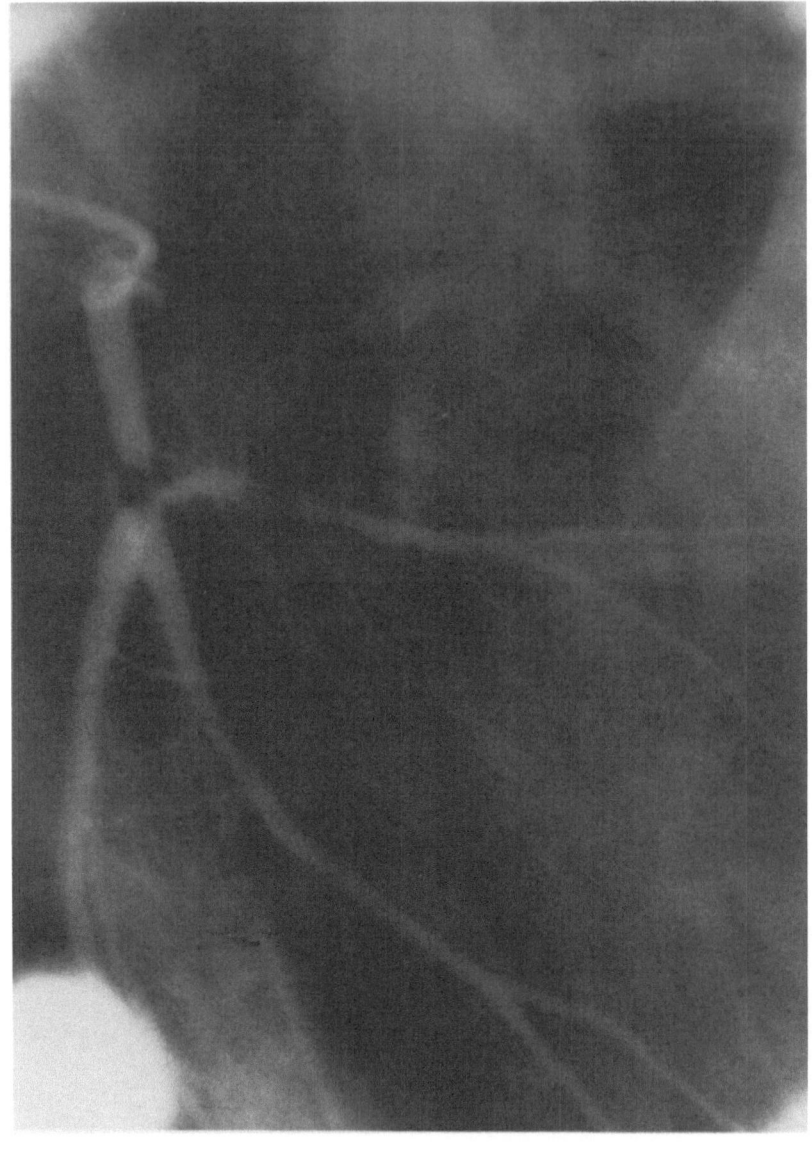

Abb. 5: Kritische Hauptstammstenose der linken Kranzarterie.

Autor		Patients (no.)	Operative survival (no.)
Feneley	(1983)	2	0
Magovern	(1985)	11	6
Tepe	(1985)	11	5
David	(1986)	15	11
Weintraub	(1986)	7	3
Rankin	(1988)	15	6
Personal experience		3	1
Total		64	32 (50 %)

Tabelle 4: OP-Ergebnisse bei Intervention wegen ischämischer Mitralinsuffizienz

Behandlung von infarktbedingten Herzwandaneurysmen

In der Literatur wird die Entstehungshäufigkeit von Einherzwandaneurysmen nach Infarkt mit 5–30% angegeben. Denton A. Cooley hat 1958 [9] als erster die Resektion eines Infarktaneurysmas mittels cardiopulmonalem Bypass beschrieben. Im Rahmen der CASS-Studie konnte eindeutig gezeigt werden, daß bei Aneurysmaentstehung nach Infarkt das Überleben im Vergleich zum Kontrollkollektiv deutlich verkürzt ist. 4 Jahre nach Infarkt mit Aneurysmabildung leben noch 71% der konservativ behandelten Patienten. Determinanten des Verlaufes waren Alter, Funktion des Restventrikels, linksventrikulärer enddiastolischer Druck (LVEDP) und Phasen von Linksherzdekompensationen in der Anamnese [14]. Heute gültige Indikationen zur chirurgischen Therapie sind: anamnestisch Episoden kardialer Dekompensation, therapierefraktäre Arrhythmien, arterielle Embolien aus intracavitären Thromben [15].

Neben der reinen Aneurysmaresektion sind häufig zusätzliche chirurgische Prozeduren gefordert. Aortocoronare Bypass Anlage, Klappenersatz und der Verschluß eines Ventrikelseptumdefektes belasten die Prognose des Eingriffs. Weitere Risikofaktoren der chirurgischen Therapie stellen fortgeschrittenes Alter und Notfallsituationen dar [10, 28, 40]. Aneurysmaoperationen aus rhythmologischer Indikation stellen ein spezielles Kollektiv dar, das im nächsten Abschnitt behandelt wird [12].

In der Literatur schwanken die Angaben zur Operations-Sterblichkeit zwischen 2% (Akins 1986 [1], 100 Fälle) und 19% (Brawley et al., 1983 [3], 145 Fälle). Cosgrove et al. [10] haben 1989 in einer Übersichtsarbeit für 3439 Behandlungsfälle zwischen 1976 und 1987 aus der Literatur eine Mortalität von 9,9% gefunden.

Behandlung von infarktbedingten lebensbedrohenden ventrikulären Rhythmus-störungen

Heutzutage steht zur Behandlung von medikamentös nicht einstellbaren lebens-bedrohenden ventrikulären Rhythmusstörungen ein breitgefächertes Instrumen-tarium, abhängig von kardinaler Grunderkrankung und Art der Rhythmusstörung, zur Verfügung.

Ischämisch induzierte Reentry-Tachykardien, die zu Kammerflimmern degene-rieren, sind die weitaus häufigste Ursache eines plötzlichen Herztodes. Meist fin-det man bei diesen Patienten eine diffuse koronare Herzerkrankung oder es ist nach ausgedehnten Infarkten zur Ausbildung von Herzwandaneurysmen gekom-men.

Kann der Elektrophysiologe bei Vorliegen von Reentry-Tachykardien im Myo-kard (meist im Randgebiet zwischen vitalem Myokard und Infarktnarbe) ein arrhythmogenes Substrat nachweisen, ist die Ablation dieser arrhythmogenen Zone Therapieziel. Neben den Verfahren der interventionellen Kardiologie stehen an chirurgischen Prozeduren die subendokardiale Resektion, die „elektrische Iso-lation" in Form der partiellen oder totalen endokardialen Ventrikulotomie oder die Kryoablation, in jüngster Zeit auch die Lasertechnik zur Verfügung. Technisch wird unter extracorporaler Zirkulation der Ventrikel über das mehr oder weniger gut abgrenzbare Aneurysma eröffnet. Die präoperative Lokalisationsdiagnostik wird durch ein intraoperatives endokardiales Mapping ergänzt. Nach Lokalisation wird die eigentliche rhythmuschirurgische Prozedur am schlagenden oder kardio-plegisch stillgestellten Herzen vorgenommen. Der Eingriff wird mit der Aneurysma-resektion beendet, bzw. Klappenersatz und Bypassanlage werden angeschlossen.

Patienten mit ischämisch induzierten Rhythmusstörungen stellen ein weiteres Hochrisikokollektiv für die chirurgische Behandlung dar. Die linksventrikuläre Funktion ist durch abgelaufene Infarkte meist deutlich eingeschränkt, häufig sind lange Intensivaufenthalte mit Reanimationen und Dauerbeatmung vorausgegan-gen. Bis zur Indikationsstellung zur operativen Behandlung waren die bettlägeri-gen Patienten nicht selten über mehrere Monate hospitalisiert, was den postopera-tiven Verlauf durch nosokomiale Infektionen und Schwierigkeiten bei der post-operativen Mobilisation belastet. Es kann aus diesen Gründen nicht verwundern, daß rhythmuschirurgische Prozeduren mit einem höheren Risiko als reine Aneu-rysmaresektionen belastet sind. Die Literaturangaben schwanken zwischen 0% (Saksena 1986, 93 Fälle) und 21% (McGriffin 1982, 123 Fälle). Eine Zusammen-stellung von 844 Rhythmusprozeduren aus der Literatur (Cox 1989 [11], Tab. 5) ergibt eine globale Letalität von 12,4%.

Tachyarrhythmien ohne morphologisches Substrat entziehen sich dem direkten chirurgischen Zugriff, obwohl auch hier erste Ansätze zu verzeichnen sind. In die-sen Fällen stellt die Implantation eines automatischen Kardioverter-Defibrillator-Systemes eine palliative Therapiemöglichkeit dar. Die Systeme der neueren Gene-ration besitzen zusätzlich eine antibradykarde Funktion und sind in der Lage,

Autor		Patients (no.)	Operative mortality (%)
Moran	(1983)	65	12
Miller	(1984)	100	9
Brodman	(1984)	22	14
Ivey	(1985)	11	9
Swerdlow	(1986)	98	17
Garan	(1986)	36	17
Krafchek	(1986)	39	10
Hammon	(1986)	32	12
Balooki	(1986)	18	16
Saksena	(1986)	24	0
Vigano	(1986)	36	8
Kron	(1987)	70	13
Ostermeyer	(1987)	93	5
Svenson	(1987)	15	13
Yee	(1987)	62	8
Mc Giffin	(1987)	123	21
Total		844	12,4

Cox 1989.79 (Suppl. I):I-163 - I-177

Tabelle 5: OP-Ergebnisse bei Intervention wegen ischämiebedingter ventriculärer Tachykardie

Kammertachykardien durch Überstimulation elektrisch zu terminieren. War früher immer eine epikardiale bzw. perikardiale Elektrodenanlage notwendig, so können neuere Systeme über einen transvenös/subcutanen Zugang implantiert werden. In Extremfällen kann auch eine Herztransplantation therapeutisch notwendig werden.

Literatur

[1] Akins, C.W.: Resction of left ventricular aneurysm during hypothermic fibrillatory arrest without aortic occlusion. J. Cardiovac. Surg. 1986; 91: 610–618.
[2] Bolooki, H.: Emergency Cardiac Procedures in Patients in Cardiogenic Shock Due to Complications of Coronary Artery Disease. Circulation 1989; 79 (suppl. I): I-137–I-148.
[3] Brawley, R.K., Magovern, G.J., Gott, V.L., Donahoo, J.S., Gardner, T.J., Watkins, L.: Left ventricular aneurysmectomy. Factors influencing postoperative results. J. Thorac. Cardiovasc. Surg. 1983; 85: 712–717.
[4] Bulkley, G.H., Hutchins, G.M.: Accelerated atherosclerosis. A morphologic study in 97 saphenous vein grafts. Circulation 1977; 55: 163–169.
[5] Califf, R.M., Harrell, F.E., Jr., Lee, K.L., Rankin, J.S., Mark, D.B., Hlatky, M.A., Muhlbaier, L.H., Wechsler, A.S., Jones, R.H., Oldham, H.N., Pryor, D.B.: Changing efficacy of coronary revascularization: Implications for patient selection. Circulation 1988; 78 (suppl. I): I-185–I-191.

[6] Campeau, L., Enjalbert, M., Lesperance, J., Bourassa, M.G., Kwiterovich, P. Jr., Wachol-
der, S., Sniderman, A.: The relation of risk factors to the developement of atherosclerosis in saphenous vein bypass grafts and the progression of desease in the native circulation. N. Engl. J. Med. 1984; 311: 1329–1332.

[7] CASS principal investigators and their associates: Coronary Artery Surgery Study
(CASS): A randomized trial of coronary artery bypass surgery; survival data. Circulation 1983; 68: 939–940.

[8] CASS principal investigators and their associates: Coronary Artery Surgery Study
(CASS): A randomized trial of coronary artery bypass surgery; quality of life in patients
randomly assigned to treatment groups. Circulation 1983; 68: 951–960.

[9] Cooley, D.A., Collins, H.A., Morris, G.C., Chapman, D.W.: Ventricular aneurym after
myocardial infarction. Surgical excision with use of temporary cardiopulmonary bypass.
JAMA 1957; 167: 557–562.

[10] Cosgrove, D.M., Lytle, B.W., Taylor, P.C., Stewart, R.W., Golding, L.A.R., Mahfood, S.,
Goormastic, M., Loop, F.D.: Ventricular Aneurysm Resection: Trends in Surgical Risk.
Circulation 1989; 79 (suppl. I): I-97–I-101.

[11] Cox, J.L.: Patient Selection Criteria and Results of Surgery for Refractory Ischemic
Ventricular Tachycardia. Circulation 1989; 79 (suppl. II): I-163–I-177.

[12] European Coronary Surgery Study Group: Prospective randomized study of coronary
artery bypass surgery in stable angina pectoris: Second interim report. Lancet 1980;
2: 491–495.

[13] Favaloro, R.: Sapenous vein autograft replacement of serve segmental coronary artery
occlusion. Ann. Thorac. Surg. 1968; 5: 335–339.

[14] Faxon, D.P., Ryan, T.J., Davis, K.B., McCabe, C.H., Myers, W., Lesperance, J., Shaw, R.,
Tong, T.G.L.: Prognostic Significance of Angiographically Documented Left Ventricular
Aneurysm From the Coronary Artery Surgery Study (CASS). Am. J. Cardiol. 1982; 50:
157–164.

[15] Frank, G., Klein, H., Lichtlen, P., Borst, H.G.: Spätergebnisse nach linksventrikulärer
Aneurysmaresektion. Münch. med. Wschr. 1978; 120: 565–568.

[16] Fuchs, J.C.A., Mitchener, J.S. III, Hager, P.O.: Postoperative changes in autologous vein
grafts. Ann. Surg. 1978; 188: 1–15.

[17] Gersh, B.J., Califf, R.M., Loop, F.D., Akins, C.W., Pryor, D.B., Takaro, T.C.: Coronary
Bypass Surgery in Chronic Stable Angina. Circulation 1989; 79 (supp. I): I-46–I-59.

[18] Green, G.E., Reed, G.E., Stertzer, S.H., Reppert, E.H.: Coronary arterial bypass grafts.
Ann. Thorac. Surg. 1968; 5: 443–450.

[19] Grondin, C.M., Campeau, L., Lesperance, J., Enjalbert, M., Bourassa, M.G.: Comparison
of late changes in internal mammary artery and saphenous vein grafts in two consecutive
series of patients 10 years after operation. Circulation 1984; 70 (suppl. I): I-208–I-212.

[20] Grondin, C.M., Campeau, L., Thornton, J.C., Engle, J.C., Cross, F.S., Schreiber, H.:
Coronary Artery Bypass Grafting With Saphenous Vein. Circulation 1989; 79 (suppl. I):
I-24–I-29.

[21] Grüntzig, A.R., Senning, A., Siegenthaler, W.E.: Nonoperative dilatation of coronary-
artery stenosis: Percutaneous transluminal coronary angioplasty. N. Engl. J. Med. 1979;
301: 61–68.

[22] Harken, A.H., Horowitz, L.N., Josephson, M.E.: Comparison of standard aneurysmectomy and aneurysmectomy with directed endocardial resection for treatment of recur-
rent sustained ventricular tachycardia. J. Thorac. Cardiovasc. Surg. 1980; 80: 527–534.

[23] Hill, J.D., Stiles, Q.R.: Acute Ischemic Ventricular Septal Defect. Circulation 1989; 79
(suppl. I): I-112–I-115.

[24] Jones, R.H.: In Search of the Optimal Surgical Mortality. Circulation 1989; 79 (suppl. I):
I-132–I-136.

[25] Kaiser, G.C., Schaff, V.H., Killip, T.: Myocardial Revascularization for Unstable Angina
Pectoris. Circulation 1989; 79 (suppl. I): I-60–I-67.

[26] Kramer, J.R., Proudfit, W.L., Loop, F.D., Goormastic, M., Zimmerman, K., Simpfendor-
fer, C., Horner, G.: Late follow-up of 781 patients undergoing percutaneous transluminal
coronary angioplasty or coronary artery bypass grafting for an isolated obstruction in
the left anterior descending coronary artery. Am. Heart. J. 1989; 118: 1144–1153.

[27] Livesay, J.J., Cooley, D.A., Hallman, G.L.: Early and late results of coronary endarterectomy. J. Thorac Cardiovasc Surg. 1986; 92: 649–660.
[28] Magovern, G.J., Sakert, T., Simpson, K., Laub, G.W., Park, S.B., Liebler, G., Burkholder, J., Maher, T., Benckart, D., Magovern, G.J. Jr.: Surgical Therapy for Left Ventricular Aneurysms, A Ten-Year Experience. Circulation 1989; 79 (suppl. I): I-102–I-107.
[29] Malone, J.M., Kischer, C.W., Moore, W.S.: Changes in venous endothelial fibrinolytic activity and histology with in vitro venous distention and arterial implantation. Am. J. Surg. 1981; 142: 178–182.
[30] Miller, D.C., Stinson, E.B., Oyer, P.E.: Long-term clinical assessment of the efficacy of adjunctive coronary endarterectomy, J. Thorac Cardiovasc Surg. 1981; 81: 21–29.
[31] Mock, M.B., Fisher, L.D., Holmes, D.R. Jr., Gersh, B.J., Schaff, H.V., McConney, M., Rogers, W.J., Kaiser, G.C., Ryan, T.J., Myers, W.O., Killip, T., and Participants in the Coronary Artery Surgery Study: Comparison of effects of medical and surgical therapy on survival in servere angina pectoris and two-vessel coronary artery disease with and without left ventricular dysfunction: A coronary artery study registy study. Am. J. Cardiol. 1988; 61: 1198–1202.
[32] Murphy, M.L., Hultgren, H.N., Detre, K., Thomsen, J., Takaro, T., and Participants of the Veterans Administration Cooperative Study: Treatment of chronic stable angina: A preliminary report of survival data of the randomized Veterans Administration cooperative study. N. Engl. J. Med. 1977; 297: 621–627.
[33] Parisi, A.F., Khuri, S., Deupree, R.H., Sharma, G.V.R.K., Scott, S.M., Luchi, R.J.: Medical Compared With Surgical Management of Unstable Angina. 5-Year Mortality and Morbidity in the Veterans Administration Study. Circulation 1989; 80: 1176–1189.
[34] Passamani, E., Davis, K.B., Gillespie, M.J., Killip, T., and the CASS principal investigators and their associates: A randomized trial of coronary artery bypass surgery: Survival of patients with low ejection fraction. N. Engl. J. Med. 1985; 312: 1665–1671.
[35] Pryor, D.B., Harrell, F.E., Jr., Rankin, J.S., Lee, K.L., Muhlbaier, L.H., Oldham, H.N., Hlatky, M.A., Mark, D.B., Reves, J.G., Califf, R.M.: The changing survival benefits of coronary revascularization over time. Circulation 1987; 76 (suppl. V): V-13–V-21.
[36] Qureshi, S.A., Halim, M.A., Pillai, R.: Endarterectomy of the left coronary system. Analysis of a 10 year experience. J. Thorac. Cardiovasc. Surg. 1985; 89: 852–859.
[37] Rankin, J.S., Hickey, M.St.J., Smith, L.R., Muhlbaier, L., Reves, J.G., Pryor, D.B., Wechsler, A.S.: Ischemic Mitral Regurgitation. Circulation 1989; 79 (suppl. I): I-116–I-121.
[38] Ross, R.: The pathogenesis of atherosclerosis. An update. N. Engl. J. Med. 1986; 314: 488–447.
[39] Scheld, H.H., Moosdorf, R., Görlach, G., Ewers, J., Hehrlein, F.W.: Coronary Endarterectomy in Patients with Diffuse Coronary Disease. Vasc. Surg. 1989; 23: 133–137.
[40] Stephenson, L.W., Hargrove, W.C. III, Ratcliffe, M.B., Edmunds, L.H.: Surgery for Left Ventricular Aneurysm. Circulation 1989; 79 (suppl. I): I-108–I-111.
[41] Takaro, T., Hultgren, H.N., Lipton, M.J., Detre, K.M., and Participants in the Study Group: The VA cooperative randomized study of srugery for coronary arterial occlusive disease. II. Subgroup with significant left main lesions. Circulation 1976; 54 (suppl. III): III-107–III-117.
[42] Tally, J.D., Jones, E.L., Weintraub, W.S., King, S.B. III: Coronary Artery Bypass Surgery After Failed Elective Percutaneous Transluminal Coronary Angioplasty. A Status report. Circulation 1989; 79 (suppl. I): I-126–I-131.
[43] Taylor, H.A., Deumite, N.J., Chaitman, B.R., Davis, K.B., Killip, T., Rogers, W.J.: Asymptomatic Left Main Coronary Artery Disease in the Coronary Artery Surgery Study (CASS) Registry. Circulation 1989; 79: 1171–1179.

Verhütung und Behandlung mentaler Risikofaktoren vor und nach Herzinfarkt

Johannes Siegrist
Institut für Medizinische Soziologie
Fachbereich Humanmedizin der Philipps-Universität Marburg

Das vergangene Jahrzehnt hat in der Stressforschung, soweit sie das Herz-Kreislauf-System betrifft, einen qualitativen Sprung erbracht. Die wichtigsten Erkenntnisfortschritte lassen sich kurz wie folgt zusammenfassen:

1. Es ist gelungen, die spezifische Qualität jener mentalen, aus dem sozio-emotionalen Erleben resultierenden Belastungserfahrungen herauszuarbeiten, die langfristig das Herz-Kreislauf-System schädigen. Nicht Stress im Sinne Selyes, das heißt eine unspezifische Alarmreaktion wirkt pathogen, sondern aktiver Distress, das heißt jene chronifizierten sympatho-adrenergen Aktivierungsprozesse, die sich aus einem wiederkehrenden Ungleichgewicht von Verausgabung und Belohnung, von Anstrengung und Kontrolle in wichtigen sozialen Situationen ergeben.

2. Es ist gelungen, verschiedene pathophysiologische Mechanismen aktiver Distress-Zustände zu belegen. Sie betreffen erstens die über fortgesetzte autonome Aktivierung eingeleiteten Dysregulationen von Blutdruck, endogenem Lipidstoffwechsel und Blutplättchen-Aggregationsneigung, zweitens zentralnervöse Einflüsse auf die Entwicklung und Progression arteriosklerotischer Prozesse, drittens schließlich, allerdings nur im vorgeschädigten Myokard, die Veränderung der Schwelle für transiente Ischämien sowie für Arrhythmien.

3. Die sozialepidemiologische und verhaltensmedizinische Forschung hat verschiedene Risikosituationen, aber auch individuelle Risikodispositionen identifiziert, die mit erhöhten Distresserfahrungen und, langfristig, mit erhöhter koronarer Erkrankungs- bzw. Wiedererkrankungsgefahr verbunden sind. Die wichtigste Risikosituation betrifft in unserer Gesellschaft den Leistungszusammenhang der Erwerbsarbeit, die wichtigste Risikodisposition die Unfähigkeit zu entspanntem zwischenmenschlichem Verhalten.

4. Aus diesen Erkenntnissen lassen sich therapeutische und präventive Maßnahmen ableiten, die heute zumindest in der Sekundärprophylaxe nach Herzinfarkt bereits deutliche Erfolge erbracht haben. Angesichts der gesundheitspolitischen Bedeutung von Herz-Kreislaufrisiken sind jedoch beim nunmehr erzielten Erkenntnisstand darüber hinaus auch primärpräventive Maßnahmen angezeigt.

In diesem Beitrag sollen neue wissenschaftliche Befunde speziell zum dritten der o.g. Punkte vorgestellt und unter dem Aspekt ihrer Bedeutung für die primäre und sekundäre Prävention diskutiert werden.

Stressphysiologische Grundlagen

Zwei Erkenntnisse standen am Anfang der modernen kardiovaskulären Stressforschung: erstens die Einsicht, daß nur langandauernde bzw. immer wiederkehrende sympathoadrenerge Aktivierungen für das initial intakte Herz-Kreislauf-
System schädlich sind, also Aktivierungen, die nicht kompensiert werden durch
gegenregulierende, stärker Parasympathikus-gesteuerte Prozesse [1]. Die zweite,
vielleicht noch wichtigere Erkenntnis betraf die Differenziertheit neuroendokriner
Reaktionen auf sensorische und symbolische Stimuli unterschiedlicher Qualität.
Umfangreiche tier- und humanexperimentelle Forschungen zeigten, daß in Situationen, die als eine Herausforderung erlebt werden, der man sich im Prinzip
gewachsen fühlt, vorwiegend das noradrenerg-medulläre System aktiviert wird
[2]. Diese Aktivierung führt zu der bereits von Walter Cannon beschriebenen
physiologischen Bereitstellungsreaktion. Dagegen wird in Situationen, die als über-
mächtig erlebt werden, in denen keine erfolgversprechenden Kontrollchancen bestehen, vorwiegend die Hypophysen-Nebennierenrindenachse aktiviert. Sie legt
Rückzug und Passivität nahe, einen Zustand, den die Forscher „passiven Distress"
nennen [3]. Für das Herz-Kreislaufsystem sind nun langandauernde Aktivierungen
bedeutsam, die auf der einen Seite die katabole Bereitstellungsreaktion provozie-
ren, vorwiegend in Situationen fortgesetzter Verausgabung, die aber auf der anderen Seite keine erfolgversprechenden Kontroll- und Belohnungschancen gewähren.
Solche Erfahrungen nennen wir „aktiven Distress" [4]. Die neurohormonelle
Dysregulation, die sich aus der simultanen Aktivierung beider Stressachsen ergibt
und der nicht kompensierte sympathoadrenerge „Drive" sind für die langfristig
pathogenen Folgen aktiver Distress-Zustände verantwortlich.

Langfristige Folgen aktiver Distress-Zustände für die Progression der Koronar-
arteriosklerose sind in einer Reihe tierexperimenteller Studien auf eindrucksvolle
Weise belegt worden. So hat eine Arbeitsgruppe unter Leitung von Jay Kaplan bei
männlichen Makaken chronische Distress-Zustände experimentell erzeugt, indem
Kleingruppen periodisch reorganisiert wurden. Durch Hinzufügen eines jeweils
dominanten neuen Alpha-Tieres verloren bisherige Führungstiere ihren sozialen
Rang [5]. Hypothesengemäß wurden langandauernde Distress-Zustände speziell
bei den dominanten, sozial deklassierten Männchen erwartet: hier sollte das
Muster von Kampf, Verausgabung und Kontrollverlust am deutlichsten ausgeprägt
sein. Die Vermessung der Koronarläsionen nach mehr als 20monatiger Intervention zeigte sowohl bei den mit atherogener Diät wie bei den mit normocholesterin-
ämischer Diät gefütterten Tieren den erwähnten Effekt: die Gruppe der dominanten, zugleich sozial instabilen Tiere wies signifikant erhöhte Intimaläsionen auf.
Selbstverständlich war das Ausmaß der Läsionen bei den mit atherogener Diät
gefütterten Tiere größer. Aber läßt sich der erzielte Effekt wirklich über neurogene
Mechanismen erklären?

In einem weiteren Experiment wurde die Zufallshälfte der dominanten Tiere
unter sonst gleichen Bedingungen mit dem Betarezeptoren-Blocker Propranolol

behandelt. Das Ergebnis war eindeutig: trotz gleicher Ernährung, trotz vergleich-
barer sozialer Verhaltensweisen und körperlicher Aktivität wies die behandelte
Gruppe hochsignifikant geringere Intimaläsionen auf [6]. Dies deutet darauf hin,
daß bestimmten Betarezeptoren-Blockern unter Umständen antiatherogene Eigenschaften zuzuschreiben sind. Nach Ablad sind diese Eigenschaften auf eine bisher
allerdings nicht genau lokalisierte Beta 1-Blockade im Zentralnervensystem zurück-
zuführen, von der eine Reduktion der Sympathikus-Aktivität ausgeht. Ihre wichtigsten Folgen sind eine Veränderung der Blutplättchen-Dynamik an der Intima,
eine erhöhte Synthese des anti-atherogenen Prostacyclins sowie eine Modulation
des endogenen Lipidstoffwechsels [7].

Da tierexperimentelle Ergebnisse nur mit Einschränkungen auf den Menschen
zu übertragen sind und da sie nur einen, allerdings zentralen pathogenetischen
Mechanismus ischämischer Herzkrankheiten, die Arteriosklerose, betreffen, müssen die zitierten Befunde mit Vorsicht interpretiert werden. Sie deuten allerdings
nachdrücklich darauf hin, daß fortgesetzte, intensive sympatho-adrenerge Akti-
vierungszustände infolge sozialer Risikosituationen (soziale Statusbedrohung) und
infolge individueller Dispositionen („Dominanzstreben") die Progression von Intimaläsionen in den Koronargefäßen direkt beeinflussen.

Gibt es, auf der Ebene epidemiologischer Beweisführung, Belege dafür, daß
auch beim Menschen aktive Distress-Zustände aufgrund einer Exposition gegenüber bestimmten sozialen Risikosituationen und aufgrund bestimmter psychischer
Risikomerkmale mit einer erhöhten Koronargefährdung einhergehen? Und wie lassen sich diese Risikobedingungen genauer definieren?

Psychomentale und sozio-emotionale Risiken im Erwerbsleben

Wie bereits einleitend erwähnt, erwarten wir die nachhaltigsten aktiven Distress-
Zustände im Erwerbsleben; denn im Erwerbsleben werden die wichtigsten und
häufigsten Verausgabungserfahrungen gemacht. Zugleich sind die Chancen erfolgreicher Kontroll- und Belohnungserfahrungen strukturell begrenzt. Allerdings
lassen sich koronargefährdende psychomentale und sozio-emotionale Belastungserfahrungen im Erwerbsleben nicht auf ganz bestimmte Berufsgruppen im Sinne
klassischer Berufskrankheiten beschränken. Vielmehr müssen mit Hilfe theoretischer Modelle spezifische Belastungsdimensionen definiert und in den jeweiligen
Tätigkeitsprofilen bzw. beruflichen Rahmenbedingungen identifiziert werden.
Im folgenden sollen zwei theoretische Modelle kurz vorgestellt werden, die aus
einer Zusammenarbeit zwischen Medizinsoziologen und Herz-Kreislauf-Epidemi-
ologen entstanden sind und die angesichts der Entwicklungstendenzen der Arbeitswelt in entwickelten Industriegesellschaften von besonderer Bedeutung sind.

Im Zentrum beider Modelle stehen psychomentale und sozio-emotionale Belastungserfahrungen am Arbeitsplatz. Diese beiden Begriffe sollen daher zunächst
definiert werden.

Psychomentale Belastungen gehen von fortgesetzten Beanspruchungen zentralnervöser Leistungen (Vigilanz, Informationsverarbeitung, Entscheidungsfindung unter Zeitdruck etc.) aus, die entweder zu einer Leistungsüberforderung oder -unterforderung führen. Unter sozio-emotionalen Belastungen verstehen wir alle affektiv getönten sensorischen oder symbolischen Erfahrungen, welche negative Rückmeldungen an das Selbstwertgefühl des Arbeitenden beinhalten. Diese negativen Rückmeldungen können das Ergebnis bzw. die Bewertung der erbrachten Leistung zum Gegenstand haben, sie können aber auch aus Konflikten mit Vorgesetzten, Kollegen, Untergebenen oder aus tiefgreifenden Statusunsicherheiten (Arbeitsplatzrisiko, Umsetzung, ungewisse Beförderungschancen) resultieren. Sowohl psychomentale wie auch sozio-emotionale Belastungen initiieren und modulieren wiederkehrende, nur bedingt bewußtseinspflichtige autonom-neuroendokrine Aktivierungen des Organismus, die von Erregungen der limbischen Strukturen im Zentralnervensystem, von hypothalamischen und hypophysären Hormonen sowie einer höherfrequenten Sympathikus-Aktivität ihren Ausgang nehmen.

Das erste Modell betrachtet fortgesetzte psychomentale und sozio-emotionale Belastungen am Arbeitsplatz als Ergebnis eines Zusammenwirkens hoher Arbeitsanforderungen (vor allem Zeitdruck) *und* geringer Entscheidungsfreiheit am Arbeitsplatz. Geringe Entscheidungsfreiheit kennzeichnet häufig Berufstätigkeiten, die begrenzte Chancen persönlicher Qualifizierung und Weiterentwicklung beinhalten. Die Belastungserfahrung ist hier also das Ergebnis einer Diskrepanz zwischen hoher (quantitativer) Anforderung und niedriger (qualitativer) Kontroll- und Steuerungschance angesichts vorgegebener Aufgaben. Nach dem sog. „job strain" (Arbeitsbelastungs)-Modell, das von dem amerikanischen Soziologen Robert Karasek entwickelt wurde, sind somit beispielsweise Orchestermusiker stärker belastet als Dirigenten, Fließbandarbeiter stärker als Industriemeister, Schalterbeamte stärker als Bankdirektoren etc. [8].

Ein zweites, in den vergangenen zehn Jahren von unserer Arbeitsgruppe entwickeltes und überprüftes theoretisches Modell definiert fortgesetzte psychomentale und sozio-emotionale Belastungserfahrungen am Arbeitsplatz als Ergebnis einer Diskrepanzerfahrung zwischen (hoher) beruflicher Verausgabung und (niedrigen) Belohnungschancen (sog. Modell beruflicher Gratifikationskrisen). Das Modell enthält, trotz gewisser Ähnlichkeiten mit dem vorhergehenden, zwei wesentliche Unterschiede: erstens wird die berufliche Verausgabung des Einzelnen nicht einfach als ein Reflex objektiver Arbeitsplatzanforderungen betrachtet, vielmehr wird sie als Produkt aus Anforderung und individueller Leistungsbereitschaft begriffen. Mit anderen Worten: erst die Kombination belastender objektiver Arbeitsanforderungen und eines individuellen Bewältigungsstils, der sich durch exzessive Verausgabungsbereitschaft auszeichnet, führt in der Regel zu jener Intensität zentralnervöser Aktivierungen, welche für das Herz-Kreislauf-System langfristig kritisch wird. Zweitens wird in diesem Modell nicht die begrenzte persönliche Kontrollmöglichkeit über die Arbeitsaufgabe als zentrales Moment betont, sondern die begrenzte Gratifikation angesichts hoher Verausgabung. Enttäuschte Belohnungserwartungen und -erfahrungen beziehen sich nicht nur auf das Einkommen, sondern auch auf die Anerkennung der Arbeitsleistung im sozialen Umfeld, insbesondere jedoch auf die Sicherung oder sogar Verbesserung des erreichten beruflichen Status. Bedingungen begrenzter sozialer Statuskontrolle wie blockierter Aufstieg, unfreiwillige Umsetzung, sozialer Abstieg, Arbeitsplatzunsicherheit modulieren, im Verein mit fortgesetzter hoher Verausgabung am Arbeitsplatz, den Effekt ungünstiger Emotionen auf die Herz-Kreislauf-Gefährdung [9].

Beide Modelle sind angesichts der gegenwärtigen Entwicklungstendenzen der Arbeitswelt von hoher Aktualität. Mit Hilfe des „job strain" Modells lassen sich gefährdete Berufsgruppen feststellen, deren Tätigkeit sich durch hohe psychomentale Belastungen und geringe Qualifikationsspielräume auszeichnet. Solche Tätigkeiten sind nicht auf die herkömmliche, arbeitsteilig organisierte Industrieproduktion beschränkt, sie finden sich auch in der Datenverarbeitung, in Büro- und Verwaltungstätigkeiten und in manchen Dienstleistungsberufen. Das Modell beruflicher Gratifikationskrisen ist bei der Identifizierung gefährdeter Beschäftigtengruppen hilfreich, die sich aus der Fragmentierung stabiler Berufsbiographien und den Folgen raschen sozio-technischen Wandels im heutigen Erwerbsleben ergeben. Aufgrund des begrenzten Raumes können hier nur kurze exemplarische Hinweise zur empirischen Bedeutung der beschriebenen Modelle gegeben werden.

Empirische Befunde

Das „job strain" Modell wurde bereits Ende der siebziger Jahre bezüglich seiner Erklärungskraft für Herz-Kreislauf-Krankheiten getestet. Aber erst die vergangenen Jahre brachten mit großen sog. prospektiven Studien überzeugende Belege. So gelang es nachzuweisen, daß Inhaber von Berufen mit hohen „job strain"-Werten auch nach statistischer Kontrolle der wichtigsten koronaren Risikofaktoren einem höheren Herzinfarktrisiko, ebenfalls einer höheren kardiovaskulären Mortalität ausgesetzt waren. Das relative Risiko liegt je nach Studie, und je nach Alters- und Geschlechtsgruppe, mit Werten zwischen 1,3 und 3,0 zwar niedrig, es ist jedoch angesichts der weiten Verbreitung gefährdender Arbeitsbedingungen von erheblicher gesundheitspolitischer Bedeutung. Neuere Studien zeigen interessanterweise, daß auch die Ausprägung des wichtigen koronaren Risikofaktors Bluthochdruck anhand des „job strain" Modells miterklärt werden kann, insbesondere dann, wenn ambulante Registriertechniken während der Arbeitszeit eingesetzt werden [10]. Zumindest eine Studie belegt ferner eine erhöhte Blutgerinnungsneigung bei Beschäftigten, die hohem „job strain" ausgesetzt sind. Neuesten Datums schließlich sind Studien, welche erhöhte Ausscheidungen von Stresshormonen ins Blut bei solchen Erwerbspersonen nachweisen [8].

Zusammengenommen schließt sich mit diesen Forschungsergebnissen eine Beweiskette, welche von der Struktur des Arbeitsplatzes über vermittelnde physiologische Mechanismen bis hin zur manifesten organischen Erkrankung führt.

Das Modell beruflicher Gratifikationskrisen ist besonders intensiv im Rahmen einer 6 1/2jährigen prospektiven Industriearbeiterstudie getestet worden. Bei 416 Metallarbeitern (25 bis 55 Jahre), die initial frei von manifester koronarer Herzkrankheit waren, wurden in vier Untersuchungswellen somatische, verhaltensgebundene und psychosoziologische Risikofaktoren konsekutiv erhoben. Das Ziel der Studie bestand darin, anhand von Komponenten des Modells beruflicher Gratifikationskrisen klassische Risikofaktoren wie Hyperlipidämie und Hypertonie zu erklären, darüber hinaus aber auch ihre möglichen direkten Effekte auf Neuerkrankungen im Beobachtungszeitraum zu analysieren. Aus den umfangreichen Ergebnissen seien hier lediglich die folgenden herausgehoben: Atherogene Blutfettwerte waren deutlich bei denjenigen Arbeitern erhöht, die unter hohem Rationalisierungsdruck und der Ungewißheit arbeiteten, ihren Arbeitsplatz erhalten zu können. Das gleiche zeigte sich für langjährige Schichtarbeit in Kombination mit subjektiver Arbeitsplatzunsicherheit. Diese Einflüsse waren statistisch unabhängig von Körpergewicht, Rauchen, Alkohol, Bewegungsarmut etc. [11]. Ferner belegte die Studie, daß die Gruppe der Industriearbeiter, welche gleichzeitig erhöhte Blutfettwerte und Bluthochdruck aufwiesen, durch blockierten beruflichen Aufstieg, aber auch durch ein hohes Maß chronischer Verärgerung sowie durch gesteigerte Wettbewerbshaltung gekennzeichnet war [12]. Schließlich waren, selbst bei Kontrolle dieser mittelbaren Wirkungen, direkte statistische Beziehungen zwischen hohen beruflichen Gratifikationskrisen und der Neuerkrankungsrate an Herzinfarkt zu beobachten. Anhand einer logistischen Regression konnte zunächst bestätigt werden, daß LDL-Cholesterin, Blutdruck und Lebensalter bei den Neuerkrankten signifikant erhöht waren. Der Einfluß von Zigarettenrauchen erwies sich aufgrund eines hohen Anteils von Exrauchern unter den Neuerkrankten als nicht signifikant, ebenso der Einfluß von körperlicher Bewegung. Das Körpergewicht war, nach statistischer Kontrolle von Blutdruck und LDL, nicht mehr positiv, sondern nunmehr sogar leicht negativ mit der Erkrankungswahrscheinlichkeit assoziiert. Interessanter ist jedoch in unserem Zusammenhang die Tatsache, daß vier zentrale Komponenten des Modells beruflicher Gratifikationskrisen mit einem erhöhten relativen Erkrankungsrisiko verknüpft waren: bei Vorliegen sog. Statusinkonsistenz, das heißt einer Diskrepanz zwischen beruflicher Stellung und Ausbildung, bei subjektiv erlebter Arbeitsplatzunsicherheit (Indikatoren begrenzter beruflicher Gratifikationschancen), bei starkem Zeitdruck am Arbeitsplatz sowie bei Vorliegen eines kritischen individuellen Bewältigungsstils, der sich durch ein übersteigertes Kontrollbedürfnis am Arbeitsplatz und eine Unfähigkeit zu innerer Distanzierung gegenüber Leistungsansprüchen auszeichnet (Indikatoren hoher Verausgabung) fand sich jeweils ein drei- bis vierfach erhöhtes relatives Risiko der Herzinfarkt-Erkrankung.

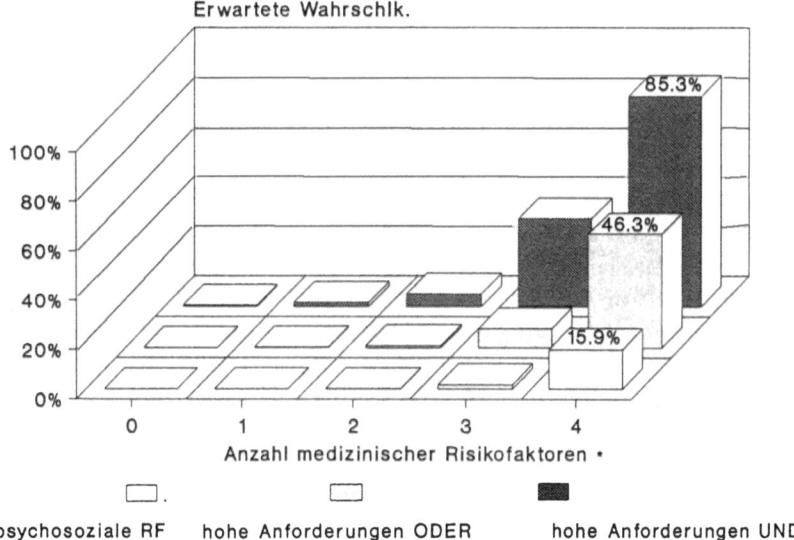

Abb. 1: Medizinische und psychosoziale Prädiktoren der Infarkt-Inzidenz (6.5 Jahre)
(N = 263 Industriearbeiter)

Die Abbildung 1 zeigt in graphischer Darstellung die Verbesserung der Modell-schätzung durch eine kombinierte Analyse klassischer somatischer und psychoso-ziologischer Risikofaktoren im Rahmen des Modells beruflicher Gratifikations-krisen. Wie man der Abbildung entnehmen kann, läßt sich die Auftretenswahr-scheinlichkeit von Herzinfarkt-Ereignissen anhand des logistischen Modells beson-ders gut schätzen, wenn Probanden mit den erwähnten somatischen Risikofakto-ren *und* mit gleichzeitig hoher Verausgabung und niedriger Gratifikation (niedriger beruflicher Statuskontrolle) betrachtet werden. Hier sagt das Modell über 85% der Herzinfarkt-Ereignisse korrekt voraus [9].

Wir können somit festhalten, daß für beide erwähnten theoretischen Modelle empirische Belege vorhanden sind und daß die kombinierte biomedizinische und psychosoziologische Betrachtung koronarer Herzerkrankungen zu einer verbesser-ten Erklärung und Vorhersage führt.

Praktische Konsequenzen

Welches sind die praktischen, sekundär- und primärpräventiven Konsequenzen aus diesen Erkenntnissen? Bei der Sekundärprophylaxe nach Herzinfarkt ist es angezeigt, aktive Distress-Zustände bei Koronarkranken durch verhaltensmedizinische Intervention in Form sog. Stressbewältigungsprogramme zu verringern, notfalls ergänzt durch eine medikamentöse Intervention. Aktive Distress-Zustände lassen sich aber auch durch mikro-soziale Interventionen verringern: durch Änderungen, deren Ziel in der Stärkung sozio-emotionalen Rückhalts in der Primärgruppe liegt [13]. Mit entspannenden Erfahrungen von Zugehörigkeit, von Liebe, Wertschätzung und Anerkennung auch außerhalb des beruflichen Leistungszusammenhangs wird ein schützendes Gegengewicht gegen Situationen berufsbedingter Daueraktivierung geschaffen. Soziales Kompetenztraining, beispielsweise in Herzgruppen im Rahmen der Langzeitbetreuung nach Herzinfarkt, veränderte Freizeit- und Vergesellschaftungsaktivitäten können hier ebenfalls hilfreich sein [14]. Bzgl. der beruflichen Rehabilitation nach Herzinfarkt ergeben sich aus den hier vorgestellten Ergebnissen verschiedene betriebs- und sozialpolitische Konsequenzen. So sollten Arbeitsplätze mit Mehrfachbelastungen und eingeschränkter Kontrollmöglichkeit zugunsten von Arbeitsplätzen, welche einen höheren Dispositionsspielraum gewähren und höhere Qualifikationsansprüche stellen, gemieden werden. Es sollte eine Begrenzung der Beschäftigungsdauer an Arbeitsplätzen mit hoher Beanspruchung bei gleichzeitiger Anpassung des Lohnniveaus bei Übergang zu Normalarbeitsplätzen durchgesetzt werden. Inner- und überbetriebliche Qualifizierungs- und Gratifikationsangebote, eine besondere personalpolitische Sensibilität bei innerbetrieblichen Umsetzungen und schließlich eine Erhöhung von Arbeitsplatzsicherheit oder allgemeiner von Chancen subjektiv befriedigender beruflicher Statuskontrolle sollten Ziele einer umfassenden Sekundärprophylaxe nach Herzinfarkt, möglicherweise sogar Ziele primärpräventiver Maßnahmen darstellen.

Zusammenfassend können wir festhalten: Psychomentale und sozio-emotionale Belastungen im Arbeitsleben wirken sich in Form aktiver Distress-Zustände über katabole, sympathoadrenerge Daueraktivierungen schädigend auf das Herz-Kreislauf-System aus. Diese Auswirkungen betreffen sowohl wichtige somatische Risikofaktoren wie die Hyperlipidämie, die Hypertonie und das Thromboserisiko, als auch die beschleunigte Entwicklung atherothrombotischer Komplikationen bereits im mittleren Erwachsenenalter (Herzinfarkt, plötzlicher Herztod). Anhand theoretischer Modelle lassen sich spezifische Belastungsdimensionen identifizieren und in den jeweiligen Tätigkeitsprofilen bzw. beruflichen Kontexten identifizieren (sog. „job strain"-Modell, Modell beruflicher Gratifikationskrisen). Nachdem in epidemiologischen Studien die Erklärungs- bzw. Prognosekraft dieser Modelle belegt worden ist, ergeben sich hieraus für die sekundäre, in Ansätzen auch für die primäre Prävention, neuartige Denkanstöße und praktische Empfehlungen. Obwohl sie über das herkömmliche Handlungsspektrum des Arztes hinausreichen, sind auch die mit individueller Prävention, Diagnostik, Therapie und Rehabilitation befaßten Ärzte aufgerufen, den dargestellten psychomentalen und sozio-emotionalen Risiken ihrer Patienten mit mehr Nachdruck als bisher Beachtung zu schenken.

Literatur

[1] Beamish, R.E., Singall, P.K., Dhalla, N.S., eds.: Stress and heart disease. Boston, The Hague, M. Nijhoff 1985.
[2] Henry, J., Stephens, P.: Stress, health, and the social environment. Berlin, Heidelberg, New York: Springer 1977.
[3] Frankenhaeuser, M.: Psychoneuroendocrine approaches to the study of emotions related to stress and coping. In: Howe D ed. Nebraska symposium on motivation. University of Nebraska Press: Lincoln 1979.
[4] Siegrist, J., Siegrist, K., Weber, I.: Sociological concepts in the etiology of chronic disease: the case of ischemic heart disease. Soc. Sci. Med. 1986; 22: 247–255.
[5] Kaplan, J.R., Manuck, S.B., Clarkson, T.B.: Psychosocial stress and atherosclerosis in Cynomolgus macaques. In: Beamish, R.E., Singall, P.K., Dhalla, N.S., eds. Stress and heart disease. M. Nijhoff Boston 1985, 250.
[6] Manuck, S.B., Kaplan, J.R., Adams, M.R., Clarkson, T.B.: Effects of stress and the sympathetic nervous system on coronary artery atherosclerosis in the Cynomolgus macaque. Am. Heart. J. 1988; 116 (1): 328–333.
[7] Ablad, B., Björkmann, J.-A., Gustafsson, D., Hansson, G., Östlund-Lindquist, A.-M., Petterson, K.: The role of sympathetic activity in atherogenesis: Effects of beta-blockade. Am. Heart. J. 1988; 116: 322–327.
[8] Karasek, R., Theorell, T.: Healthy work. New York: Basic Books 1990.
[9] Siegrist, J., Peter, R., Junge, A. et al.: Low status control, high effort at work and ischemic heart disease: prospective evidence from blue-collar men. Soc. Sci. & Med. 1990; 31: 1127–1134.
[10] Schnall, P.J., Pieper, C., Schwartz, J.E. et al.: The relationship between "job strain" workplace, diastolic blood pressure, and left ventricular mass index. J. Am. Med. Ass. 1990; 263: 1929–1935.
[11] Siegrist, J., Matschinger, H., Cremer, P., Seidel, D.: Atherogenic risk in men suffering from occupational stress. Atherosclerosis 1988; 69: 211–218.
[12] Siegrist, J., Peter, R., Georg, W. et al.: Psychosocial and biobehavioral characteristics of hypertensive men with elevated atherogenic lipids. Atherosclerosis 1991; 86: 211–218.
[13] House, J.S., Ladis, K.R., Umberson, D.: Social relationships and health. Science 1988; 241: 540–545.
[14] Ornish, D., Brown, S.E., Scherwitz, L.W. et al.: Can lifestyle changes reverse coronary heart disease? Lancet 1990; 336: 129–133.

POSTER PRESENTATIONS

Effects of oral treatment of SHR with enalapril and hydrochlorothiazide (A light- and electronenmicroscopical study)

H. Arnold-Schmiebusch
Anatomisches Institut (II)
Albert-Ludwigs-Universität Freiburg i.Br.

Our previous research on the pathological reaction of the vessel wall to arterial hypertension (stages of hypertension: Ischijima, 1969) and its dependence on age and vessel in SHR has included EM studies on the walls of the aorta, and the coronary, basilar, renal, femoral and testicular arteries. Differences dependent upon age and region were found in all layers of the vessel wall.

Our present aim is to determine whether different drug-specific reactions can be established which might be of clinical significance for human patients.

The following were investigated:

1. The morphology of hypertension-damaged vessel walls after subsequent treatment with enalapril and hydrochlorothiazide.
2. The action of these drugs on different layers of the vessel wall (intima, media) and different vessels (aorta, coronary and renal arteries).

Animals and Treatment: 10 controls = normotensive Wistar-Kyotorats (WKY), 10 untreated Spontaneously hypertensive rats (SHR), 10 treated SHR (30 mg enalapril) and 10 treated SHR (25 mg hydrochlorothiazide) per kg body weight per day were added to the drinking-water for a total of 6 weeks. Age of the animals: over 1 year.

Results: Both drugs (enalapril, HCT) reduce the blood pressure. In the more advanced stages of the pathological process, the coronary arteries show only a limited tendency to return to normal after treatment with either drug. The aorta reacts well to HCT. More weibel-palade-bodies appear in the endothelium. The smooth muscle cells of the media which have already begun to show signs of osmiophilia, and/or focal cytoplasmic necroses seem to be irreversibly damaged and even with antihypertensive treatment, the latter show a tendency to calcify.

Reference

Ischijima, K.: Morphological studies on the peripheral small arteries of SHR. Jap. Circulat. J. 33, 785–833 (1969).

Transplant Arteriopathy

Similarities to atherosclerosis in morphology, immunohistochemical characterization of cells and distribution of Apolipoproteins

S. Blasius, E. Vollmer, A. Fahrenkamp, K.-H.* Dietl, A. Roessner, W. Boecker
Gerhard-Domagk-Institute of Pathology, *Department of Surgery
University of Münster

Until now the pathogenesis of transplant arteriopathy has not been explained. The lesions of the vascular wall in transplant arteriopathy resemble the stages of atherosclerosis on morphological evaluation. Immunological damage, either cellular or humoral, to the endothelium is considered to be the initiating event in development of transplant arteriopathy. Morphologically intimal edema with cytoplasmic swelling and a distinct cellular infiltrate consisting mainly of T-lymphocytes can be detected. In severe cases the endothelium is completely lost and platelets and neutrophils adhere to the subendothelium, sometimes forming mural thrombi. The lesions resembling lipid-rich intimal plaques and fibrosclerotic plaques are made of foam cells, spindle shaped cells and collagens, elastin and proteoglycans of the extracellular matrix in varying amounts.

Using immunohistochemical standard procedures (APAAP-method) the cellular composition and the distribution of Apolipoproteins (APO) in arteries of explanted renal allografts was investigated with monoclonal antibodies against antigens of smooth muscle cells (Actin, Desmin, Vimentin) and mature macrophages (25F9) as well as monocytes (27E10) and with antibodies against APO A1, A2 and B.

Foam cells located in luminal and external areas of the intima and also some spindle-shaped cells are of macrophage nature immunohistochemically, whilst only some monocytes can be found in the intimal lesions. Other spindle-shaped cells express Actin revealing their smooth muscle cell nature (Fig. 1a). Whereas cells in the media show a strong positivity with the antibody against Desmin, those in the plaque-like lesions only show a weak reaction (Fig. 1b). In contrast there is a constant finding with the antibody against Vimentin throughout the whole vessel wall (Fig. 1c).

These findings show, that there is a loss of differentiation antigens in proliferating smooth muscle cells. Analogous findings are reported in atherosclerosis [1, 2]. At least the main cellular constituents of the vascular wall lesions are monocytes/macrophages and "transformed" smooth muscle cells in atherosclerosis as well as in transplant arteriopathy.

Immunohistochemical staining reveals intracytoplasmic deposits of Apo A1 (Fig. 2a) and A2 (Fig. 2b) predominantly in foam cells and in extracellular position. Deposits of Apo B (Fig. 2c) are located mainly extracellularly. This distribu-

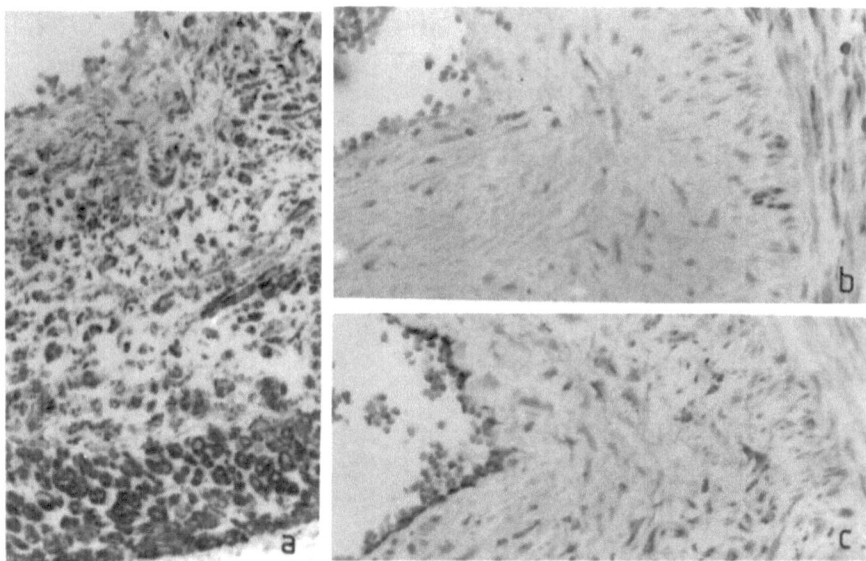

Figure 1: Immunohistochemical detection of muscle specific-actin isotype (a), Desmin (b) and Vimentin (c) in a fibrosclerotic plaque in transplant arteriopathy, with an evident loss of Desmin expression in intimal smooth muscle cells.

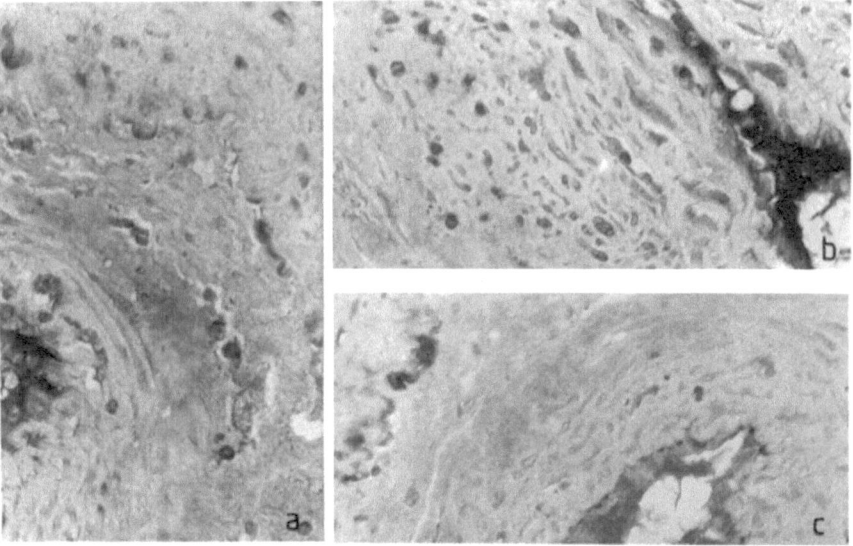

Figure 2: Immunohistochemical detection of extracellular and intracellular deposits of Apolipoprotein A1 (a), A2 (b) and of mainly extracellular depots of Apolipoprotein B (c) in transplant arteriopathy.

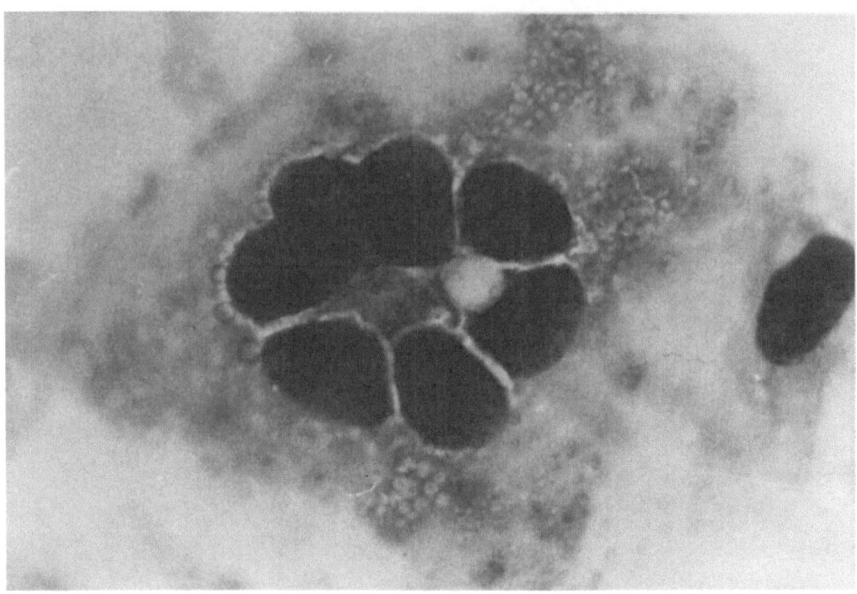

Multinuclear giant cell from a human coronary artery. Frozen-Häutchen preparation, H & E, x 700
(Figure belongs to Bürrig et al., p. 203 f.)

tion of Apolipoproteins in lesions of transplant arteriopathy is similar to that found in atherosclerosis [3–5]. These findings suggest the alteration in lipoprotein metabolism to be a prominent feature in the development of transplant arterio-pathy probably in a corresponding manner to the process of atherosclerosis.

Thus there are striking morphological and immunohistochemical similarities between transplant arteriopathy and atherosclerosis. A main difference is the often rapid progression of transplant arteriopathy within a few weeks. That re-quires a severe and/or repeated kind of endothelial or intimal likely immunologi-cal damage with subsequent extraordinary dysfunction.

References

[1] Kocher, O., Gabbiani, G. (1986): Cytoskeletal features of normal and atheromatous human arterial smooth muscle cells. Hum. Pathol. 17: 875–880.
[2] Osborn, M., et al. (1987): Intermediate filament expression in human vascular smooth muscle and in arteriosclerotic plaques. Virchows Arch. A 411: 449–458.
[3] Vollmer, E., et al. (1989): Immunhistochemische Untersuchungen zur Verteilung von Apolipoproteinen in der arteriosklerotischen Gefäßwand menschlicher Arterien. Verh. Dtsch. Ges. Path. 73: 445.
[4] Carter, R.S., et al. (1987): Immunohistochemical localization of apolipoproteins A1 and B in human carotid arteries. J. Pathol. 153: 31–36.
[5] Niendorf, A., et al. (1990): Morphological detection and quantification of lipoprotein(a) deposition in atheromatous lesions of human aorta and coronary arteries. Virchows. Arch. A 417: 105–111.

Giant cells in the endothelial layer indicate persistent injury and are a heterogenous subpopulation

K.F. Bürrig[1], D. Dominik[1], S. Zink[2], R. Oestreich[2], P. Rösen[2],
W. Sandmann[3]
[1] Institute of Pathology, [2] Diabetes Research Institute,
[3] Dept of Vascular Surgery,
Heinrich-Heine-University, Düsseldorf, Germany

Mono- or multinuclear giant cells (defined as cells with a surface area of $800\,\mu m^2$ or more) are regular constituents of the endothelial layer of arteries in elderly humans. However, only little is known about the natural history of these cells. In order to determine factors which promotes the appearance of such giant cells we have studied various locations of the arterial system (aorta, carotid and coronary arteries in humans, subhuman primates, cattles, and rats) by the use various me-thods (en-face and scanning electron microscopy, Häutchen preparations, cell culture, histo- and immunocytochemistry). Giant cells were usually found in regions of disturbed flow at the carotid bifurcation, in sclerotic plaques and in coarcted aortas. In contrast, giant cells were usually not found in non-sclerotic coronaries of humans and subhuman primates or very old rats. Furthermore, in senescent cultures of bovine aortic endothelium giant cells are always present. In such cultures the spectrum of the synthesized prostaglandins is changed and the production of the von Willebrand-factor is reduced. In humans about one third to one half of the giant cells contain unspecific esterase or tartrat-resistant acid phosphatase or α-1 anti-chymotrypsin or express CD68 (mab KP1, DAKO). This indicates that the giant cells in parts are derived from monocytes/macrophages but not from endothelial cells. From our study it is concluded that giant cells are a heterogeneous subpopulation in the endothelial layer and can be considered as a result of an increased regeneration and advanced senescence probably attributable to sustained injury as a result of flow irregularities.

Supported by the Deutsche Forschungsgemeinschaft (SFB 242, B3)

Characterisation of α-Adrenoceptors of Porcine Aorta: Differences between Vascular Smooth Muscle and Cultured Vascular Wall Cells

W. Erdbrügger, P. Vischer, H.J. Bauch, W.H. Hauss
Institut für Arterioskleroseforschung an der Universität Münster

Introduction

Several in vitro studies with cultured aortic cells showed that catecholamines alone or in combination with other serum factors act as mitogens and thus might contribute to the development of arteriosclerosis [1, 2, 3]. Although direct characterization of α-adrenoceptors by radioligand binding studies is well established, there is only limited information on whether or not and in what amount α-adrenoceptors are present on cultured vascular wall cells. We therefore investigated the binding characteristics of the α_1-antagonist [^{3}H]prazosin and the α_2-antagonist [^{3}H]yohimbine to porcine medial aortic membranes and compared the results with those obtained with membranes from cultured porcine aortic smooth muscle and endothelial cells.

Methods

Preparation of Medial Aortic Membranes

Medial aortic segments were prepared from porcine aortas. The segments were homogenized in a 4-fold excess (w/v) of sucrose-medium (5 mM Tris; 0.25 M sucrose; 2 mM $MgCl_2$; 2 mM $CaCl_2$; 1 mM PMSF; ph .7.6) using a Polytron homogenizer and centrifuged at 1000 g for 5 minutes. The supernatant was collected and centrifuged again at 100,000 g for 60 minutes. The pellet, a crude particulate fraction, was washed twice with assay buffer (50 mM Tris, pH 7.25, for the α_1-assay and 50 mM Tris, pH 7.75, for the α_2-assay, respectively) and suspended in an aliquot of the same buffer (1 ml buffer/g fresh weight). Membrane suspensions were frozen in liquid nitrogen and stored at $-20\,°C$ until use.

Preparation of Membranes from Cultured Vascular Wall Cells

Porcine aortic smooth muscle and endothelial cells were seeded in 25 ml DMEM at a density of 4.5×10^6 and 3.5×10^6 cells per cell culture plate (22.5 cm × 22.5 cm). 4–5 culture plates were kept at $37\,°C$ in an atmosphere containing 5% CO_2 until the cells reached confluency $(1-1.4 \times 10^8$ cells). Isolation of membranes from cultured vascular wall cells was performed according to Teitel [4].

Assay Conditions

200 µl of membrane suspension (250 µg protein) was incubated with the appropriate concentrations of radioligands in the absence or presence of 10^{-4} M noradrenaline. The total assay volume was 300 µl.

Competition binding studies were performed by incubating a constant concentration of radioligand (0.1 nM of [^{3}H]prazosin or 1 nM [^{3}H]yohimbine, respectively) and 200 µl of membrane suspension with rising concentrations of competitor.

The assays were stopped after incubation for 30 minutes at room temperature by diluting with cold assay buffer. Then the samples were filtered through Whatman GF/C glass fiber filters and were washed subsequently with 15 ml of cold buffer. The radioactivity retained on the filters was determined by liquid scintillation counting.

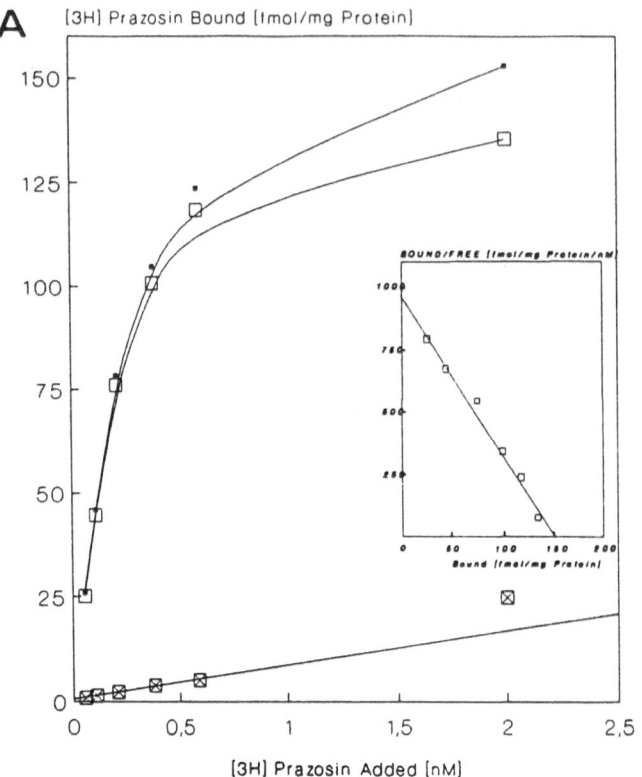

Figure 1: A) [^{3}H]prazosin binding to medial aortic membranes as a function of increasing concentration of [^{3}H]prazosin in the absence (points) or presence of 10^{-4} M noradrenaline (filled squares).
Insert: Rosenthal (Scatchard) Plot of [^{3}H]prazosin-specific binding (open squares).
B) Comparison of binding characteristics of [^{3}H]prazosin to medial aortic membranes and membranes derived from cultured vascular wall cells. Media: medial aortic membranes; SMC: membranes from cultured aortic smooth muscle cells; EC: membranes from cultured aortic endothelial cells.

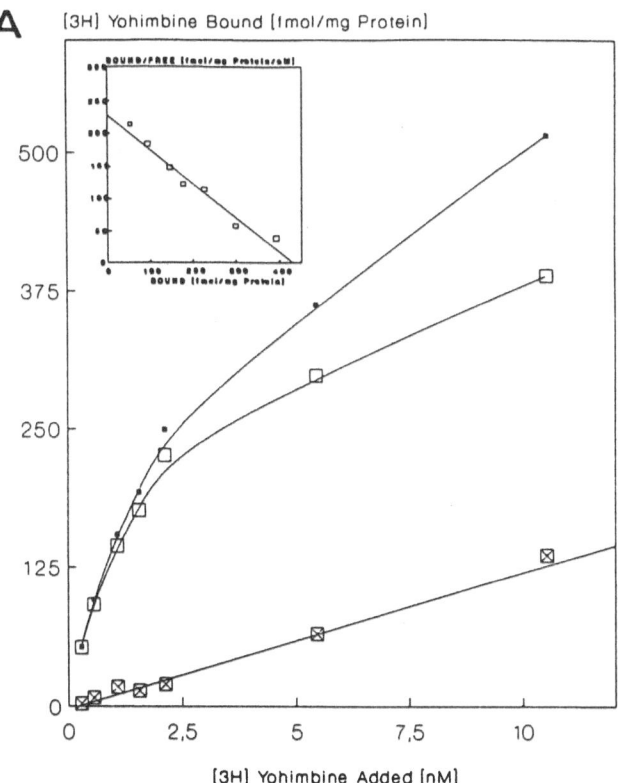

A [3H] Yohimbine Bound [fmol/mg Protein]

[3H] Yohimbine Added [nM]

B	KD	B$_{max}$	B$_{max}$
	[M]	[fmol/ mg Protein]	[Receptors/ Cell]
Media	1.83	372.2	1770
SMC	4.50	10.0	1096
EC	1.20	2.3	435

Figure 2: A) [^{3}H]yohimbine binding to medial aortic membranes as a function of increasing concentrations of [^{3}H]yohimbine in the absence (points) or presence of 10^{-4} M noradrenaline (filled squares).
Insert: Rosenthal (Scatchard) Plot of [^{3}H]yohimbine-specific binding (open squares).
B) Comparison of binding characteristics of [^{3}H]yohimbine to medial aortic membranes and membranes derived from cultured vascular wall cells. Media: medial aortic membranes; SMC: membranes from cultured aortic smooth muscle cells; EC: membranes from cultured aortic endothelial cells.

Results

With medial aortic membranes high affinity saturable binding was obtained for the α_1-antagonist [^{3}H]prazosin (Fig. 1A), yielding a K_d of 0.182 nM and a Bmax of 145 fmol/mg protein (Fig. 1B). High affinity saturable binding was also obtained with these membrane preparations for the α_2-antagonist [^{3}H]yohimbine (Fig. 2A), which yielded a K_d of 1.83 nM and a Bmax of 372 fmol/mg protein (Fig. 2B).

As shown by competition binding studies the [^{3}H]prazosin binding site exhibited α_1-adrenergic receptor specifity (order of potency: prazosin > phentolamine > yohimbine > adrenaline > noradrenaline >> phenylephrine), whereas the [^{3}H]yohimbine binding site exhibited α_2-adrenergic receptor specifity (order of potency: yohimbine > phentolamine > adrenaline > phenylephrine > noradrenaline > prazosin).

No obvious differences in the K_d values were found for membrane preparations from cultured porcine aortic smooth muscle cells (SMC) and membrane preparations from porcine medial aortic cells (see above). K_d values were 0.181 nM for the binding of [^{3}H]yohimbine (Fig. 2B) to α_2-adrenoceptors. The densities of α-adrenoceptors, however, were reduced in cultured SMC. Bmax values of α_1-adrenoceptors only reached 4.5 fmol/mg protein, corresponding to 238 α_1-receptors/cell (Fig. 1B), and 10 fmol/mg protein for α_2-adrenoceptors, corresponding to 1096 α_2-receptors/cell (Fig. 2B).

Saturation analysis with membranes from cultured porcine aortic endothelial cells (EC) revealed no significant specific binding of [^{3}H]prazosin (Fig. 1B), indicating that these cells lack α_1-adrenoceptors. Only α_2-adrenoceptors were present on membranes from cultured EC. The K_d for [^{3}H]yohimbine binding was 1.2 nM, and the Bmax 2.3 fmol/mg protein corresponding to 435 α_2-receptors/cell (Fig. 2B).

Conclusions

α-adrenergic receptors are present only in small amounts on membranes obtained from cultured SMC (Fig. 1B and Fig. 2B), when compared with membranes from the media of porcine aortas (Fig. 1B and Fig. 2B). On membranes derived from cultured porcine EC only α_2-adrenoceptors, but no α_1-adrenoceptors were found.

From these data we conclude, that α-adrenoceptors are downregulated in cultured porcine aortic cells. In the case of aortic SMC this might be due to the modulation of phenotype from the contractile state in the aorta to the synthetic state in culture [5].

References

[1] Blaes, N., Boisel, J.-P. (1983): J. Cell. Physiol. 116: 167–172.
[2] Sherline, P., Mascardo, R. (1984): J. Clin. Invest. 74: 483–487.
[3] Bauch, H.-J., et al. (1987): Exp. Pathol. 31: 193–204.
[4] Teitel, J.M., et al. (1986): J. Cell. Physiol. 128: 329–336.
[5] Chamley-Campbell, J., et al. (1979). Physiol. Rev. 59 (1): 1–61.

Comparison of several HDL parameters in discriminating between subjects with different risk for myocardial infarction

C. Gens, A. Klement, S. Gehrisch, M. Menschikowski, W. Jaross
Institute of Clinical Chemistry and Laboratory Diagnostics,
Medical Academy "C.G. Carus", Dresden

The aim of the study was to evaluate the power of several HDL parameters for discrimination of younger survivors of MI with normal or moderate elevated risk profile especially in respect to serum lipids from healthy controls.

Methods

A group of male patients (n = 100), surviving a myocardial infarction at least 4 months before investigation aging less than 51 years at time of the event was involved in the study. The criteria for selection were triglycerides < 3.1 mmol/l and cholesterol < 6.8 mmol/l, absence of metabolic diseases, blood pressure RR < 180/100, smoking < 20 g tabaco/d. A normal age matched group of 115 probands served as a reference group.

Blood samples were taken after overnight fasting by venipuncture and the following parameters were determined: TC (automated variant of Liebermann-Burchard-reaction, AB.GDR), TG (AB.GDR), HDLC (phosphotungstate precipitation and cholesterol determination, AB.GDR), Apolipoprotein (Apo)A-I, ApoA-II, ApoB, ApoC-II, ApoC-III, ApoD, ApoE (rocket immunelectrophoresis with own produced rabbit antisera).

LDLC was calculated according the FRIEDEWALD-Formula, VLDLC was calculated from TG (mmol/l)/2.2.

The different lipoproteins were fractionated by density gradient ultracentrifugation (Beckman) into the fractions U-HDL, U-HDL2, U–HDL3, U–LDL, U-VLDL. Cholesterol and main apolipoproteins were determined in these fractions.

Discrimination analysis on the basis of WILKS' lambda was used to estimate the value of parameters mentioned.

Results

The lipid parameters TG, TC, U-LDLC, U-VLDLC, P-VLDLC, apoB and apoE did not show any significant differences between the two groups, whereas several HDL-parameters did (Table 1).

The ratios of apolipoproteins A-I and A-II to cholesterol in HDL and HDL subfractions HDL-2 and HDL-3 differ significantly between the MI group and the

Table 1: HDL

	Patients $x \pm (s)$		Control $x \pm (s)$
P-HDLC (mmol/l)	1.50 (0.36)	$p < 0.05$	1.61 (0.36)
U-HDLC (mmol/l)	1.72 (0.53)		1.67 (0.44)
Apo A-I (g/l)	1.56 (0.27)	$p < 0.01$	1.65 (0.26)
Apo A-II (g/l)	0.49 (0.11)		0.48 (0.08)
U-HDL2C (mmol/l)	0.70 (0.42)		0.73 (0.31)
U-HDL3C (mmol/l)	1.02 (0.26)	$p < 0.05$	0.94 (0.24)
HDL2-ApoA-I (g/l)	0.26 (0.22)	$p < 0.01$	0.32 (0.16)
HDL2-ApoA-II (g/l)	0.06 (0.05)	$p < 0.001$	0.09 (0.04)
HDL3-ApoA-I (g/l)	0.74 (0.20)		0.70 (0.19)
HDL3-ApoA-II (g/l)	0.24 (0.10)		0.24 (0.08)
Apo D (mg/l)	81.3 (34.5)		78.3 (20.7)

Figure 1: Ratio apolipoprotein/cholesterol in HDL and HDL-subfractions, $\bar{x} \pm s$.

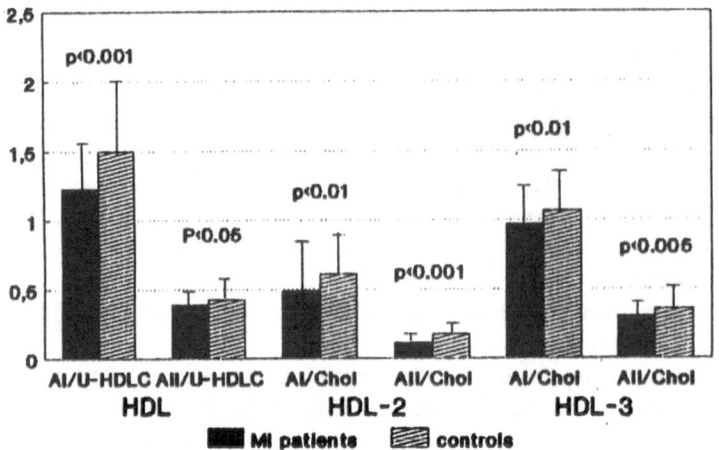

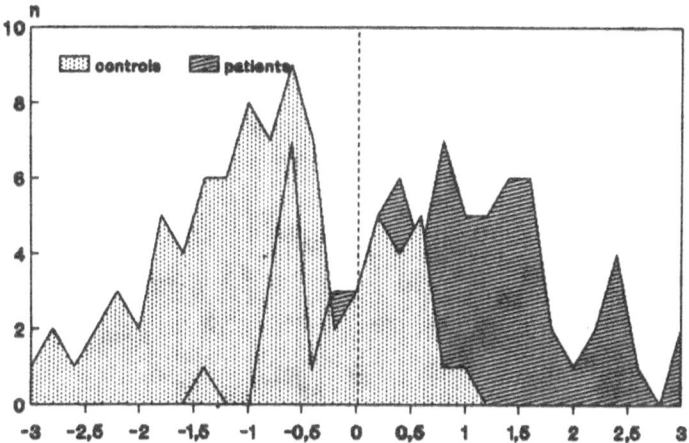

Figure 2: Discrimination analysis (WILKS' lambda), HDL-parameters.

control group, showing a higher cholesterol load of HDL in patients than in controls (Figure 1).

Discrimination analysis (WILKS'lambda) using only HDL-parameters resulted in a correct classification of about 75% for each group (see Figure 2).

As shown in Table 2 the ratio HDL2-ApoA-II/HDL2-Cholesterol has the highest discriminating value, being greater than that of ApoA-I serum concentration and much greater than HDL-cholesterol.

Table 2: Value of special HDL parameters for differentiation

1. HDL2-A-II/HDL2-C ratio
2. Apo A-I in serum
3. U-HDL3-C
4. Apo D in serum
5. U-HDL 2
6. HDL2-A-I/HDL2-C ratio
7. U-HDL-C

Conclusions

In subjects without strongly elevated TC and TG different HDL parameters are informative for discrimination between high and low atherogenic risk. Beside the wellknown differences of HDLC and apo A-I the ratios of apolipoproteins A-I and A-II to cholesterol as well in HDL as in the HDL subfractions are sufficient discriminators between the groups. The cholesterol reverse transport capacity might be impaired in the group of MI patients indicated by an overload of HDL with cholesterol. The reasons for these facts must be subject of further investigation.

Lipid-lowering therapy with garlic tablets
Comparison with other lipid-lowering drugs

J. Grünwald, W.D. Hübner, D. Laudahn, V. Schulz

Medical Department, Lichtwer Pharma GmbH, Berlin

The prophylactic use of garlic preparations against arteriosclerosis is widely accepted within the German population. The best documented and mostly used preparation "Kwai" garlic tablets (600 mg garlic powder/daily) had last year 2.43 mill. regular users in Germany.

In addition, a higher dosed garlic preparation (Sapec, 900 mg garlic powder/daily) has been recognized as prescription lipid-lowering drug by the health authorities in mild and moderate cases of hyperlipidaemia and is reimbursed by the health insurance system.

More than one dozen clinical trials proove the cholesterol- and triglyceride-lowering action of Kwai/Sapec in a doserelated manner. After a 1–4 months lasting therapy with 600–900 mg garlic powder daily, a mean cholesterol-lowering of about 11% and a mean triglyceride-lowering of about 13% was shown.

Other lipid-lowering natural substances are either less or only partially effective, have to be used in rather high dosages and are generally more expensive than garlic.

Other synthetic, lipid-lowering drugs have generally more side-effects, the wide majority is more or much more expensive, but they are partially more effective.

Table 1: Median daily dose and lipid-lowering effectiveness

Preparations (in alphabetical order)	Dose (g/d)	Lowering effect (%) Cholesterol	Triglyceride
A. Synthetic remedies:			
Ion exchange resins	8–16	20–25	0
Fibrate group	0.5– 2	5–15	25–60
HMG-CoA reductase inhibitors	0.04	20–40	5–25
Nicotinic acid group	2– 6	15–25	20–40
Anti-oxydants	1	5–15	0
B. Natural remedies:			
Garlic (dried)	0.6–1.2	5–15	10–20
Omega-3-oils (fish oil)	3–10	5–10	20–50
Phospholipides (soybean)	1– 3	5–10	7
Phytosterol preparations	6	5–15	0

Table 1 summarises the different dosage levels and lipid-lowering effects of synthetic and natural lipid-lowering drugs. Two other important factors like the costs and the side effects are not listed. In general, garlic powder tablets are the lowest in price. Virtually, no real side-effects occur and the compliance of the patients is generally very good.

Therefore, garlic powder tablets should be the first step of a lipid-lowering therapy, if diet alone is insufficient. The ideal patients for garlic therapy have starting cholesterol levels between 220–300 mg/dl. For these patients, a moderate lipid-lowering of 10–15% with a side-effect free medication is advisable. For patients with higher lipid-levels, other forms of lipid-lowering drugs should be used, according to the recommendation in Table 2.

Table 2: Recommendations relating to cholesterol-lowering treatment

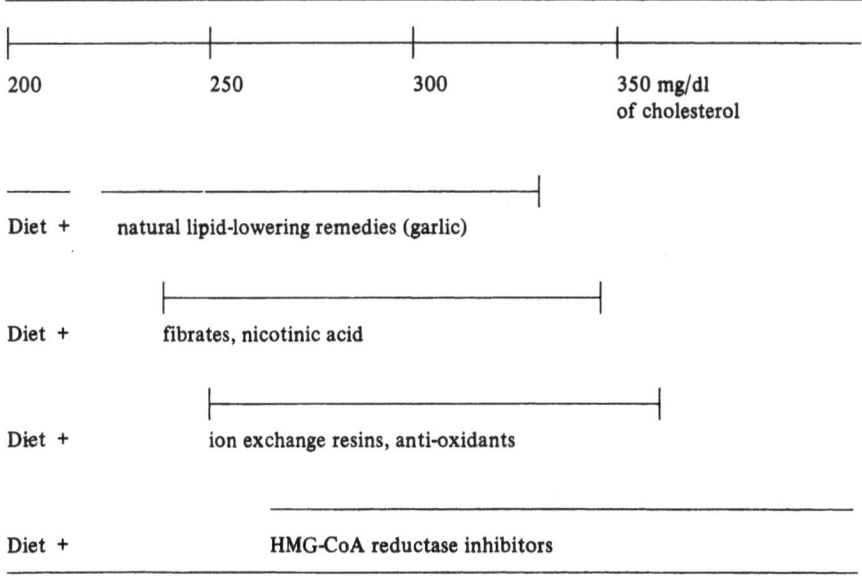

| 200 | 250 | 300 | 350 mg/dl of cholesterol |

Diet +   natural lipid-lowering remedies (garlic)

Diet +   fibrates, nicotinic acid

Diet +   ion exchange resins, anti-oxidants

Diet +   HMG-CoA reductase inhibitors

Cardiac Stress in Everyday Life versus During Coronary Group Therapy

H.-Ch. Heitkamp, A. Hipp, H.-H. Dickhuth
Medizinische Klinik V, Sportmedizin, Universität Tübingen

Introduction

General practitioners often refrain from recommending patients to join coronary outpatient groups. They argue that cardiac stress is higher than in everyday life due to higher pulse rate and higher blood pressure, thus increasing the rate-pressure product and myocardial oxygen demand. ST-depression as a sign of oxygen deficit is equally well documented by modern Holter monitoring and conventional 12-lead ECG in bicycle or treadmill ergometry [2, 3, 8]. Cardiac stress during unrestricted daily activity and sport therapy was investigated by Holter monitoring over 24 hours.

Method

12 coronary patients (age 60 ± 6 years, height 172 ± 10 cm, weight 77 ± 12 kg) joined the study after being informed about the risks. The duration of coronary disease was 68 ± 56 months. They had taken part in coronary group therapy for 40 ± 32 months. Cardiac history included 7 anterior wall infarctions, 3 posterior wall infarctions and 2 documented coronary artery diseases. Bypass surgery was performed on 4 patients and all had stable angina.

An incremental upright bicycle ergometry was performed before Holter monitoring. Maximum work load was 1.5 ± 0.3 W/kg. Signs of ischemia occurred earlier: The pulse limit of 102 ± 11/min was set at that workload without any symptoms (1.1 ± 0.2 W/kg). Holter monitoring was performed with a 2-channel, digitized system (Epicardia, Hellige, Freiburg, FRG). Periods of heart frequency above the pulse limit and of ischemia were printed out and optically controlled. ST depression of $\geqslant 0.1$ mV and of a duration of $\geqslant 1$ minute was considered significant.

Patients kept diaries during monitoring with emphasis on angina.

Results

One patient did not pass the pulse limit, 4 others remained below during group therapy and 3 others during everyday life. The pulse limit was exceeded by 7% (range 2–23) during group therapy and by 11% (range 1–32) during everyday life, the difference not being significant. The limit was passed more often during everyday life ($p < 0.05$; Fig. 1).

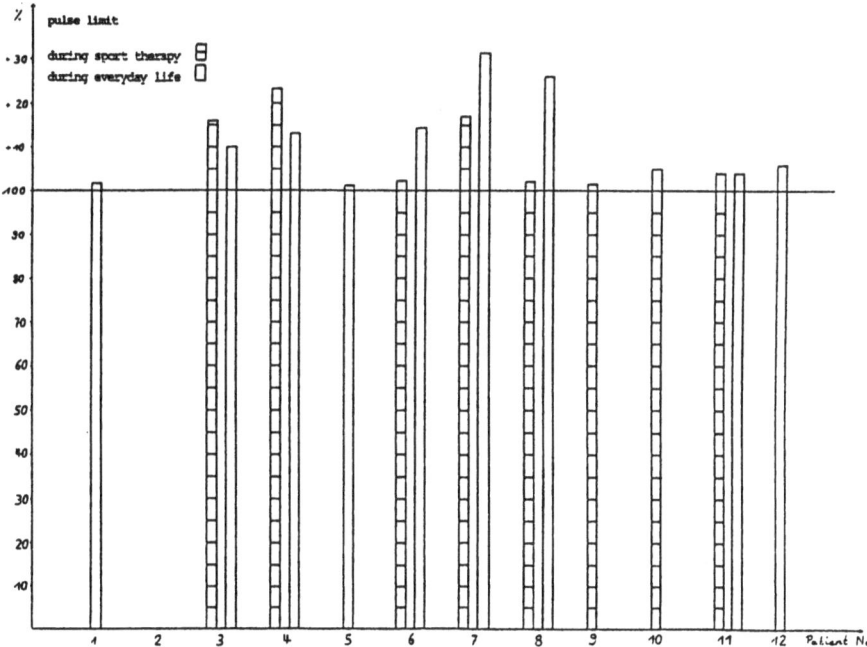

Figure 1: 11 coronary patients exceeding the pulse limit during sport therapy or everyday life. Patient 2 did not pass the limit.

Ischemic ST depression only was detected in 2 patients and 5 patients reported chest pain only and one patient boths. The ischemic episodes were all but one during everyday life.

Discussion

Studies comparing coronary patients during sport therapy and everyday life are rare. In most instances they were studied during ergometry in comparison to ambulatory monitoring. In agreement with our results, ST-depression was more often discovered during Holter monitoring than in treadmill testing [5], opposed by other results when 70% of the patients showed ischemia in the Holter ECG compared to 86% on the bicycle ergometer [4]. The use of transient ST depression in continuous monitoring was documented to be valuable only in patients with proved coronary artery disease [1].

Our earlier investigations had shown that the pulse limit is often exceeded during group therapy [6, 7]. Coronary patients seem to overexert not only during outpatient therapy, but more often during everyday life, exceeding the limit by the same amount. Coronary patients must be guided not to pass the pulse limit by counting pulse and by learning to avoid physical or mental stress before signs of ischemia.

References

[1] Deanfield, J.E., Shea, M., Ribiero, P., de Landsheere, C.M., Wilson, R.A., Horlock, P., Selwyn, A.P.: Transient ST-segment depression as a marker of myocardial ischemia during daily life. Am. J. Cardiol. 1984, 54: 1195–1200.

[2] Eggeling, Th., Osterspey, A., Kochs, M., Jansen, W., Günther, H., Höher, M., Hombach, V.: Bewertung der ST-Streckenanalyse im Langzeit-EKG. Dtsch. med. Wschr. 1988, 113: 88–90.

[3] Egstrup, K.: The relationship between ST segment deviation projected to the front of the chest during exercise and simultaneous Holter monitoring. Eur. Heart J. 1988, 9: 412–417.

[4] Hausmann, D., Nikutta, P., Daniel, W.G., Hartwig, C.-A., Wenzlaff, P., Lichtlen, P.R.: Wertigkeit von Belastungs- und Langzeit-EKG in der Diagnostik der stummen Myokard-ischämie bei Patienten mit koronarer Herzkrankheit. Z. Kardiol. 1988, 77: 282–290.

[5] Levy, R.D., Shapiro, L.M., Wright, C., Mockus, L., Fox, K.M.: Haemodynamic response to myocardial ischaemia during unrestricted activity, exercise testing, and atrial pacing assessed by ambulatory pulmonary artery pressure monitoring. Br. Heart J. 1986, 56: 12–18.

[6] Schmitt-Kip, R.B., Heitkamp, H.-Ch., Jeschke, D.: Energieumsatz und kardiale Belastung bei Übungs- und Trainingsgruppenteilnehmern einer ambulanten Herzgruppe. In: Sport Rettung oder Risiko für die Gesundheit, Deutscher Ärzteverlag 1989.

[7] Schuberth, S., Jeschke, D., Brühl, G.: Energieumsatz bei Übungs- und Trainingstherapie in ambulanten Koronargruppen. In: Stellenwert der Sportmedizin in Medizin und Sport-wissenschaft, Springer-Verlag 1984.

[8] Tzivoni, D., Benhorin, J., Gavish, A., Stern, S.: Holter recording during treadmill testing in assessing myocardial ischemic changes. Am. J. Cardiol. 1985, 55: 1200–1203.

The thrombocyte function inhibiting effect of garlic: a randomized, placebo-controlled, double-blind parallel group investigation

H. Kiesewetter, F. Jung, G. Pindur, E.M. Jung, C. Mrowietz, E. Wenzel
Department of Clinical Haemostasiology and Transfusion Medicine,
University of the Saarland, Homburg/Saar

Introduction

Since the drugs used for thrombocyte aggregation inhibition in the treatment of arterial occlusive disease have side effects – especially in high doses – the patients may refuse the intake of these preparations. Thus, the intake of coated tablets of garlic could be a well tolerated alternative as serious side effects are not known after the intake of coated tablets of garlic [7]. The aim of the study was to investigate if the intake of garlic powder (800 mg/d) can normalize an initially disturbed thrombocyte function.

Design of Study

The study is performed as double-blind, placebo-controlled parallel group investigation. Only participants with constantly increased spontaneous thrombocyte aggregation are included; it is required, that two of the three controls must present a disturbed thrombocyte function. The participants receive 800 mg of garlic powder (4 coated tablets Kwai forte®, Lichtwer Pharma GmbH) or 4 coated tablets of placebo (identical preparation). Further measurements are made on the 14th, 21st, 28th and 35th day after inclusion. A total number of 140 volunteers had to be examined to determine and include 60 participants with constantly disturbed thrombocyte function. 3/5 of the participants in the placebo/active substance group smoked, 1/0 were overweight, 12 of the 20/10 of 21 women took contraceptives. There were no other cardiovascular risk factors or medications.

Methods

Spontaneous thrombocyte aggregation was determined according to the method of Breddin [3]. For the description of the transmission curve the angle of ascent $\alpha 2$ was chosen.

Additionally, the thrombocyte function was evaluated by the test modified by Grotemeyer et al. [5]. The test procedure is based on the dissolution of platelet aggregates (existing in vivo or caused by the withdrawal of blood) in ethylenediaminetetraacetic (EDTA) but immediate fixation in EDTA formalin. With the EDTA-formalin-test, the number of platelets in the supernatant is reduced by the number of platelet aggregates. The results of both tests can be indicated as quotient. If the result from the EDTA formalin test is chosen as denominator the quotient increases with the number of aggregates. A PR value greater than 1.05 is suspicious, values over 1.2 highly pathological.

Results

At the onset of the study both groups are structurally homogenous. The double-blind design ensured also homogeneity of observation thus statistical comparison of the groups is permissible [9]. During the five weeks of investigation the placebo group presents a slight increase in spontaneous thrombocyte aggrea-

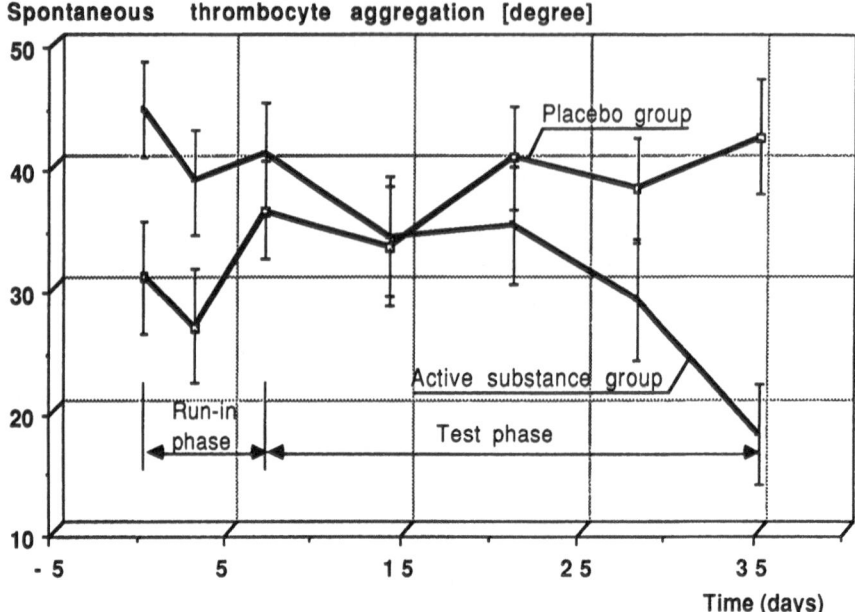

Figure 1: Spontaneous platelet aggregation before and 4 weeks after garlic or placebo respectively

Figure 2: Platelet reactivity index before and after 4 weeks of garlic or placebo respectively

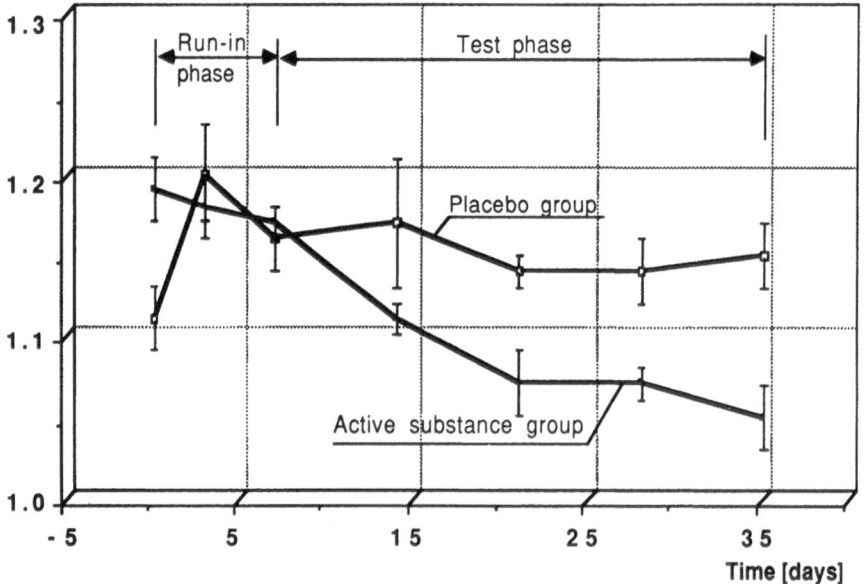

tion; the seven samples are not from the same parent population ($p < 0.0042$). In the active substance group there is a considerable decrease in spontaneous thrombocyte aggregation; the seven samples are not from the same parent population ($p < 0.0004$).

While the circulating thrombocyte aggregates in the placebo group did not change significantly during the five weeks of investigation (the seven samples are from one parent population, $p < 0.062$) there is a marked decrease in the active substance group (the seven samples are not from the same parent population, $p < 0.0001$).

Discussion

Besides the primary control of haemorrhage and activation of the plasmatic coagulation system thrombocytes are an important factor of atherogenesis. After attachment to the vascular endothelium they release mitogenic factors to the endothelial cells thus producing an increased proliferation which can lead to a constricted lumen and a reduced blood flow. In a prospective study with diabetics Breddin could show that the constantly increased thrombocyte aggregation represents a risk factor concerning vascular occlusions [PARD study].

In the study presented here only participants with constantly increased thrombocyte aggregation were included in order to investigate the influence of garlic on the disturbed thrombocyte function. It turns out, that the intake of 800 mg of garlic powder per day leads to a progressive decrease in elevated spontaneous thrombocyte aggregation as well as to a decrease in circulating thrombocyte aggregates. Concerning this significant reduction of the disturbed thrombocyte function different mechanisms are discussed:

For the first time, Vanderhoeck could demonstrate that the inhibition of platelet aggregation is produced by means of the blockage of the arachidonic acid metabolism [10] which leads to a reduced production of prostaglandins and thromboxane in the thrombocytes [4]. Besides an inhibition of induced thrombocyte aggregation, Srivastava [8] demonstrated an inhibition of the thromboxane production from exogenic arachidonic acid, an inhibition of the lipase activity, an inhibition of thromboxane synthesis and lipoxigenase products from marked arachidonic acid and an inhibition of the incorporation of arachidonic acid in platelelet phospholipides. This suggests that garlic can inhibit thrombocyte aggregation in different stages. Furthermore, an increase in the synthesis of prostacyclin (PGI_2) by garlic is described also leading to an inhibition of thrombocyte aggregation and a dilatation of the vessels [6].

References

[1] Bordia, A.: Atherosclerosis 30, 355–360 (1978).
[2] Bordia, A., Verma, S.K.: Artery 7, 428–437 (1980).
[3] Breddin, K., Grun, H., Krzywanek, H.J., Schremmer, M.M.: Thromb. Haemostas. 48, 261–272 (1975).
[4] Doutremepuich, C., Gamba, G., Refauvelet, J.: Ann. pharm. franc. 43, 273–280 (1985).
[5] Grotemeyer, K.-H., Viand, R., Beykirch, K.: Dtsch. med. Wschr. 108, 775–778 (1983).
[6] Mohammed, S.F., Woodward, S.C.: Thromb. Res. 44, 793–806 (1986).
[7] Reuter, H.D.: Spektrum Allium sativum. Aesopus Verlag, Zug (1988).
[8] Srivastava, K.C.: Biomed. Bioc. 43, 335–346 (1984).
[9] Trampisch, H.J.: Angio Archiv 13: 9–13 (1986).
[10] Vanderhoeck, J.Y., Makheja, A.N., Bailey, J.M.: Bioch. Pharm. 29, 3169–3173 (1980).

Prevalence of Autoantibodies to Glycated LDL in Diabetic and Normal Subjects

T. Koschinsky, C.E. Bünting, U. Glahn, and J.L. Witztum*
Diabetes Research Institute Düsseldorf, F.R. Germany
*University of California, San Diego, CA, USA

Modifications of the chemical structure of low density lipoproteins can affect their biological properties and may increase their atherogenic potential [1]. In diabetes, related research has focused on both short- and longterm nonenzymatic glycation of LDL which has been implicated for example in the pathogenesis of macrovascular complications [2]. But the detailed mechanisms how these glycated LDL affect the development of diabetic complications is still incompletely understood. During the course of these studies we noted that nonenzymatic glycation resulted not only in abnormal functional properties of LDL, but also rendered so modified LDL immunogenic [3]. This has been proven in animals studies [4]. Serumautoantibodies to nonenzymatically glycated LDL had been described also in a few diabetic patients and normal subjects, but prevalence data have been still missing.

The aim of this study was to examine the prevalence of autoantibodies vs. short-time glycated (Glc-)LDL and advanced glycated endproducts (AGE-)LDL in sera from type I and type II diabetic patients and normal subjects within the age range of 10–80 years.

Methods

Therefore, sera from 281 diabetic patients (age range: 11–85 years, 142 Type 1, 139 Type 2, 132 male, 149 female) and 169 normal subjects (10–80 years, 82 male, 87 female) were tested by dilution and competition RIA for binding to the following antigens: LDL from normal subjects incubated with glucose (80 mM) for 7 days (glc-LDL) and for 2–3 months to generate advanced glycation endproducts (AGE-LDL).

To determine the titer of antisera to a given antigen a solidphase radioimmuno assay was used. Microtiter plates were coated with the glycated proteins at a final concentration of 50 ng/well. After postcoating with human albumin various dilutions of the serum antibodies ± the competing antigen were added and incubated for 18 hours. The amount of immunoglobulin bound was than quantitated by use of 125 I-labelled, affinity purified goat antihuman immunoglobulin that reacted with all immunoglobulin classes. In addition, for every sample and at every dilution tested a control value was obtained from wells that contained the postcoat protein, but no antigen. This control value was subtracted from the respective binding data, obtained when the antigen was present. A positive titer is defined as the reciprocal of the highest dilution of serum that gave absolute binding at least twice that of controls.

Results and Discussion

As there have been no detectable differences between males and females in diabetic and normal subjects as well as between the groups of type I and type II diabetic patients their data have been combined into one group each. Normal subjects and diabetic patients showed a similar pattern of antibody titer distribution vs. glc-LDL: about 50% of the sera from each group showed specific antibodies to glc-LDL with a titer range between 4 and 2048, and a mean value at the titer of 256. The other sera did not contain detectable titers of antibodies vs. glc-LDL. There was no difference between both groups.

Normal subjects and diabetic patients showed a similar pattern of antibody titer distribution vs. AGE-LDL: about 30% of the sera from each group showed specific antibodies to AGE-LDL with a titer range between 4 and 2048 and a mean value at the titer of 256. More than 2/3 of the sera of both groups did not contain detectable titers of antibodies vs. AGE-LDL. Again, there was no difference between both groups.

Under standardized conditions using only one concentration of competing antigen (short- and longterm glycated LDL), competition results varied over a wide range (20–100% competition) but could be demonstrated in diabetic and normal sera against both antigens.

In diabetics as well as in normal subjects the antibody titers did not correlate between the 2 forms of glycated LDL. Instead, 4 groups could be identified: 1) with no antibodies vs. both antigens, 2) and 3) with antibodies, of variable titers vs. only the short or the longterm glycated LDL form and 4) with antibodies of variable titers vs. both antigens.

In normal subjects, there was no age dependent increase of antibody containing sera vs. short and longterm glycated LDL. In contrast, in diabetic patients the percentage of antibodies containing sera vs. both glycated forms of LDL increased significantly with age. But the existence of antibodies vs. glycated LDL did not depend on diabetes duration, clinical complications or metabolic control expressed as HbA_{1c} value.

While we have shown for the first time prevalence data for autoantibodies vs. glycated LDL, autoantibodies f.e. vs. glucitol human serum albumin in diabetic and normal subjects have been already demonstrated [5]. In this paper, higher titers have been found to be more prevalent in 29 type 1 diabetic patients vs. 20 normal subjects. The difference to our results is probably related to the rather small number of patients and controls compared to the nearly tenfull higher numbers of our sera.

The antibodies described here may be natural antibodies, as their presence in normal subjects and relative low affinity could suggest. An increased concentration of glycated LDL in diabetic patients may result in an enhanced production and clearance of specific antibodies. The binding of these antibodies to glycated LDL, whether circulating or bound, f.e. within the vascular wall, would lead to increased formation of immune complexes. An increased deposition of immune complexes of unknown origin in blood vessels has been described already in diabetes previously [6–8]. LDL-containing immun complexes lead to increased intracellular cholesterol accumulation and foam cell formation [9]. In the diabetic aorta, we could demonstrate in preliminary experiments by using antibodies raised vs. FFI-LDL, a characteristic compound of AGE, an increased concentration of FFI-epitopes.

From these results we conclude that specific antibodies to glc- and AGE-LDL are present in both normal subjects and diabetics. Such autoantibodies could be involved in the pathogenesis of late complications including arteriosclerosis, as well as in the aging process.

References

[1] Witztum, J.L., Koschinsky, T.: Metabolic and immunological consequences of glycation of low density lipoproteins. Progr. Clin. Biol. Res. 304: 219–234 (1989).
[2] Brownlee, M., Cerami, A., Vlassara, H.: Advanced glycosylation end products in tissue and the biochemical basis of diabetic complications. N. Eng. J. Med. 318: 1315–1321 (1988).

[3] Steinbrecher, U.P., Witztum, J.L., Kniemi, Y.A., Elam, R.: Comparison of glycosylated LDL with methylated or cyclohexandione-treated LDL in the measurement of receptor-independent LDL catabolism. J. Clin. Invest. 71: 960–964 (1983).

[4] Witztum, J.L., Steinbrecher, U.P., Fisher, M., Kesaniemi, A.: Nonenzymatic glucosylation of autologous LDL, and albumin, render them immunogenic in the guinea pig. Proc. Natl. Acad. Sci. 80: 2757–2761 (1983).

[5] Mangili, R., Viberti, G.C., Vergani, D.: Antibodies to human albumin epitopes in type 1 (insulin-dependent) diabetes mellitus. Diabetologia 31: 639–649 (1988).

[6] Larsson, O.: Studies of small vessels in patients with diabetes: the result of the immunofluorescent localization of G-globulin in small dermal blood vessels. Acta. Med. Scand. 480: 47 (1967).

[7] Cohn, R.A., Mayer, S.M., Barbosa, J., Michael, H.F.: Immunofluorescence studies of skeletal muscle extracellular membranes in diabetes mellitus. Lab. Invest. 39: 16 (1978).

[8] Irvine, W.J., Di Mario, U., Guy, K., Iavicoli, M., Pozzilli, P., Lumbroso, B., Andreani, D.: Immune complexes and diabetic microangiopathy. J. Clin. Lab. Immunol. 1: 187 (1978).

[9] Tertov, V.V., Orekhov, A.N., Kacharava, A.G., Sobenin, I.A., Perova, N.V., Smirnov, V.N.: Low density lipoprotein-containing circulating immune complexes and coronary atherosclerosis. Exp. Mol. Pathol. 52: 300–308 (1990).

Foam cells of early Atherosclerosis: are they Macrophages or smooth Muscle Cells?

J. Kulka, M. Hubay*, A. Kádár
2nd Department of Pathology and *Department of Forensic Medicine, Semmelweis University of Medicine, Budapest, Hungary

The 2nd Department of Pathology and the Department of Forensic Medicine of the Semmelweis University of Medicine have been participating in the international PBDAY (Pathobiological Determinants of Atherosclerosis in Youth) study organised by the WHO.

Materials collected from standard sites of the thoracic and abdominal aorta, the coronary arteries and heart muscle during autopsies performed within 24 hours following death on subjects from the 5–34 years age group are studied in the Reference Centers.

Beside the standard procedure our Center have the possibility to collect materials for further investigation and comparison with the background informations obtained from questionnaires completed in each case with the help of a computer.

Acting both as a Collaborating and as a Reference Center, we performe GAG and macrophage studies on frozen aortic specimens. As a pilot study the cellular elements of the intimal proliferation seen in the thoracic and abdominal aorta — with special emphasis on the foam cells of fatty streaks — were investigated by light- and electron microscopy and by immunfluorescence method.

A series of 50 autopsies were performed within the study between January 1987 and June 1990. The aortic specimens were investigated by the following methods:

— light microscopy: HE, Orcein, PAS, Alcian blue, Azan trichrome, Sudan IV and Toluidine blue.

— Electron microscopy.

— Immunfluorescence method: monoclonal mouse antibodies to human Vimentin and Desmin (DAKO) and monoclonal anti-macrophage antibody (AMERSHAM), performed on six aortas.

There is still some controversy in the literature concerning the origin of the foam cells in early atherosclerosis. Recently investigations were focused on the role of macrophages in the process of atherogenesis.

The majority of the lipid containing cells (Fig. 1a, b) of the intimal thickening (macroscopically observed as fatty streak) in our cases show the ultrastructural and immunohistochemical characteristics of activated smooth muscle cells (Fig. 2a, b). Only few anti-macrophage antibody positive cells were found.

Our results seem to indicate that important role can be attributed to the smooth muscle cells in early atherogenesis, but further studies are necessary to demonstrate the role of macrophages.

References

[1] Gerrity, R.G. (1981): The role of the monocyte in atherogenesis. I. II. Am. J. Pathol. 103: 181–200.

[2] Allard, C., van der Wal, Pranab, K. Das, David Bentz van der Berg, Chris, M., van der Loos, Anton E. Becker (1989): Atherosclerotic lesions in humans. Lab. Invest. 61 (2): 166.

[3] Malcolm, J., Mitchinson, Keri, L.H. Carpenter, Richard, Y. Ball: The role of macrophages in human atherosclerosis. In: Pathobiology of the human atherosclerotic plaque. Eds.: Seymour Glagov, W.P. Newman, Sh. A. Schaffer, Springer-Verlag 1990.

[4] Atherosclerosis: Cellular aspects. In: Diseases of the arterial wall. Eds.: J.-P. Camilleri, C.L. Berry, J.-N. Fiessinger, J. Bariéty, Springer-Verlag 1988.

[5] Wissler, R.W., Vesselinovitch, D., Komatsu, A., Bridenstine, R.T.: The arterial wall and atherosclerosis in youth. In: Biology of the arterial wall — Satellite Meeting, 8th International Sympsium on Atherosclerosis, Siena, 1988.

[6] Campbell, G.R., Campbell, J.H., Manderson, J.A., Horrigan, S., Rennick, R.E. (1988): Arterial smooth muscle cell. Arch. Pathol. Lab. Med. 112: 977.

[7] Yoshida, Y., Mitsumata, M., Yamane, T., Tomikawa, M., Nishida, K. (1988): Morphology and increased growth rate of atherosclerotic intimal smooth muscle cells. Arch. Pathol. Lab. Med. 112: 987.

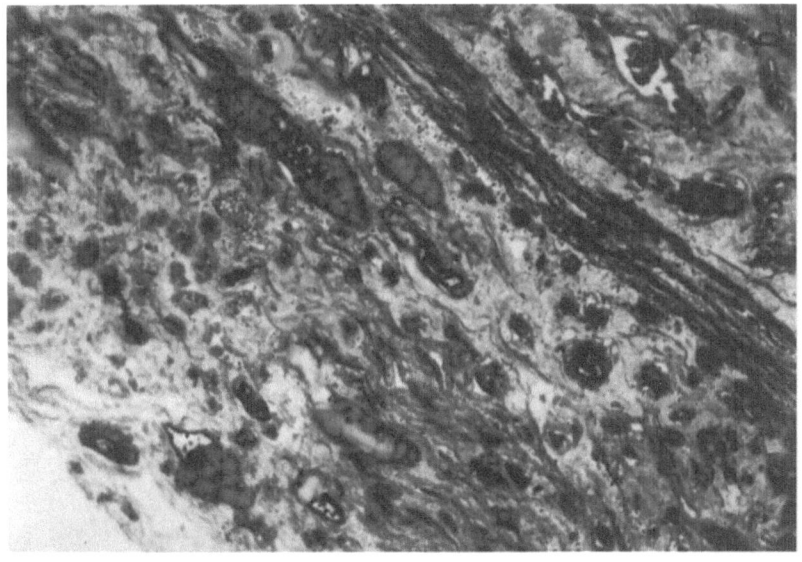

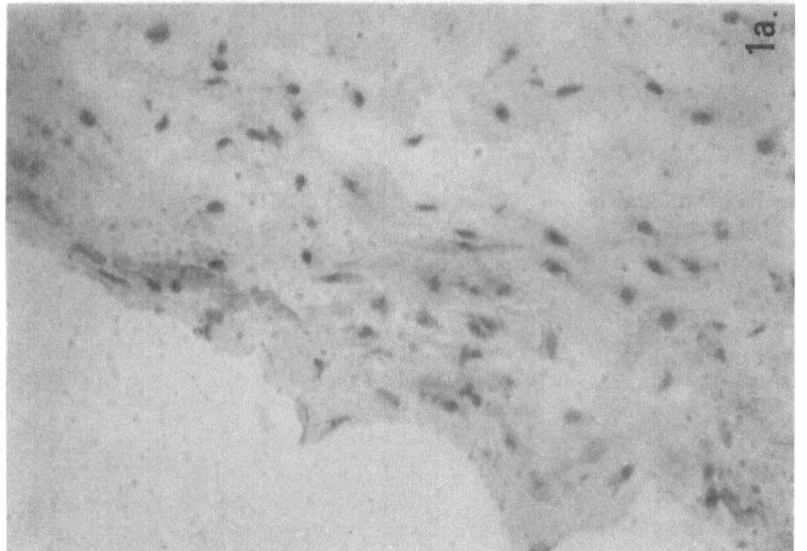

Figure 1a: Sudan positive cells in aortic intimal thickening. (Sudan IV, x600)
b: The cytoplasm of the cells contains lipid droplets. (Toluidine blue, x600)

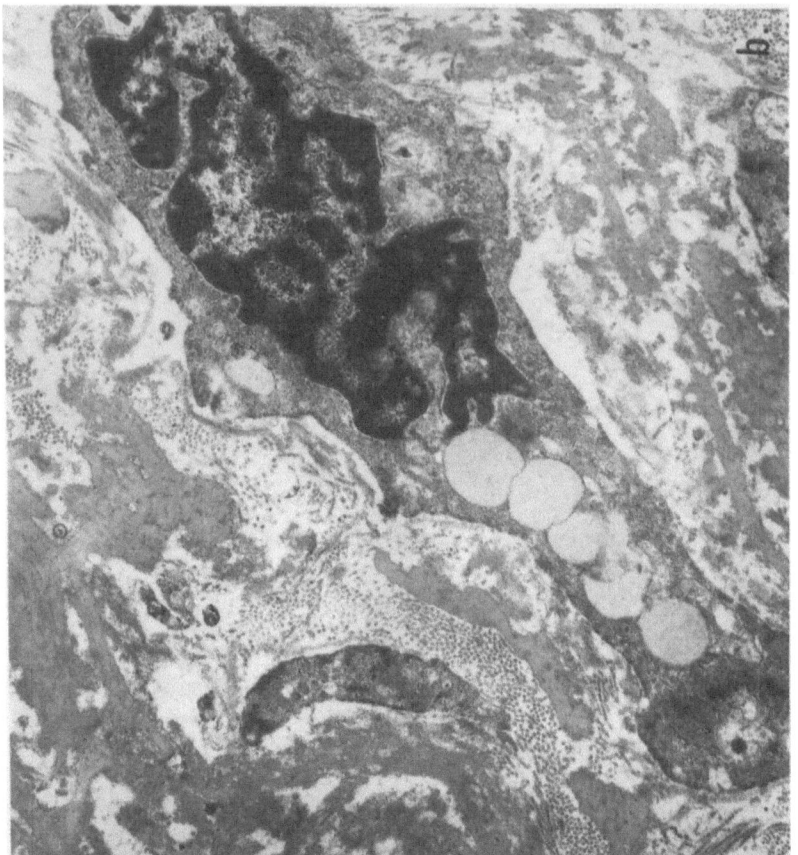

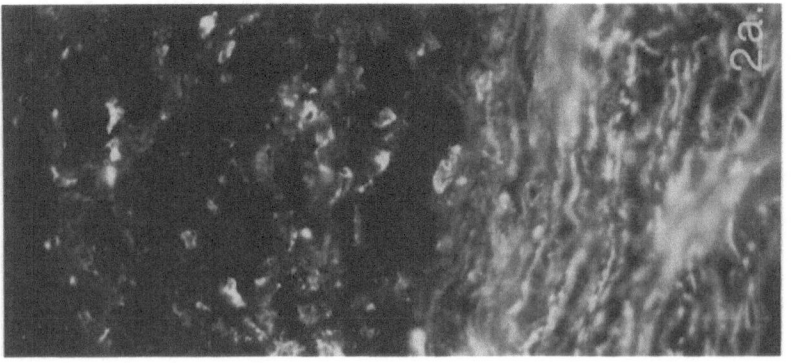

Figure 2a: Vimentin positive cells in the intimal thickening. (x600)
b: Ultrastructurally the lipid laden cells have the characteristics of smooth muscle cells. (UaPb, x10600)

Prognosis for patients after ischemic stroke: Hemorheological aspects

F. Meier, G. Grohmann, R. Thiele, A. Brandstätt
Department of Internal Medicine, Friedrich Schiller University Jena

The investigations were carried out on 81 patients with acute ischemic stroke, 38 women and 43 men. At the start, no more than 6 hours were allowed to have elapsed since this event. During the first 30 minutes after hospitalization, the patients received 250 ml of low-molecular dextran, followed by a further continuous administration of 1000 ml within 24 hours during a period of 5 days.

For the assessment of prognostically valid parameters, two patient groups were compared: these who survived after 21 days (n = 39) and these who deceased in the first 21 days (n = 42).

The deceased had a significantly higher age (74.2 ± 8 and 69.2 ± 10.5 years, respectively, $p < 0.05$) and a significantly higher myocardial insuffiziency (83.3% versus 48.7%, $p < 0.001$).

Although 50% of the patients were subjected to a rheologically effective treatment with low-molecular dextranes as early as within the first hour, the comparison of the first 6 hours revealed no advantages in the lethality for those patients with early onset of treatment. An early start of therapy was also in the survivors of no influence upon a possible improvement in their neurological deficiencies. On the first three days after stroke, the mean hematocrit values were not significantly different between both groups. But with regard to the hematocrit of the first day, the patients with a value of ≤ 0.45 were significantly more often found among the deceased ($p < 0.05$). All deceased had higher fibrinogen values, on the 3rd day after stroke this difference was significant (4.7 ± 1.6 g/l vs 3.9 ± 1.3 g/l, $p < 0.05$).

A presumable relationship between higher hematocrit values (essential parameter of whole blood viscosity) and a bad prognosis cannot be confirmed.

At a generally older age and in a high percentage of patients with myocardial insufficiency, lower hematocrit levels with a reduced oxygen transport rate rather suggest a restricted oxygen saturation of the brain and other vital organs. A detrimental influence was merely observed for the fibrinogen having an impact on plasma viscosity. The results might suggest that the plasma viscosity is of greater importance for (cerebral) microcirculation than assumed thus far. Low-molecular dextrans, however, elevates the plasma viscosity.

Quantitative Determination of Total Cholesterol, Free Cholesterol and Different Cholesteryl Esters in Serum Samples Using RP-HPLC and UV-Detection

G. Petersen, H.-J. Bauch, U. Wahrburg, G. Assmann
Institut für Arterioskleroseforschung an der Universität Münster

Introduction

The composition of dietary fat is important for the etiology and pathogenesis of atherosclerotic vascular diseases. Since the distribution of fatty acids in blood cholesteryl esters reflects the pattern of fatty acid consumption, the direct estimation of different blood cholesteryl esters may be of clinical, physiological and dietetic interest. This has been shown already in particular for linoleic acid consumption, which correlates well with the content of linoleic acid in the different blood lipid fractions like phospholipids, triglycerides and cholesteryl esters [1].

Usually the fatty acid composition in cholesteryl esters is determined indirectly using capillary gas chromatography. This procedure is rather laborious and time consuming, because it involves the isolation of cholesteryl esters by thin layer chromatography as described by Glatz et al. [2].

Therefore, this paper describes a new rapid and simpler method allowing the direct and precise determination of free cholesterol and the main cholesteryl esters in serum and other biological fluids. This method employs a solid phase extraction procedure for the isolation of serum lipids combined with HPLC-UVD for their separation and quantitative determination.

Patients

Serum lipids of 37 patients suffering from hypercholesterolemia (373 ± 81 mg/dl, LDL-cholesterol 293 ± 70 mg/dl) were analyzed and compared with the lipid composition of sera from 39 healthy volunteers (cholesterol 173 ± 25 mg/dl, LDL-cholesterol 95 ± 25 mg/dl).

Methods

0.5 ml of a 0.9% NaCl solution were added to 0.5 ml serum and the mixture was applied to an Extrelut 1-column (Merck) together with cholesteryl heptadecanoate (1 mg/sample) as the internal standard. After an equilibration time of 15 minutes, serum lipids were eluted with 25 ml n-hexane/isopropanol (3/2). The lipid extract was dried over Na_2SO_4 and taken to dryness under a stream of nitrogene. The residue was reconstituted in 1.0 ml dibutylether/n-heptane (1/1) and filtered (pore size 0.45 µm, Millipore).

Free cholesterol and cholesteryl esters were separated by reversed phase (RP-) HPLC using a 5 µm Ultrasphere reversed phase column (2.0 × 250 mm; Beckmann) and an isocratic system consisting of a M 112 pump (Beckmann), an auto-sampler with a 5 µl loop (Beckmann), a column thermostat (Beckmann) and a variable wavelength UV-detector M 165 (Beckmann). The mobile phase consisted of acetonitrile/isopropanol/n-heptane (50/35/15) and the flow rate was 0.22 ml/min. The analyses were carried out at 27 °C. Free cholesterol and the different cholesteryl esters were detected at 206 nm and the different cholesteryl esters were detected at 206 nm and quantified by external standard calibration using the peak height method and the System Gold Software (Beckmann).

Results

The HPLC conditions given above allowed the separation (Fig. 1 A) and quantitative determination of free cholesterol and several cholesteryl esters with short and long chain fatty acids (Fig. 1 B). Using this method the five cholesteryl esters, cholesteryl linoleate, cholesteryl arachidonate, cholesteryl oleate, cholesteryl palmitate, and cholesteryl stearate, and free cholesterol could be identified in sera of patients and healthy volunteers (Fig. 2 A and B). This blood lipid analysis showed that about 85% of circulating blood cholesterol was esterified with various fatty acids, whereas only 15% of total cholesterol remained unesterified.

Table 1: Relative distribution of cholesterol and cholesteryl esters in patients with hypercholesterolemia (n = 37) and healthy volunteers (n = 39)

Parameter / Substance	Patients [n = 37]	Healthy Volunteers [n = 39]	Significance level*
Total Cholesterol (mg/dl)	373 ± 81	173 ± 25	$p < 0.001$
% Free Cholesterol	17.4 ± 2.5	16.6 ± 1.5	n.s.
% Esterified Cholesterol	82.6 ± 2.5	83.4 ± 1.4	n.s.
% C-Arachidonate	18.6 ± 3.4	16.7 ± 2.3	$p < 0.01$
% C-Linoleate	40.7 ± 5.0	41.8 ± 4.1	n.s.
% C-Oleate	13.6 ± 1.8	14.3 ± 1.9	n.s.
% C-Palmitate	8.9 ± 1.3	10.1 ± 4.0	n.s.

* Student's t-test

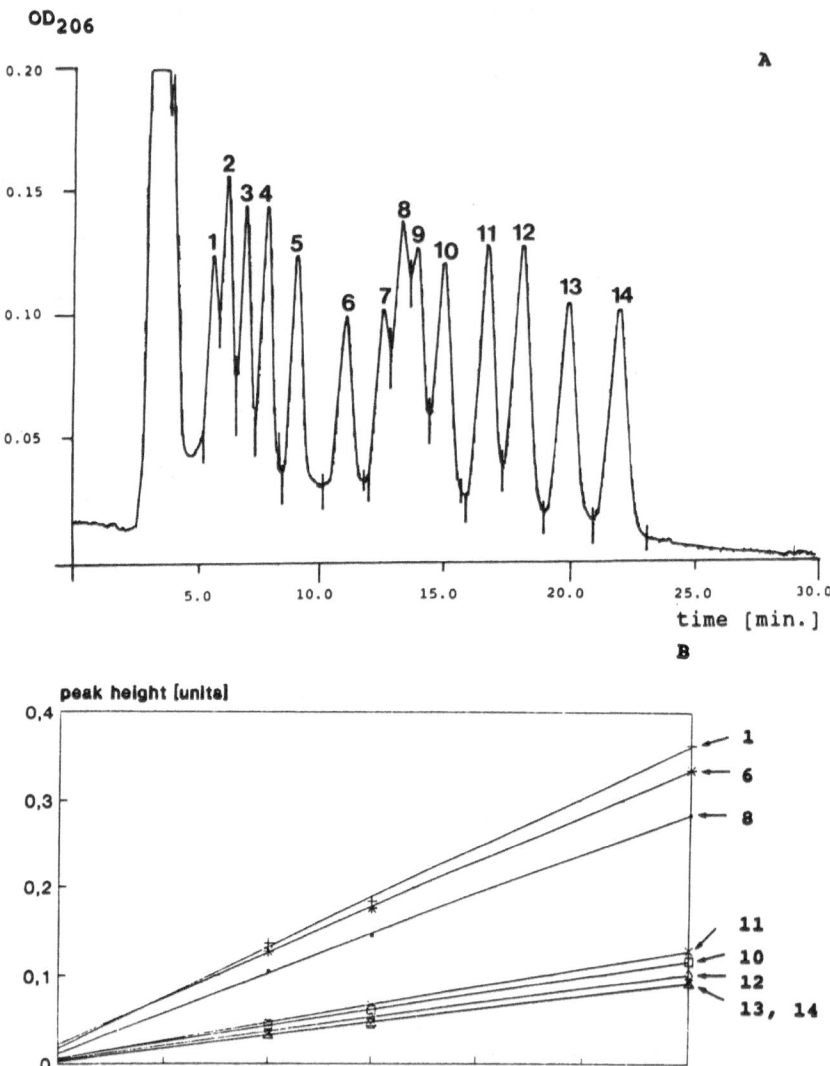

Figure 1:
A) Chromatogram of a standard mixture consisting of cholesterol (1), chol.-acetate (2), chol.-butyrate (3), chol.-hexanoate (4), chol-octanoate (5), chol-arachidonate (6), chol.-laurate (7), chol.-linoleate (8), chol.-palmitoleate (9), chol.-myristate (10), chol.-oleate (11), chol.-palmitate (12), chol.-heptadecanoate (13) and chol.-stearate (14).
B) Standard calibration curves for the quantitative determination of 1, 6, 8, 10, 11, 12, 13 and 14.

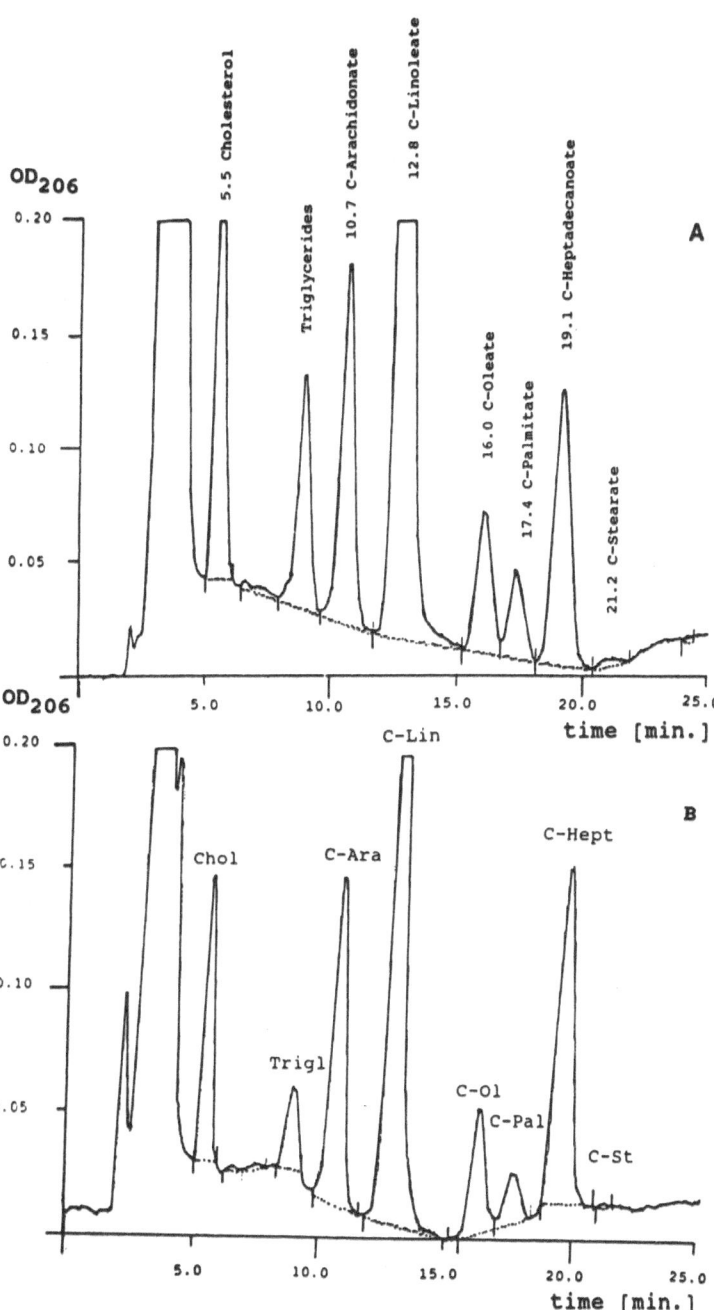

Figure 2: Representative chromatograms of serum lipids isolated from serum of a hyper-cholesterolemic patient (A) and a healthy volunteer (B).

Linoleic acic is the main fatty acid incorporated into blood cholesteryl esters, whereas palmitic acid for example only appears in minor amounts (Fig. 2 A and B).

In the blood of patients suffering from hypercholesterolemia, only the relative proportion of cholesteryl arachidonate of total cholesterol was found to be statistically significantly elevated when compared to that of healthy volunteers ($p < 0.01$, student's t-test). But no significant difference was found for the relative amount of cholesteryl linoleate, cholesteryl oleate and cholesteryl palmitate between those two groups (Table 1).

The total analytical recovery of free cholesterol and the different cholesteryl esters was 98.5% ± 1.0% (mean ± S.D.). The precision for the quantitative determination of free cholesterol and the cholesteryl esters using this method, expressed as the intraassay variance, was clearly better than 5% for all evaluated substances.

Discussion

The solid phase extraction procedure combined with reversed phase HPLC and UV-detection is a rapid and simple method allowing the precise quantitative determination of blood lipids like free cholesterol and the cholesteryl esters, cholesteryl arachidonate, chol.-linoleate, chol.-oleate, chol.-palmitate and chol.-stearate.

Our investigations further show that the relative amount of cholesteryl arachidonate is significantly enhanced in the metabolic pattern of blood cholesteryl esters in hypercholesterolemic patients. As arachidonic acid is a direct biogenetic precursor of prostaglandin metabolites and thromboxane, those findings may indicate that prostanoid formation might be altered in the hypercholesterolemic patients when compared with healthy volunteers. This hypothesis is supported by the scientific work of Habenicht et al. showing the onset of prostaglandin formation from cholesteryl arachidonate in cultured fibroblasts and smooth muscle cells coupled with LDL receptor activation [3]. Further investigations in patients suffering from disorders in lipid metabolism are necessary to support this hypothesis.

References

[1] Houwelingen, A.C., Kester, A.D.M., Kromhout, D., Hornstra, G.: Comparison between habitual intake of polyunsaturated fatty acids and their concentrations in serum lipid fractions, European Journal of Clinical Nutrition 43 (1989), 11–20.
[2] Glatz, J.F.C., Soffers, A.E.M.F., Katan, M.B.: Fatty acid composition of serum cholesteryl esters and erythrocyte membranes as indicators of linoleic acid intake in man, American Journal of Clinical Nutrition 49 (1989), 269–276.
[3] Habenicht, A.J.R., Salbach, P., Goerig, M., Zeh, W., Janssen-Timmen, U., Blattner, C̆., King, W.C., Glomset, J.A.: The LDL receptor pathway delivers arachidonic acid for eicosanoid formation in cells stimulated by platelet-derived growth factor, Nature 345 (1990), 634–636.

Pattern of fatty acids in childhood and the consequences of an unfavourable nutrition in newborns for the cardiovascular risk in later life

E. Petrich, U. Spahn, L. Richter
Department of Pediatrics, University of Jena

The fatty acid composition of infant nutrition are important for many functions of metabolism. The highly unsaturated fatty acids are essential for the prevention of metabolic disorders and cardiovascular diseases. Especially the n-3 and the n-6 highly unsaturated fatty acids are essential components of the structure lipids of every cells and in this form they are the starting material of many mediators and effectors of the cell membrane e.g. the prostaglandins. The metabolism of cholesterol will also be influenced by the pattern of fatty acids in the food. The input of these essential fatty acids is very different in nursed and formula fed infants. In the past a great part of infants was artificial nourished and the extent of the increased risk in later life is not known so far.

In a longitudinal investigation over 10 years of two groups of 41 breast fed and 55 formula fed infants the lipid parameters (triglycerides, total cholesterol, HDL- and LDL-cholesterol, apoprotein A 1 and B) were examined. The pattern of serum fatty acids of phosholipids, cholesterol-esters and triglycerides were analysed by gas liquid chromatographie of each 10 nursed and formula fed infants. There

Table 1: Pattern of important fatty acids of phospholipids of breast and formula fed infants for 10 years

Age	Feeding	18:1	n-6 fatty acids 18:2	20:3	20:4	n-3 fatty acids 18:3	20:5	22:6
3 d	breast	16:0	10:5	2.7	15.5	0.27	0.49	4.7
	formula	17.7	10.6	2.4	15.5	0.24	0.50	4.0
3 m	breast	15.1	21.7	2.6	8.1	0.51	0.40	3.3
	formula	12.5**	29.5**	2.3*	7.4*	0.61*	0.27*	1.5**
1 y	breast	14.6	25.1	2.7	6.9	0.33	0.71	1.3
	formula	15.2	23.9*	2.2*	6.3	0.59*	0.49*	1.4
3–5 y	breast	11.8	21.2	2.1	9.5	0.39	0.81	4.1
	formula	13.7	22.3	3.3	8.9	0.57*	1.15*	3.9
10 y	breast	13.8	19.4	2.9	10.3	0.16	0.88	3.3
	formula	14.1	24.2*	3.0	9.6	0.14	0.90	2.5

* $p < 0.05$ ** $p < 0.01$

are significant differences in the important fatty acid composition in all serum lipid classes of the two groups in the first months of life. But these differences are lasting for a long time by the same nutrition in both groups. Table 1 shows the most important fatty acids of phospholipids. Results of cholesterolesters and triglycerides are similar but the differences are a bit higher. The dynamic of the essential fatty acids during childhood indicates different requirements in human development. The high value of docosahexaenoic acid (22 : 6) at birth demonstrates its importance for the membrane function. It is, however, not found in artificial formulae, but human milk continues sufficient amounts (0.6–2.3% of fatty acids, w/w).

The effect of different nutrition in the first months of life after 10 years of age with regard to the cardiovascular risk are shown in table 2. Only small differences are existing in the mean of lipidparameters between the two groups. But the excess over the borderlines adequate to the age of all parameters are significant and the higher risk of the artificial nourished infants are demonstrated. The best model how to feed young infants is breast milk.

Table 2: Lipidparameters and Apoproteins A 1 and B of children of 10 years of age

	breastfed	formula	borderline	excess %	
				breast fed	for- mula
	N = 41	N = 55			
TG mmol/l	0.99 ± 0.38	0.98 ± 0.39	> 1.5	4.9	12.7
t-Chol mmol/l	4.19 ± 0.60	4.28 ± 0.79	> 4.8	10.8	21.5
HDL-Chol mmol/l	1.18 ± 0.21	1.07 ± 0.24	< 0.9	5.0	16.7
LDL-Chol mmol/l	2.42 ± 0.41	2.77 ± 0.46	> 3.4	8.3	17.4
APO A 1 g/l	1.37 ± 0.16	1.40 ± 0.21	< 1.1	0	10.4
APO B g/l	0.92 ± 0.21	0.99 ± 0.24	> 1.1	10.3	19.7

Differential Regulation of Collagen Synthesis and Collagenase Activity in Cultured Smooth Muscle Cells by Growth Factors

Wolfgang Schlumberger, Ulrich Falken, Michael Thie, Jürgen Rauterberg, Horst Robenek
Institut für Arterioskleroseforschung an der Universität Münster

Introduction

In the course of atherogenesis artery stenoses are characterized by intimal thickening. Intimal thickening may be the response of vascular SMC to injury causing them to migrate from the media into the intima, to proliferate and to produce large amounts of extracellular matrix, especially collagen [1, 2]. The molecular mechanisms for the modulated cell behaviour are not known, but growth factors are believed to play an important role in this process. Adhesion of platelets to the subendothelium at sites of injury and intimal infiltration of monocytes may be key events in the formation of stenoses. In this regard, platelets and activated macrophages are known to secrete a number of growth factors, and it is well established that these substances are able to regulate many cellular functions.

We examined the role of TGF-β, EGF and bFGF on protein synthesis, collagen production and collagenase activity in cultured SMC. SMC were cultured as monolayers on plastic and in collagen lattices and the mutual influence of soluble growth factors and insoluble extracellular matrix components on the synthetic activity of the cells were studied.

Methods

Cell culture: SMC were obtained from thoracic aortas of female pigs by an enzymatic digestion [3]. In passage 4 cells were used for experiments by cultivating within collagen lattices or as monolayer cultures [4].

Collagen synthesis and protein synthesis: Confluent monolayer cultures and retracted collagen lattices cultured for 5 days were preincubated with bFGF (20 ng/ml), TGF-β, EGF or TGF-β + EGF (5 ng/ml each) in medium containing 1% serum for 24 h. Cells were further incubated with growth factors and [^{14}C]proline for 24 h. Collagen and total protein synthesis were determined as previously described [5]. Briefly, cell and medium samples were dialyzed against 0.1 M acetic acid, hydrolyzed for 24 h at 110 °C with 6 N HCl and subjected to ion exchange chromatography for separation of proline and hydroxyproline.

Collagenase activity: The cell cultures were incubated for 24 h in medium without serum in the presence of the growth factors. Latent collagenase was activated by trypsin. Samples were assayed for active collagenase by measuring the release of radioactivity from [^{14}C]-type I collagen coated into microtitre plates.

Results

Protein synthesis and collagen synthesis: Protein synthesis in SMC cultured in collagen lattices was reduced to 20% compared with SMC in monolayer culture. In both culture systems protein synthesis in SMC treated with bFGF was slightly decreased, whereas it was increased approx. 2-3-fold after treatment with TGF-β.

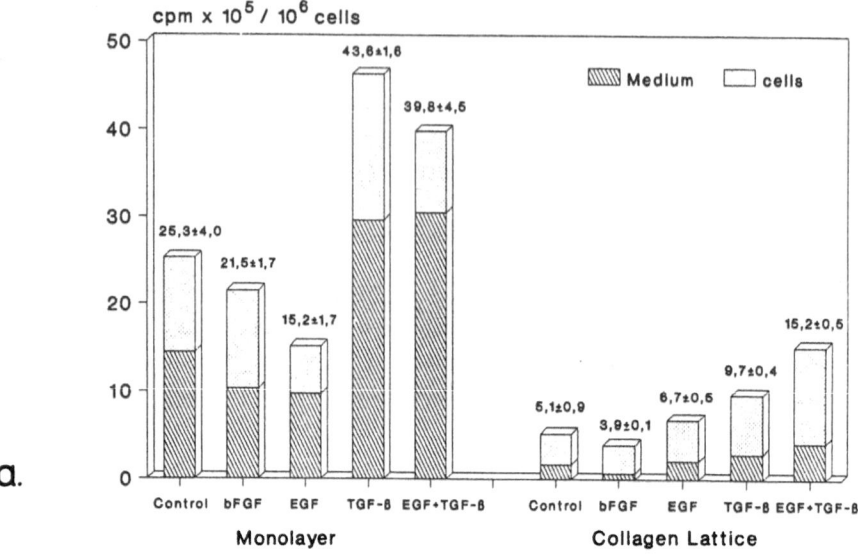

a.

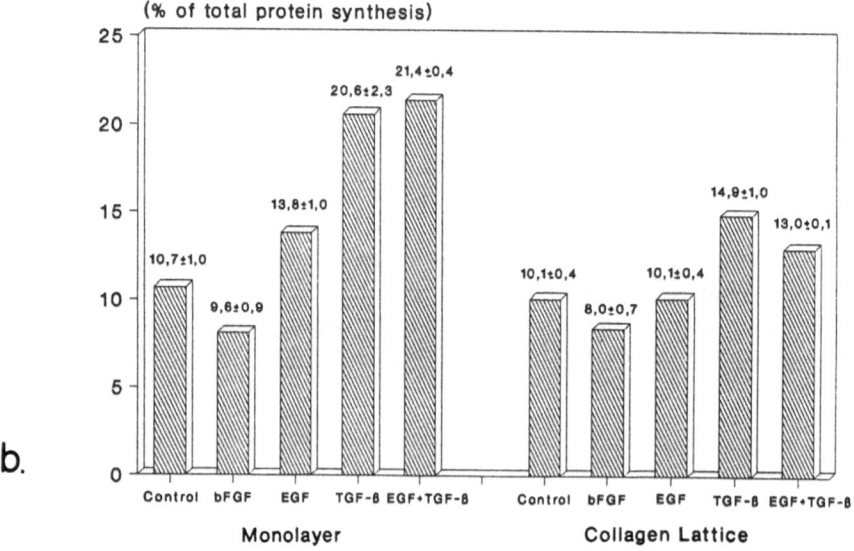

b.

Figure 1: Protein synthesis (a) and proportion of collagen in total proteins synthesized (b). Incorporation of radiolabeled non-dialyzable proline and hydroxyproline served as an index for total protein synthesis. The proportion of collagen in total proteins synthesized was calculated from the relation of radiolabelled non-dialyzable proline and hydroxyproline.

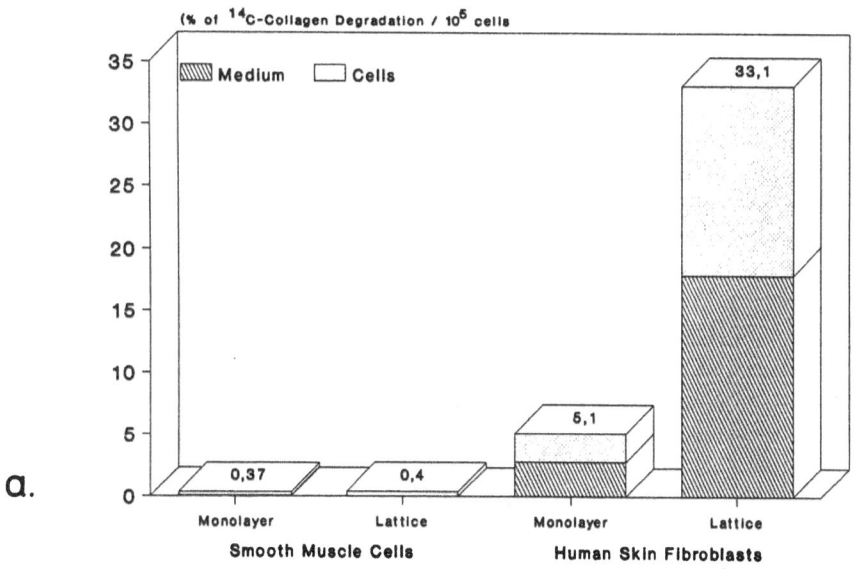

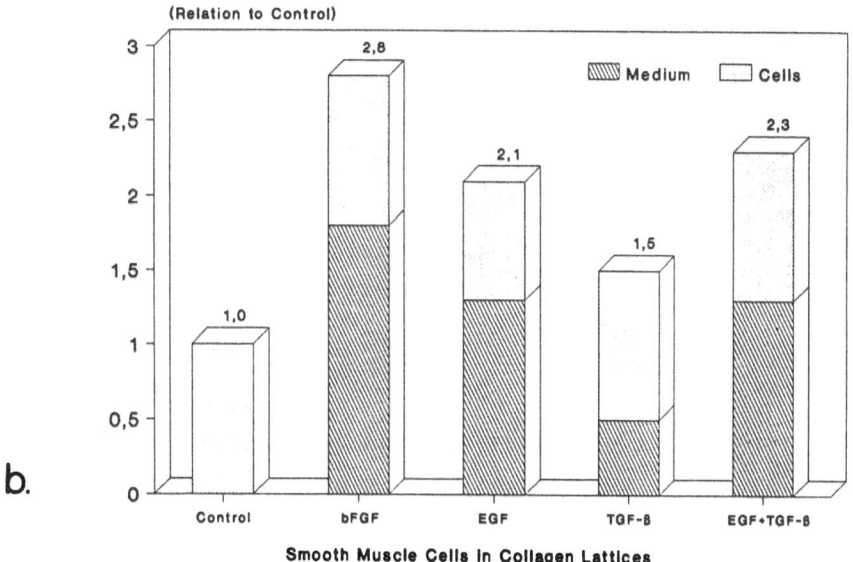

Figure 2: Collagenase production in SMC and human skin fibroblasts cultured as monolayers or in collagen lattices. Enzyme activity was determined in a radiolabeled fibril assay. Collagenous activity is expressed as percentage gel lysis by reference to 100% digestion caused by clostridial collagenase (a) or in relation to control (b).

Synergistic effects of TGF-β and EGF were only observed in SMC cultured in collagen lattices (Fig. 1a).

After incubation with growth factors, the collagen proportions in the two culture systems differed markedly. These differences indicate a mutual influence of the effects of growth factors and extracellular matrix components on collagen synthesis. Incubation of cells with TGF-β not only resulted in a stimulation of protein synthesis but also in a specific increase of collagen synthesis suggesting different mechanisms for the modulating action of TGF-β. The specific effect of TGF-β on collagen synthesis was more distinct in monolayer cultures than in collagen lattices. Treatment of cells with bFGF decreased the collagen proportion by approx. 20% (Fig. 1b).

Collagenase production: In comparison to fibroblasts SMC produce only low amounts of collagenase. Moreover, cultivation of SMC in collagen lattices did not stimulate collagenase production as it is observed in fibroblasts (Fig. 2a). Among the growth factors tested, EGF and bFGF were most effective resulting in a doubled and tripled collagenase production, respectively (Fig. 2b).

Discussion

The extracellular matrix mediates the attachment of cells to their substratum and participates in the regulation of cell differentiation, proliferation and migration. Changes in matrix composition could alter the physiological functions of cells. We demonstrate that TGF-β and bFGF modulate the production of collagen and collagenase by SMC. Overexpression of proteases like collagenase could facilitate the migration of SMC into the intima, overexpression of matrix molecules like collagen could contribute to the observed excessive matrix deposition during atherogenesis. Our results strongly support the hypothesis that TGF-β and bFGF are important pathophysiological regulators of collagen metabolism during intimal thickening in the vessel wall.

References

[1] Ross, R.: The pathogenesis of atherosclerosis – An update. New Engl. J. Med. 1986; 314: 488–499.

[2] Barnes, M.J.: Collagens in atherosclerosis. Collagen Rel. Res. 1985; 5: 65–97.

[3] Chamley-Campbell, J.H., Champbell, G.R., Ross, R.: Phenotype-dependent response of cultured smooth muscle cells to serum mitogens. J. Cell. Biol. 1981; 89: 379–383.

[4] Schlumberger, W., Thie, M., Rauterberg, J., Kresse, H., Robenek, H.: Deposition and ultrastructural organization of collagen and proteoglycans in the extracellular matrix of gel-cultured fibroblasts. Eur. J. Cell. Biol. 1989; 50: 100–110.

[5] Thie, M., Schlumberger, W., Rauterberg, J., Robenek, H.: Mechanical confinement inhibits collagen synthesis in gel-cultured fibroblasts. Eur. J. Cell. Biol. 1989; 48: 294–302.

Influence of Type I and Type III Collagen on the Biosynthetic Properties of Vascular Smooth Muscle Cells

Michael Thie, Wolfgang Schlumberger, Jürgen Rauterberg, Horst Robenek
Institute for Arteriosclerosis Research, University of Münster

Introduction

It is well established that collagens represent the major extracellular product in the atherosclerotic arterial wall. Type I and type III collagen together constitue most, probably 80–90%, of the total collagen present in this tissue (Barnes, 1985). The proportion of these collagen types is supposed to be modified during atherosclerosis. Cultivated cells obtained from atherosclerotic plaques, i.e. smooth muscle cells (SMC), synthesize relatively more type I collagen as compared to type III collagen than cells from the intact vessel wall (McCullagh et al., 1980; Rauterberg et al., 1977). Since any alteration in the composition and arrangement of the extracellular matrix may influence the behaviour of mesenchymal cells (Thie et al., 1989; Schlumberger et al., 1989), we analyzed the capacity of migration, the rate of proliferation, the level of biosynthetic activity and the ultrastructure of SMC cultured within three-dimensional matrices of either type I or type III collagen.

Materials and Methods

SMC from swine as well as human skin fibroblasts were used for the experiments. SMC were isolated from the aortic media by collagenase digestion (Chamley-Campbell et al., 1981), fibroblasts were kindly provided by Prof. Kresse (Münster). For experiments, cells were cultivated within hydrated collagen lattices from type I or type III and as monolayer on plastic in culture medium, supplemented with 10% fetal calf serum. Collagen lattices were prepared as previously described (Thie et al., 1989).

The cells in collagen lattices and monolayer cultures were counted using a Thoma chamber after Trypan blue staining. Collagen and total protein synthesis were measured after 24 h incubation of cultures with ^{14}C-proline (Thie et al., 1989).

For electron microscopy, samples were fixed with Karnovsky's reagent, embedded in Epon 812 and examined with a Philips EM 410.

a)

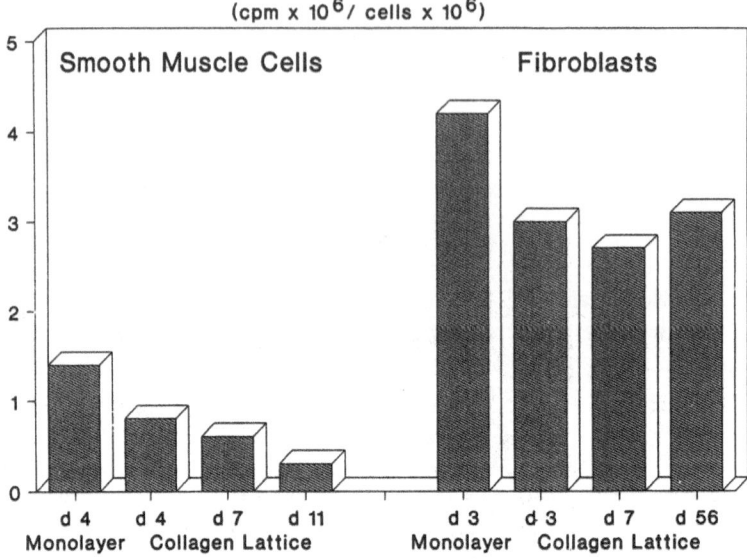

b)

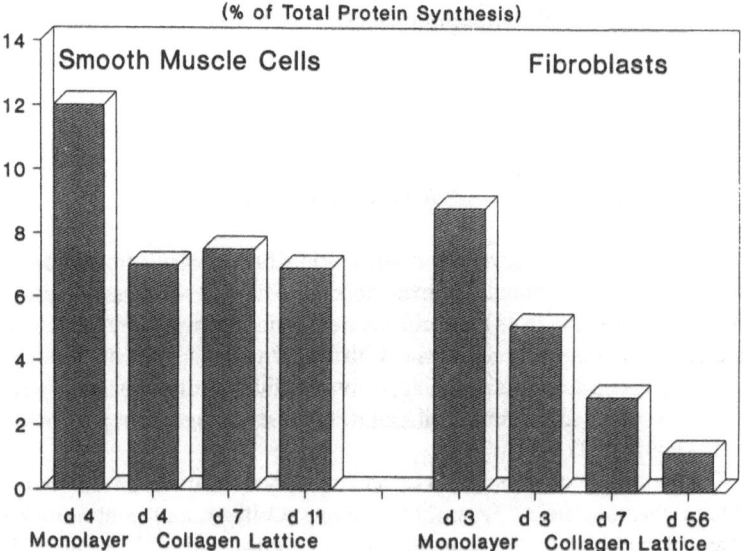

Figure 1: Effect of a three-dimensional network of type I collagen on total protein synthesis (a) and collagen synthesis (b) of vascular smooth muscle cells and skin fibroblasts. Cells were either cultured as monolayer on plastic or within collagen lattices in medium supplemented with 10% fetal calf serum for various days (d3, d4, d7, d11, d56).

a)

Percent of Outgrowth

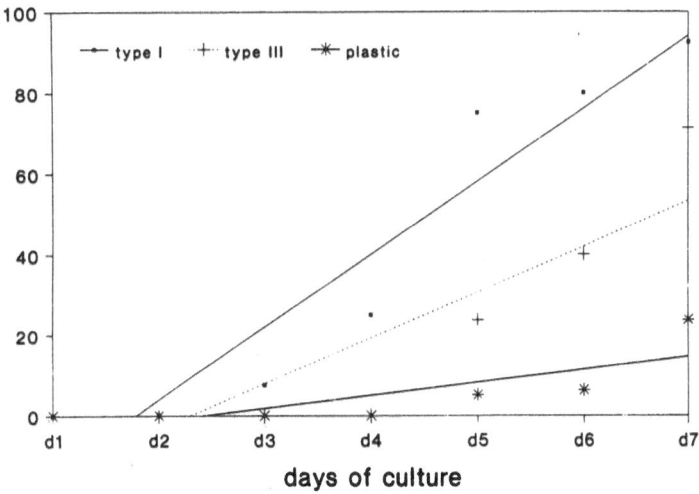

b)

Cell Number

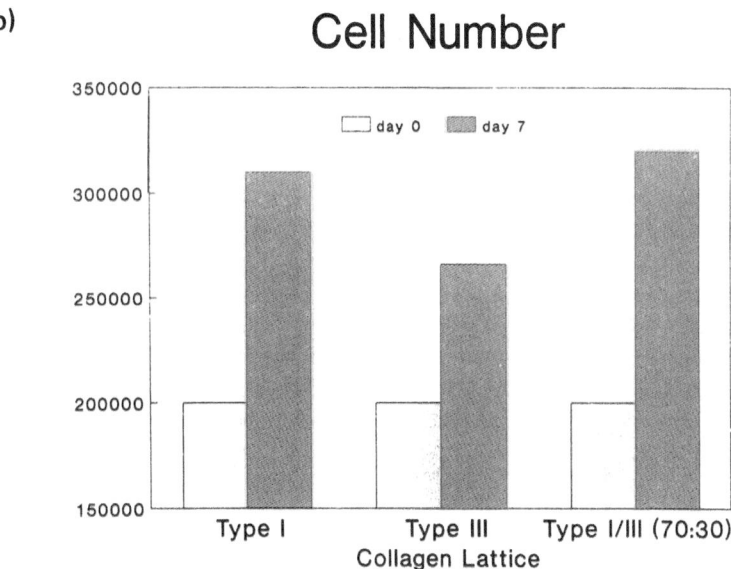

Figure 2: Effect to a three-dimensional network of type I, type III and type I/III (70:30) collagen on outgrowth of media explantats (a) and on cell proliferation (b) of lattice cultured SMC. Cell number was determined on day 0 and day 7 of culture.

Results

Ultrastructure and Biosynthetic Activity

The ultrastructure of SMC cultured within type I and type III collagen lattices was characterized by its high proportion of rough endoplasmic reticulum and Golgi complex on the one hand and by a scarcity of myofilament bundles on the other hand. The ultrastructure of entrapped SMC was comparable to that of monolayer cultured cells. With regard to morphological features SMC were comparable to cultured fibroblasts.

The amount of total protein and collagen synthesized by SMC embedded in type I collagen lattices was lowered as compared to monolayer cultures. Whereas total protein synthesis decreased continuously during the culture period, the proportion of collagen synthesis remained at a constant level (Fig. 1). In fibroblasts cultured in collagen lattices, total protein synthesis as well as collagen synthesis were reduced as compared with monolayer cultures. With prolonged culture time collagen synthesis decreased, whereas total protein synthesis remained constant (Fig. 1).

The amount of total protein synthesized by SMC embedded in type III collagen lattices was lowered as compared to type I collagen lattice cultures. In SMC cultured in type I/III (70:30) collagen lattices, total protein synthesis was enhanced as compared to type I and type III collagen lattices. The relative level of collagen synthesis was not influenced by the type of collagen used.

Migration assay, Proliferation and Lattice Contraction

Explantats of the aortic media of swine were embedded into type I or type III collagen lattices. In comparison to monolayer cultures on plastic, outgrowth of explantats was enhanced in type I collagen lattices (Fig. 2).

In comparison to type I and type I/III (70:30) collagen, SMC cultured in type III collagen lattices showed reduced proliferation (Fig. 2).

The decrease of lattice diameter showed a biphasic pattern, i.e. a rapid contraction during the first days of culture, followed by a slow contraction during the residual culture period. SMC contracted type III collagen more rapid than type I and type I/III(70:30) collagen.

Discussion

Our results show that SMC cultivated within type I or type III collagen remain in a viable state with marked suppression of total protein synthesis, collagen synthesis and rate of proliferation. However, cells in type III collagen exhibit much more reduced activities than those cultured in type I collagen. Thus, the different types of collagens in the extracellular matrix of the vessel wall (Mayne, 1986) could influence the behaviour of SMC in a type-specific manner. Our experiments indicate that the collagens themselves and changes in the proportion of the collagen types might be involved in pathogenesis of atherosclerosis.

References

[1] Barnes, M.J.: Collagens in atherosclerosis. Collagen Rel. Res. 1985; 5: 65–97.
[2] Chamley-Campbell, J.H., Campbell, G.R., Ross.: Phenotype-dependent response of cultured aortic smooth muscle to serum mitogens. J. Cell. Biol. 1981; 89: 379–383.
[3] Mayne, R.: Collagenous proteins of blood vessels. Arteriosclerosis 1986; 6: 585–593.
[4] McCullagh, K.G., Duance, V.C., Bishop, K.A.: The distribution of collagen types I, III and V (AB) in normal and atherosclerotic human aorta. J. Pathol. 1980; 130: 45–55.
[5] Rauterberg, J., Allam, S., Brehmer, U., Wirth, W., Hauss, W.H.: Characterization of the collagen synthesized by cultured human smooth muscle cells from fetal and adult aorta. Hoppe Seylers Z. Physiol. Chem. 1977; 358: 401–407.
[6] Schlumberger, W., Thie, M., Rauterberg, J., Kresse, H., Robenek, H.: Deposition and ultrastructural organization of collagen and proteoglycans in the extracellular matrix of gel-cultured fibroblasts. Eur. J. Cell. Biol. 1989; 50: 100–110.
[7] Thie, M., Schlumberger, W., Rauterberg, J., Robenek, H.: Mechanical confinement inhibits collagen synthesis in gel-cultured fibroblasts. Eur. J. Cell. Biol. 1989; 48: 294–302.

In Situ Localization of Apolipoproteins A_1, A_2, and B in Arteriosclerotic Vessels

E. Vollmer[1], J. Brust[1], A. Roessner[1],
B. Käsberg[2], B. Harrach[2], H. Robeneck[2], W. Böcker[1]
[1] Gerhard-Domagk-Institut für Pathologie,
[2] Institut für Arterioskleroseforschung
der Westfälischen Wilhelms-Universität Münster

The connection between serum lipoproteins and the development of arteriosclerosis is currently undisputed. High plasma levels of low-density lipoproteins (LDL) represent an increased risk of atherosclerosis, while an antiatherogenic potential is attributed to high-density lipoproteins (HDL). The main structural proteins of HDL are apolipoprotein (Apo) A_1 and A_2, the structural protein of LDL is Apo B. Contrary to most investigations focused mainly of the serum distribution of lipoproteins, the present study analysed their distribution, quantity and composition on the site, i.e. in the affected tissue of atherosclerotic vessels.

65 specimens of arteriosclerotic vessels (elastic and muscular type) were analysed histochemically. The specimens comprised all stages of arteriosclerosis, from
very discrete intimal changes to complicated lesions. The atherosclerotic changes
were labelled with antibodies against human Apo A_1, A_2, and B using alkaline
phosphatase techniques.

Apolipoprotein can be demonstrated already in the earliest stage of arteriosclerosis and is found to increase with the progression of disease. In that initial
stage, Apo is found first in the lumen-adjacent strata, and will be evident in the
deeper layers of the wall with advancing sclerosis. Arteries of muscular type show
this accumulation of Apo in an earlier stage (or in greater quantity at the same
stage) than do arteries of elastic type. At the same stage, the amount of Apo A_1
always dominates that of A_2 and B. In the intima, Apo B is higher than Apo A_2,
the media contains hardly any Apo B, and the adventitia has less Apo B than A_2.
Within the intimal layer, the location of Apo A_1 and A_2 is either intracellular
(mainly in foam cells) or extracellular, according to the respective stage of atherosclerosis (Fig. 1a). Apo B is almost exclusively extracellular (Fig. 1b); only the
severe cases of advanced arteriosclerosis show some intracellular deposits mostly
in foam cells. In the media, Apo A_1 and A_2 are accumulated in intracellular deposits, extracellular storage of Apo A_1, A_2 and B occurring only in case of severest
damage (Fig. 2).

The rather loose adventitial tissue, however, shows no noticeable alteration
of its Apo deposit pattern during the entire progression of atherosclerosis in contrast to the more tightly structured strata of the intima, and media who receive
an unimpeded spreading of apolipoproteins from the serum which is largely independent of the arteriosclerotic development.

Our investigations have shown that influx of LDL into the arterial intima may
occur at a very early stage of atherosclerotic change. Macrophages will take up
cholesterol esters via receptor-mediated endocytosis; these esters undergo a continuous cycle of hydrolysis and re-esterification. For maintenance of cellular
cholesterol homeostasis, macrophages have to rely on effective cholesterol receptors like LDL in their environment. If these fail, they are transformed to foam
cells. The mechanism allows for intervention by way of the "reverse cholesterol
transport" mediated by macrophages secreting Apo E. Whether Apo A_1 and A_2
are entered into the plaque passively or by active transport, is still unclear, and so
is the question whether these Apo deposits in the arterial wall might be able to
delay the development of arteriosclerosis. In view of a detailed functional and
morphologic assessment of local metabolic pathways and their potential disorders
we have started immunoelectron microscopic investigations of the atherosclerotic
plaque from which we expect further insight into the pathogenesis of arteriosclerosis.

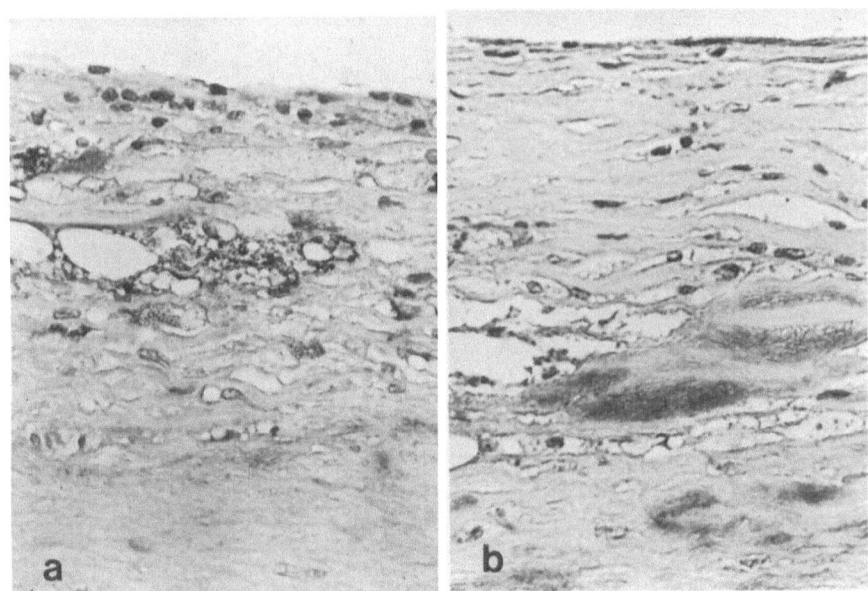

Figure 1: Intimal layer of the arterial wall with
a) intra- and extracellular deposits of Apo A.
b) solely extracellular deposits of Apo B.

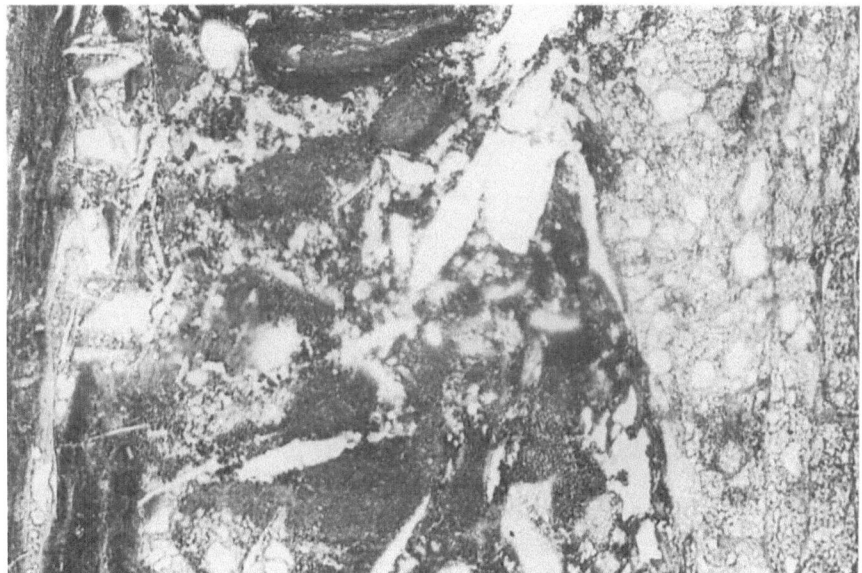

Figure 2: Severe case of atherosclerosis with intra- and extra-cellular deposits of apolipo-proteins in the media.